Roman North Africa

Social Worlds of Late Antiquity and the Early Middle Ages

The Late Antiquity experienced profound cultural and social change: the political disintegration of the Roman Empire in the West, contrasted by its continuation and transformation in the East; the arrival of 'barbarian' newcomers and the establishment of new polities; a renewed militarization and Christianization of society; as well as crucial changes in Judaism and Christianity, together with the emergence of Islam and the end of classical paganism. This series focuses on the resulting diversity within Late Antique society, emphasizing cultural connections and exchanges; questions of unity and inclusion, alienation and conflict; and the processes of syncretism and change. By drawing upon a number of disciplines and approaches, this series sheds light on the cultural and social history of Late Antiquity and the greater Mediterranean world.

Roman North Africa

Environment, Society and Medical Contribution

Louise Cilliers

Amsterdam University Press

Cover illustration: Ruins of the Antonine Baths in Carthage © Dreamstime Stockphoto's

Cover design: Coördesign, Leiden
Typesetting: Crius Group, Hulshout

ISBN 978 94 6298 990 0
e-ISBN 978 90 4854 268 0
DOI 10.5117/9789462989900
NUR 684

Table of contents

List of figures

Acknowledgements

This book came into being after many years of fruitful collaboration with François Retief, whose medical knowledge helped me to, for instance, suggest possible reasons for the death of Cleopatra, Alexander the Great, the Caesars, and the Popes, to discuss some of the epidemics that swept the Mediterranean world, poisons and poisoners, and so on. In brief, to solve some of the medical conundrums of the ancient world. This resulted in numerous articles. It greatly widened my knowledge of the medical history of ancient Greece and Rome and has helped immensely in my research for the present book; I therefore owe him a debt of gratitude.

I would also like to record my thanks to Dr. Cornelis van Tilburg for his expert compilation of the Index and for his assistance in many other respects, and to my Dutch colleague, Prof. Manfred Horstmanshoff, for valuable advice after having read the manuscript, and for his friendship over many decades.

To the members of the Amsterdam University Press who accompanied me on my visit to Roman North Africa and patiently guided me all the way, my sincere thanks, also for their meticulous work in the production of this book.

Last but not least, I would like to express my deep appreciation to my husband, Johan, who has been most supportive of my efforts over many years.

Preface

North Africa was the most prosperous province during the late Roman Empire and experienced a flowering in all fields, but especially in science and medicine. A great number of medical texts produced in this period in the Roman Empire at large originated in North Africa. Four outstanding physicians/medical authors in late fourth- and early fifth-century North Africa immediately attract our attention: Helvius Vindicianus, Theodorus Priscianus, Caelius Aurelianus and Cassius Felix.

It is my intention to envision these four authors in their own environment and time frame. The first chapter thus deals with Roman North Africa in general – its rise and its fall after three waves of foreign invaders had swept across the country; the development and demise of some of the cities, especially Carthage, where Vindicianus would have had his seat as proconsul, and Cirta, the home town of Cassius Felix; the people who inhabited these cities, each with their own language and culture; and some famous contemporary Classical and Christian authors.

The health facilities available so many centuries ago are astounding. The aqueducts, the massive bath complexes and the Cloaca Maxima, a sewer in which an ox wagon could turn around, are only a few examples of the amazing level of architectural and technological knowledge of the Roman engineers. Yet the cities were deficient in disposing of human waste, which must have led to many diseases. Hospitals, a Christian initiative, were only established in the fourth century.

Various epidemics for which there were no cures swept through North Africa in the fourth and fifth centuries, killing thousands of people. It is interesting to note the changing views of the reasons for these epidemics in the course of centuries.

The question then arises what the standard of health services was. Not only was the lack of antibiotics and antiseptics, discovered some 1500 years later, a problem, but also the fact that diagnoses and operations were done with little knowledge since there was a veto on dissection. The absence of a health board to supervise the standard of physicians meant that any quack could present himself as a doctor. And yet doctors were trained as well as was possible at that stage, with an impressive curriculum and modern didactic techniques, in highly developed institutions in, *inter alia*, Carthage and Alexandria.

The discussion of the contributions of the four physicians/medical authors forms the core of the book. The remarkable physician Vindicianus, who was proconsul and attained the prestigious post of Count of the Medical Board of Doctors in Rome, was the first to translate the works of the Greek masters of old into Latin, realising that since the knowledge of Greek was becoming extinct in the West, these works would be lost forever. Vindicianus' student, Theodorus Priscianus, followed in his footsteps and also translated Greek works, of which his *Gynecology*, a textbook containing recipes for drugs and therapies for women's diseases (*inter alia* for abortion and hysterical suffocation), is best known. Caelius Aurelianus, considered to be one of the greatest Latin medical authors in Antiquity, also wrote a *Gynecology*, basing his work on that of the famous first/second-century physician Soranus; it represented ancient gynecological and obstetrical practice at its height. Caelius' work *On acute diseases* and *On chronic diseases* is a complete handbook for pathology, therapy and pharmacology. Cassius Felix, a much-loved Christian physician, discusses 82 diseases with suggested treatments in his book *On medicine*; this text was used throughout the Middle Ages.

The Church also had a great interest in medicine. This is exemplified by the Church Father St. Augustine, who had an amazing knowledge of medical sciences. The question of how the (sometimes obligatory) conversion of the population to Christianity in the fourth century influenced the practice of contemporary physicians is discussed.

Finally, the important role played by our four authors in the preservation and transmission of medical knowledge is looked at. The foreign invasions that caused many citizens to flee the country were, paradoxically, the reason the precious works of the old Greek masters were saved from oblivion, since the translations taken along had in this way reached Italy and Spain, whence they were disseminated through Europe. The reader will find some repetition since every chapter is, as it were, a unit on its own, especially in the last chapter, where all the strands are pulled together to present an integrated picture.

The circle must be closed. The history of Roman North Africa encapsulates within half a millennium the rise from the ashes of a burnt city to become the most prosperous province in the Roman Empire, and its demise after three waves of foreign invaders had swept over the country – to disappear completely from the radar. It is indeed an extraordinary phenomenon that after some 500 years of rule (146 BCE–439 CE) hardly a trace of Rome's influence was left. However, the fact that the shipment of the erudite Arab merchant Constantine the African in the eleventh century did not contain the usual drugs and spices that he transported to Italy, but learned Arab medical books, affirms that Kairouan, the new capital of North Africa, where he probably studied medicine, was an important centre of Islamic scholarship and learning. Thanks to the immense medical contribution of Constantine, North Africa thus did flourish again after the fall of Carthage, albeit not in a Roman way.

The foregoing overview of the content of this book may have enlightened the perceptive reader as to its aim, which is to envision the four authors and Augustine in their own environment and time frame. Roman North Africa was their home country. Carthage, or Hippo Regius (now Bône), was the city where they would have spent most of their time as practicing physicians or medical writers, or as a bishop or proconsul. Some of them would have been alive to witness the Vandal invasion and the destruction of Carthage in 439 – Augustine died while the Vandals were besieging Hippo, close to Cirta, the home town of Cassius Felix. In Carthage they would have been educated in an excellent school, being taught not only Greek to the extent of becoming thoroughly bilingual (Theodorus Priscianus' Greek was so good that it is thought that it was his first language), but also Classical literature, as is evident from Vindicianus' knowledge of Latin authors in his letter to Valentinian and from his being asked to adjudicate a literary contest.

We may imagine them functioning in the political and social milieu of the late fourth and early fifth centuries. In daily life they would have rubbed shoulders with Phoenicians, Berbers and Greeks – Cassius and Muscio later even with Vandals – and heard the cacophony of all the different languages in the streets. They would have watched the games in the arena, visited the Baths, and smelled the sewers while walking through the filthy streets of the city. As physicians they would have had to cope with patients whose problems were due to inadequate health services – patients who would have contracted contagious diseases from unclean water in the Baths, or from contaminated water, or from buying food infested with flies from street vendors. We can envision Cassius, the surgeon, with his precise Latin, making instruments for his operations, educating his senior medical students, and impressing them with many Greek synonyms for Latin terms.

We may have empathy with the delicate health of Augustine, plagued in later life with hemorrhoids that sometimes totally incapacitated him, and we may smile on reading that the bishop had to tone down his grandiloquent rhetorical style (which his noisy middle-class congregation could not understand) and cut his sermons short since his audience, standing throughout, would become tired and impatient. We can understand Vindicianus' frustration with fellow physicians, even among the *archiatri* at the court, who were not well trained. We will admire a medical writer like Muscio and a physician like Theodorus Priscianus, who each devoted a whole book to recipes for drugs and therapies to cure female diseases. Vindicianus will gain our respect for his expertise, exemplified in the authoritative tone of his letter to the emperor, and evident from his contact with the famous medical centre in Alexandria, where he would probably have acquired the Greek manuscripts that he translated into Latin. In addition, despite his important post, he still found time to act as mentor for the young Augustine. Finally, we cannot but agree with Temkin's remark that the efforts of these North African writers 'to salvage the tremendous treasures of the past can be seen as the historical achievement of the millennium', and that it accurately reflects the magnitude of their contribution.

1. History, environment, population and cultural life

The history of the western part of ancient North Africa is to a great extent the history of foreign invaders who conquered the country and imposed their language and culture on the inhabitants. Apart from the Berbers, who were the indigenous inhabitants of North Africa west of the Nile Valley, the Phoenicians, Romans, Vandals, Byzantines, Arabs, Turks and French all made their presence felt in the centuries gone by. In modern times, independent states – Libya, Tunisia, Algeria, Morocco and Mauritania – have replaced the region known as North Africa in ancient times.

The period during which the Romans held sway over North Africa (146 BCE–439 CE) in particular interests us, since it presents a remarkable phenomenon: not only does this period encapsulate within some 500 years the rise and fall of a country, but equally amazing, in the aftermath it appears that not a trace of Rome's influence on the region remained, even after half a millennium of rule. Only ruins as a sad reminder of a remarkable period in world history.

A brief overview of the history of Roman North Africa

Approximately 3000 years ago the Phoenicians were the first to discern and exploit the strategic possibilities of a promontory in the Mediterranean Sea just across from Sicily. Ships crossing the sea from east to west and back all had to pass through the 320 km strait between the present-day Sharīk Peninsula and the western tip of Sicily, which made it a valuable strategic asset to the country controlling it. According to legend, the Phoenicians, Semitic colonists from Tyre (in modern Lebanon), founded a city on this promontory (near modern Tunis) in c. 800 BCE; they called it Quart-hadasht ('Carthago' in Latin), which means 'New City', implying that it was a 'new Tyre'. By the sixth century BCE Carthage had grown to one of the most important Phoenician settlements on the North African coast, especially after the influx of immigrants from the mother city, Tyre, after it had been conquered by the Babylonian king, Nebuchadnezzar. Carthage now became a serious rival to the Greek settlers in Sicily and Corsica. This led to a long and bitter war in Sicily itself and also in North Africa. One of the first battles took place at Alalia just off the coast of Corsica between 540

Figure 1.1 Tophet (burial place) in Carthage where small children were buried (eighth century BCE)

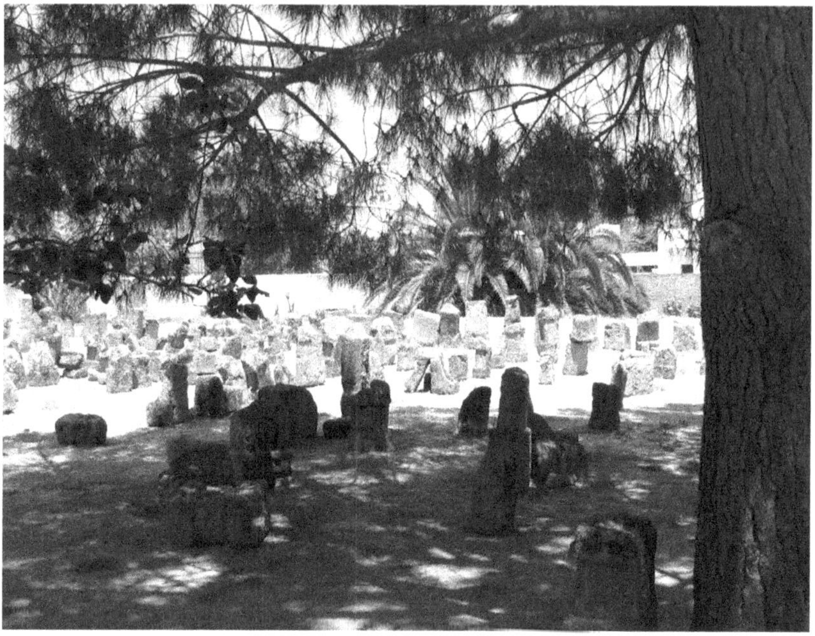

and 535 BCE, when a fleet of Phoenicians and their allies, the Etruscans, joined battle with a Greek fleet consisting of Phocaeans who had previously planted a colony in Alalia. Although the Greeks drove the allied forces off, they lost almost two-thirds of their fleet and had to evacuate Corsica and withdraw to Italy. During this battle (as in other crises), hundreds of small Phoenician children were sacrificed to appease the gods.[1] The Greeks, though defeated, left an enduring influence on the culture of the Carthaginians.

By the third century BCE Carthage had become one of the largest states in the ancient Mediterranean and was increasingly viewed by Rome as a threat to her growing influence and territorial expansion. It led to three Punic[2] wars between these two superpowers. The outcome of the first war in the middle of the third century BCE was undecided; the Carthaginians

1 Most archaeologists agree that infant sacrifices did occur. The remains of infants and children were unearthed in great numbers in, *inter alia*, a Tophet (burial place) in Carthage. It is not certain, however, what the motive for the sacrifices was, whether a religious rite, population control or a request to the gods to grant a favour. See Xella *et al.* (2013, 1191–1199), who summarized the textual, epigraphical and archaeological evidence for Carthaginian infant sacrifice.

2 From *Punicus*, Latin for Phoenician.

Figure 1.2 Tombstone of a child

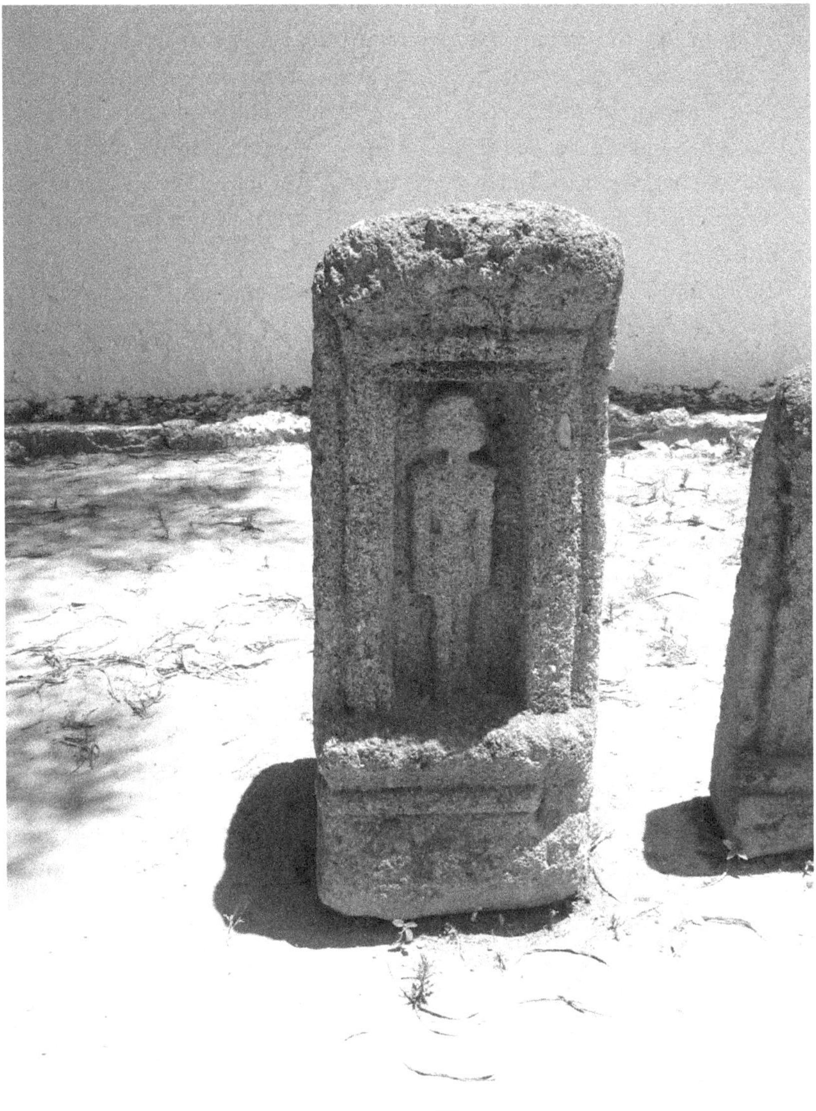

were eventually driven back to Spain, where they extended their power. In the Second Punic War (218–202) the Romans were pitted against the brilliant young African general Hannibal, who, against all odds, crossed the Alps from Spain with his army and a corps of elephants. Once in Italy, he inflicted some crushing defeats on the Romans. He remained in Italy for another thirteen years, but failed to accomplish anything of importance, since he lacked resources, and the Italian allies did not defect to him as he had hoped. He was thus recalled to Africa, where the final battle took place at Zama in 202. The Roman historian Livy states that before the battle began, the 'two greatest soldiers of their time' met in the middle of the battlefield, each attended by an interpreter, and 'for a minute mutual admiration struck them dumb and they looked at each other in silence'.[3] However, negotiations failed, the battle began, and Scipio (later called Africanus in honour of his victory) put an end to Phoenician power in the Mediterranean – for the time being.

By the middle of the second century BCE the economic revival of Carthage led to renewed fear among the Romans of a resurgence of Punic political power, and, incited by the censor Cato's paranoid exclamation *Carthago delenda est* ('Carthage must be destroyed'), with which he concluded every speech in the Senate, the Third Punic War began. After a two-year-long siege of Carthage, the war was ended in 146 when Scipio Aemilianus, adopted grandson of Scipio Africanus, finally destroyed Carthage. The site of the city was declared accursed, and the Romans created a new province called Africa out of the rest of the Carthaginian territory.

Colonisation of the new region started slowly, but the strategic location of Carthage led Julius Caesar to re-found the city in 46 BCE, extending its territory to the south. Colonisation then increased rapidly, and many Italians and war veterans were settled there, especially during the reign of the emperor Augustus (r. 27 BCE–14 CE). He handed the administration of North Africa over to the Senate and a proconsul was appointed to rule the province (hence the name Africa Proconsularis), with the new Carthage as capital. One legion was allocated to the province, the Legio III Augusta. To the west, Mauretania was reconstituted as a kingdom, with the young Roman-educated Numidian prince Juba II as client-king. The emperor Caligula (r. 37–41 CE), however, had Juba's son and successor, Ptolemy, executed for the sake of the kingdom's treasure. He also annexed Mauretania, claimed it as a province, and divided it into Mauretania Caesariensis, with Caesarea as its capital, and Mauretania Tingitana, with Tingis (now Tangiers) as its capital. By the end of the first century CE the population of North Africa had increased to about five million. Revolts by semi-nomadic Berber tribes still occurred, but by the second century the greater part of the province was Romanized and urbanized.

From the middle of the second century until deep into the fourth century, North Africa experienced a period of great prosperity (this will be discussed

3 Liv. 30.30. Translations are my own unless otherwise stated.

Figure 1.3 Old Carthage with new city in the background

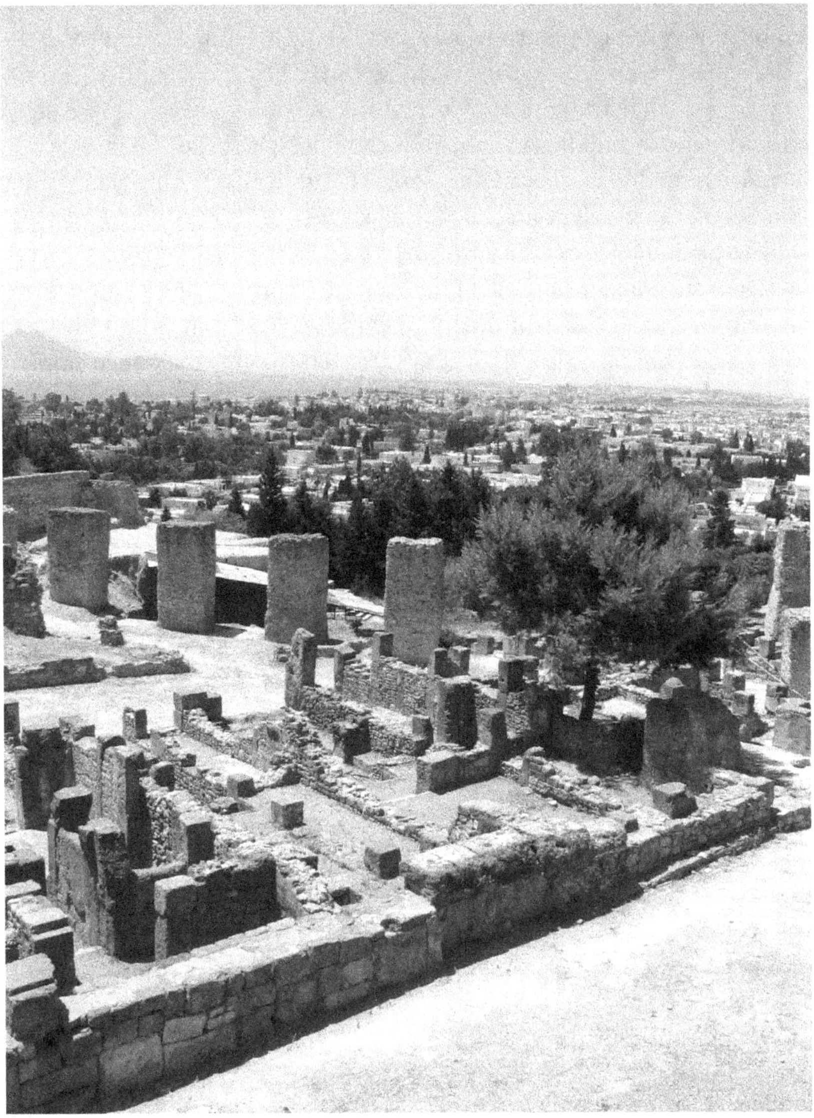

in greater detail later in this chapter). This was based largely on agriculture – the export of grain and olive oil to Rome and the provinces brought great wealth. Romanization left its imprint in many respects, especially in the architecture of the cities and towns, which all had at least a *curia* or senate house, statues of the gods and worthies, a forum, public baths and triumphal arches.

In the second half of the second century, Christianity reached North Africa and with it the persecutions. The intensity of the persecutions varied from emperor to emperor; the names of many martyrs are linked to this province. The fourth century is characterized by the Donatist/Catholic schism, which led to violent conflicts and much bloodshed. However, we also witness the building of numerous churches with beautiful mosaics; the century is further marked by the works of some brilliant Christian writers, like Tertullian, St. Cyprian and St. Augustine.

The period of prosperity in North Africa stands in strong contrast with the situation in the rest of the Roman Empire during a half-century of anarchy (235–284): from without came waves of barbarian invaders; within the empire, no less than 26 army generals were proclaimed emperor in the provinces (some not even reaching Rome), and epidemics ravaged the country. Africa was not greatly affected by these crises, but its prosperity was brought to an abrupt end in the early fifth century by the Vandals, who were in Spain at that point in time. The entire tribe – about 80,000[4] – migrated *en masse* to Africa under the leadership of Geiseric and invaded Africa.[5] Although they failed to capture the chief cities, they overran the country and were soon besieging Hippo Regius. After negotiations with the Romans, peace was concluded, but in 439 Geiseric broke the peace terms and seized Carthage in a surprise coup. The city was partially destroyed; Roman aristocrats were dispossessed in favour of Vandal overlords and many were exiled. The independence of the Vandal kingdom was recognized by the western emperor, Valentinian III, in 442, but in 455 Geiseric again broke the truce when the Vandals crossed to Italy and sacked Rome; fortunately, they only plundered it and did not wantonly demolish its buildings and monuments. Back in Africa, Geiseric defeated an attempted invasion by the Byzantines. At his death in 477 he was the undisputed master of the western Mediterranean: the Vandal kingdom included all of Roman Africa, Corsica, Sardinia and the Balearic Islands.

4 According to Victor of Vita (1992, c. 1.2), this number represents the total number of people, not of warriors.

5 According to Procopius (*Vandal War* c. 1.3), the Byzantine *Comes* (Count) Bonifacius, governor of Africa Proconsularis, found himself the victim of political intrigues in the court in Constantinople and, rather than face possible execution, asked the support of the Vandals, who were then in Spain. Schwartz (2004, 52) doubts this explanation on the grounds that the Vandals had already pillaged the coast of Mauretania under Gunderic, a former leader; he also points out that there is no indication of an accord between Bonifacius and Geiseric.

However, the Vandal regime lasted less than a century: in 533 the emperor Justinian sent a second expedition to conquer North Africa, against strong opposition from his officials, who feared the Vandals, remembering their recent defeat. But Roman rule was re-established when the Byzantines, under the leadership of Justinian's renowned general, Belisarius, defeated the Vandals under their new leader, Gelimer. Shortly after the beginning of the battle, Gelimer was informed of the death of his brother; overcome with grief, he left his forces in order first to bury his brother. Carthage was left undefended, and Belisarius simply walked into the city. During the break the Vandals regrouped, while Belisarius had the walls of Carthage rebuilt. In the final battle, the Byzantines again gained the upper hand; Gelimer went into hiding for a few months, but at last surrendered. He was taken to Constantinople to walk in Belisarius' triumphal procession, after which Justinian gave him a large estate in Galatia, where the former Vandal king retired and eventually died of old age. After the last battle, the Vandals simply disappeared – some were absorbed into the population and others fled to Spain.

The Vandal period is no longer regarded as one of universal decline. The word 'vandalism' was used for the first time in the eighteenth century by the Bishop of Blois in a dispute with revolutionaries who destroyed churches and their works of art, and the word 'vandal' was soon incorporated into daily use in a pejorative sense. Raven remarks that this saddled the Vandals with a reputation for wholesale destruction that they did not deserve.[6] They did not come to Africa to destroy, but to settle and enjoy the benefits of the Roman amenities; despite their greed for booty they did, for instance, not wantonly cut down the olive trees or the vineyards (in fact, the agricultural communities found Vandal rule less oppressive than that of the Romans). Roman administrative systems that were found effective were retained. Many of the Vandals eventually converted to Christianity; Latin remained the official language. The Greek-Byzantine historian Procopius stated that the Vandals rapidly adopted with enthusiasm the ways of life, the pastimes and the pleasures of the Romans.[7] However, no Vandal word survived in Latin or in the Berber languages. The only really far-reaching damaging action was their

6 Raven 1993, 213. See also George (2004, 134 n.4): 'The destruction of the Roman cities and imperial buildings of North Africa was not the work of the Vandals, but of their Byzantine conquerors and the African tribes during the expulsion of the Vandals in 534, and by the Arabs in later centuries.'

7 Procop. *Vand.* 2.6.5–9.

Figure 1.4 Great Mosque in Kairouan, or Mosque of Uqba, established in 670 CE; one of the oldest places of worship in the Islamic world

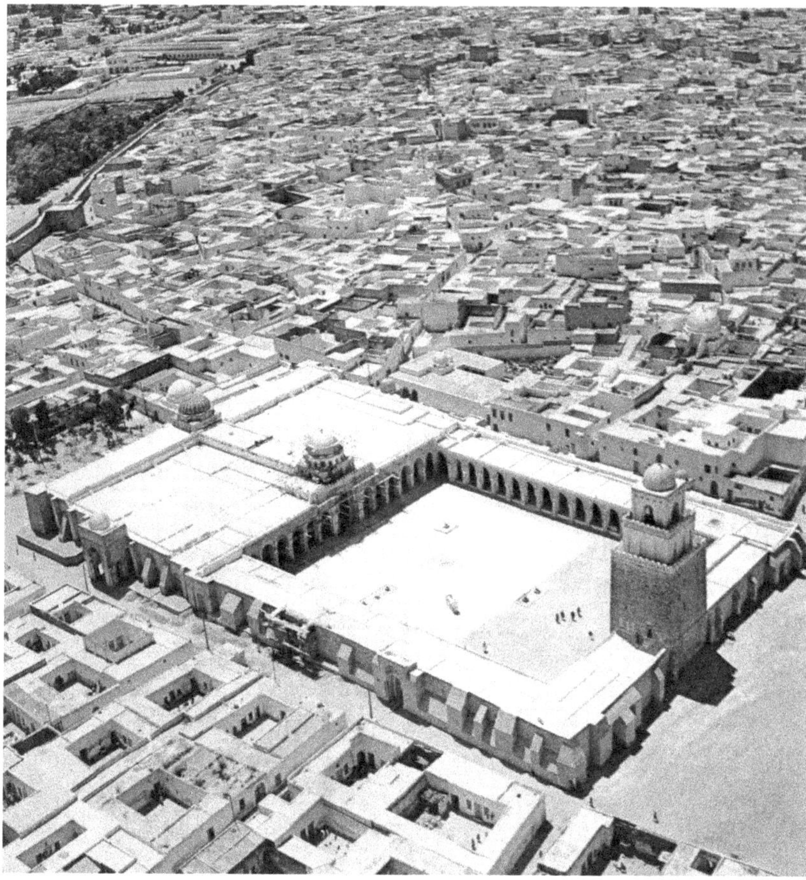

leader's order that the cities dismantle their protective walls, which left them prey to future incursions.

The Berbers had grown audacious during Vandal rule, and when the Byzantine army had left, there were several serious barbarian uprisings. Justinian ordered Belisarius' successor in the province to repair the walls of the cities and build fortresses, and it was in doing this that the greatest damage was done to Roman monuments in North Africa – it was quicker to use the masonry of the splendid but now neglected monuments as building blocks than to build the walls anew. A huge civic building program was begun, new towns were founded, aqueducts were repaired; in short, the region experienced a brief renaissance, even in the field of learning and art. Yet the cost was heavy and many African inhabitants were worse off than during Vandal rule. Corrupt administration of the Byzantines led to civil discontent; more uprisings followed and people sought refuge in fortified towns and huddled around churches and fortresses. There was a brief respite in the beginning of the seventh century when Heraclius was emperor; during these 30 years of peace even agriculture flourished again.

The revival under Byzantine rule, which lasted little more than a century, postponed but did not avert the final demise of Roman North Africa. Yet it had the benefit that the high level of civilisation of the previous centuries was maintained, with the result that the Arabs' inheritance was not that left by the Vandals and Berbers, but that of cultured people who could still read and write and remembered what the Romans had taught them. Raven rightly remarks that the Byzantines formed a link between two civilisations, and that, unlike the Vandals, the Romans' successors in North Africa made their own contribution.[8]

At the death of the Byzantine emperor Heraclius in 641, a few generations after the death of Muhammad, the Muslims had already started their drive to the West and made Palestine and Syria provinces of Arabia. It took them only half a century to swallow up North Africa. In 647 the region was invaded and an army consisting of the remnants of the Byzantine army and Berber reinforcements was annihilated. In 698 Carthage was taken and reduced to ruins. The few remaining Byzantine garrisons in what was Africa Proconsularis were taken. The Byzantines now vanished from history. To the newcomers, the Berbers were their real enemies. The Muslim general, Okba, founded a city, Kairouan, near the ruins of Carthage; the Great Mosque built by him made the city one of Islam's holy places.

With the fall of Carthage in the late seventh century we have come full circle: very soon not a trace of Rome's influence – after half a millennium's rule – was to be seen, and North Africa was lost to Christianity for good. Today the countries of the Maghreb (see note 9 below) are completely Islamicized and largely Arab-speaking.

8 Raven 1993, 229.

Figure 1.5 Map of the Mediterranean in the early Empire

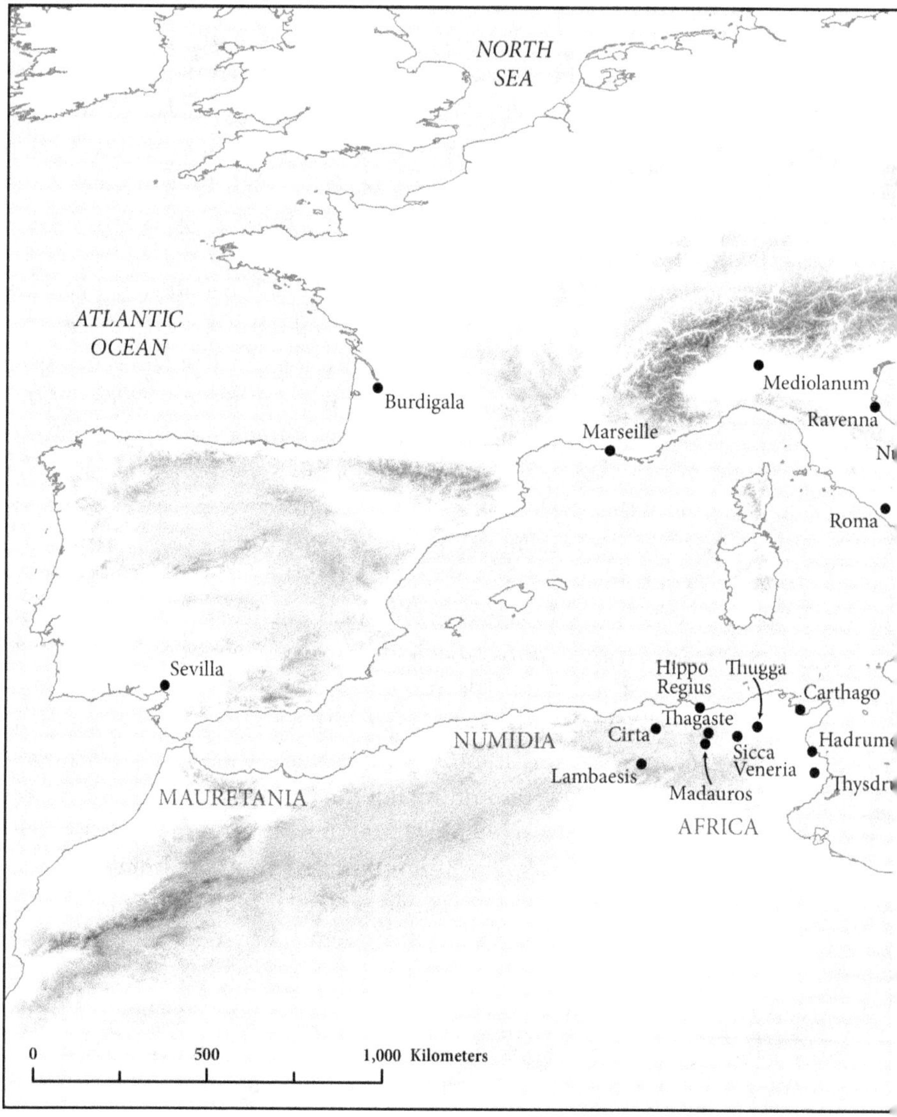

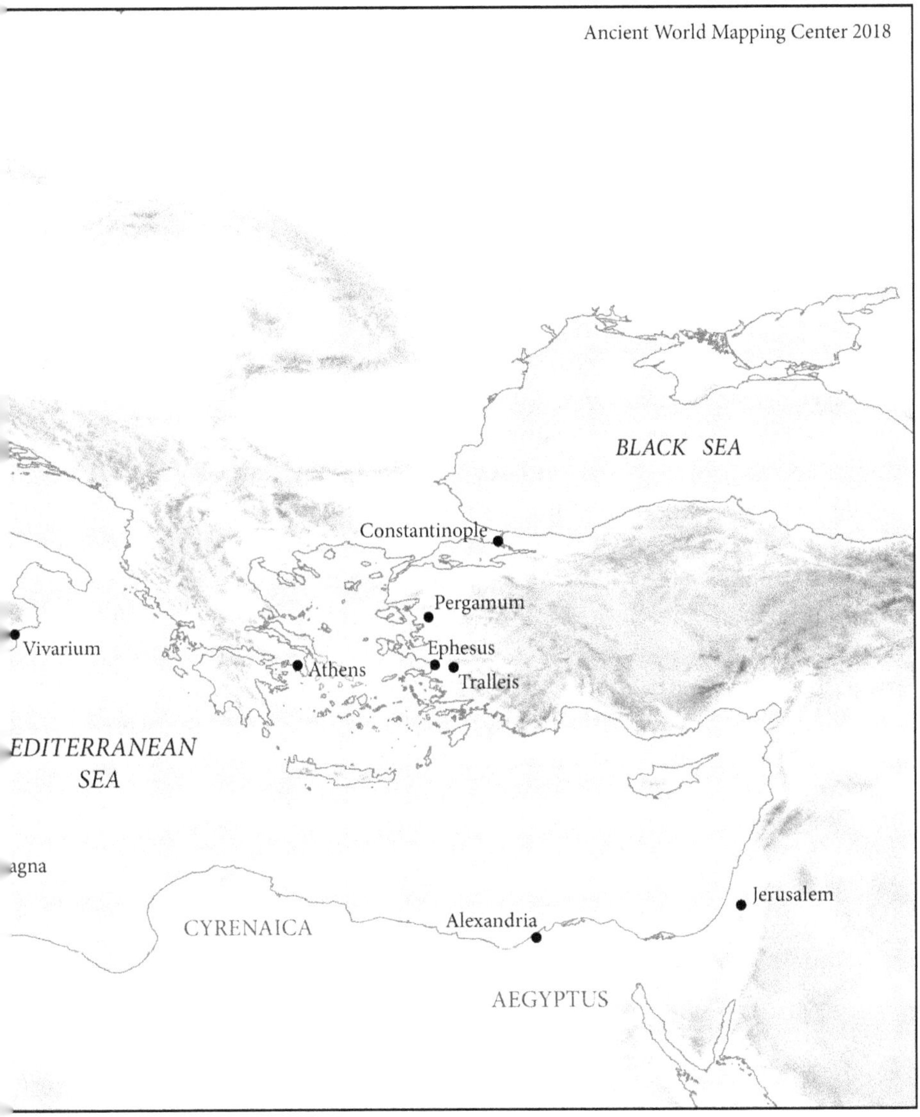
Ancient World Mapping Center 2018
BLACK SEA
Constantinople
Pergamum
Vivarium
Ephesus
Athens
Tralleis
EDITERRANEAN
SEA
agna
Jerusalem
CYRENAICA
Alexandria
AEGYPTUS

The environment

Geography

One tends to think of Roman North Africa as a whole, but at no stage did the African provinces constitute a unity.[9] One should keep in mind that the coastline of Roman North Africa is approximately 2600 km (as the crow flies), the distance from Paris to Moscow. There was a great regional disparity: agricultural and commercial activities varied considerably from one region to the next.[10] The degree of Romanization also played an important role: there was on the one hand the rich, pacified, Romanized zone of the plains of Numidia, Byzacene (the southern part of Africa Proconsularis), Carthage, Mactar and Lambaesis, and on the other the rather primitive but invincible Berber cities in the Mauretanias. Among the indigenous peoples too there were differences. It has been pointed out that in the 'old' part around Carthage, urban life had already been established before the Roman conquest, but that beyond this the indigenous tribes responded to the influence of Rome in different degrees and at different times.[11] In Numidia, for instance, flourishing cities like Cirta (now Constantine) developed, while Thamugadi (now Timgad) and Lambaesis, originally military camps, only gradually became the centres of cities, and other tribal centres developed into villages over a period of time. Farther westward and inland there were fewer cities, and in the Mauretanian mountains there were still 'enclaves of unsubdued barbarism', untouched by Roman civilization.[12]

9 Roman North Africa in the first century CE was divided into various regions. From West to East: Mauretania Tingitana (modern Morocco), Mauretania Caesariensis (the western half of Algeria), Numidia (the eastern half of Algeria), Africa Proconsularis (modern Tunisia), together with the fertile strip along the coast of Libya and Cyrenaica (called Tripolitana). This whole area was later known as the 'Maghreb' (an Arabic word meaning 'where the sun sets'), whereas eastern North Africa (Libya and Egypt) was known as the 'Mashrig' (meaning 'where the sun rises'). Dunbabin 1978, 15.

10 Lepelley 1979, 37.

11 Dunbabin 1978, 15.

12 Dunbabin 1978, 15.

The wealth of North Africa

The granary of the empire

The coastal areas and the eastern part of Roman North Africa have, on the whole, a favourable climate; this ensured reliable harvests. Even before Roman times the Phoenicians had learned the principles of crop rotation and irrigation and had great harvests, but they used this to feed their own population, not for export purposes. Italy's agriculture, on the other hand, had fallen on bad times in the late Republic and early Empire, and small farmers who could not make a living flocked to Rome, where they clamoured for food. From the first century CE Rome thus increasingly depended on the import of grain from Egypt and Africa. In fact, every year for 300 years North Africa sent half a million tons of corn to Rome to feed the masses.[13] For these exports the province received no credit – it was regarded as their annual tribute to Rome. There must therefore have been a sizeable surplus if, after the tax collectors had taken their share, there still remained enough to sell abroad and make a profit.

In order to encourage the cultivation of corn in Africa but also to protect the small farmers in Italy who grew olives and grapes, the emperor Domitian (r. 81–96) placed a restriction on the cultivation of the olive and vine in Africa. This was reversed by Hadrian (r. 117–138) after his visit to Africa in 125, with the stipulation that all land not yet under cultivation should be opened up. North Africa thus reverted to its former 'mixed economy' – growing wheat, olive trees and vines and providing pastures for sheep, goats and cattle, and game for hunting. The so-called Dominus Julius mosaic, found near Carthage, gives a good idea of the affluent agricultural scene in the fifth century CE: we see the house of the master, turreted at the corners with a domed bath house behind it; the living quarters are on the first floor for protection; around the house is a garden with cereal crops and olive trees, domestic animals and poultry, servants and farm labourers.[14]

The great expansion under the emperors Trajan (r. 98–117) and Hadrian caused Tertullian, the early Christian writer from Africa (c. 160–c. 240), to describe this period as follows: 'Smiling estates have replaced the famous deserts, cultivated fields have conquered the forests, flocks of sheep have put wild beasts to flight [...] certain proof of the increase of mankind!'[15]

13 Raven 1993, 88

14 Raven 1993, 165.

15 Tert. *De anima* 30.3.

Figure 1.6 Dominus Iulius mosaic

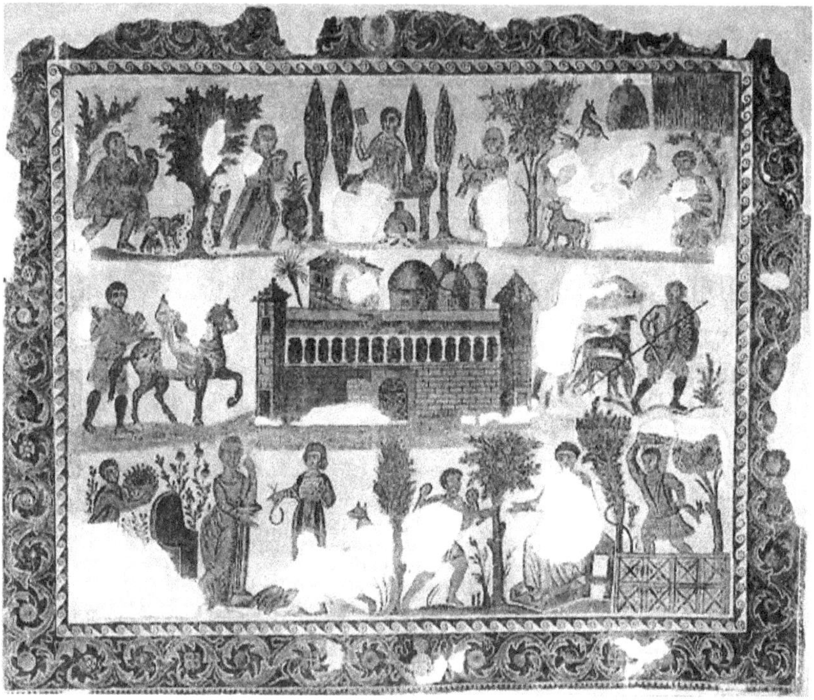

The olive culture

North Africa's greatest wealth, however, derived from the export of olives and olive oil, an industry that was especially flourishing in the third and fourth centuries. Olive oil was used for numerous purposes all over the empire – for instance, to cook, make soap and perfume and, importantly, to use as fuel for lighting. A remark made by St. Augustine (354–430) throws light on just how valuable this export from Africa was: he states that the room that he was renting in Milan at that time was rather dark, since the continued use of oil lamps was a luxury that only rich people in Italy could afford, whereas in Africa he could study at night with an oil lamp (of which archaeologists found innumerable examples) without worrying about excessive cost.[16]

The value of the olive is illustrated by the anecdote about a farmer in Sufetula (seventh century CE): when asked by the commander of the Arabs who had captured the city and was amazed at the amount of

16 Aug. *De ordine* 10.1.3. See also *Sermon* 177.10, *Patrologia Latina* 38–39, 959.

Figure 1.7 Amphitheatre in Thysdrus

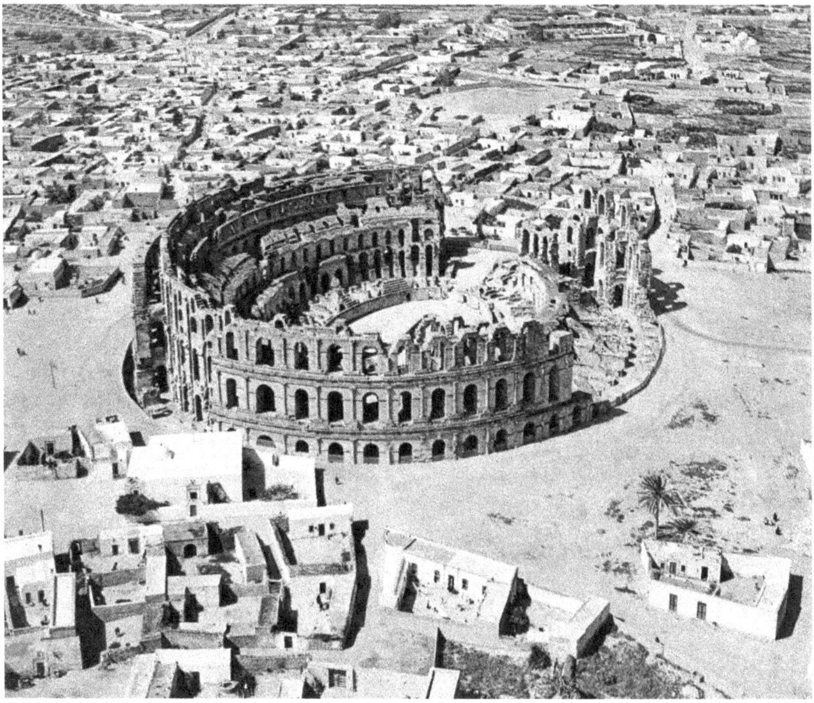

treasure that had fallen into his hands, the farmer looked about him as if in search of some hidden object, and then picked up an olive and, laying it before the commander, told him that this little fruit was the cause of their prosperity.[17]

The wealth resulting from the oil production was the reason the Vandal leader, Geiseric, after having travelled through Gaul, Spain and Mauretania, wanted to settle in North Africa.[18] A contemporary, the African bishop Victor of Vita (b. circa 430), states that the Vandals saw Africa as 'a peaceful and quiet province, the beauty of the whole region bright with colours everywhere'.[19] Salvian, a Christian writer of the fifth century, also became lyrical about the wealth of Africa – according to him, the Vandals 'captured the soul of the empire'.[20]

17 Ibn Abd el Hakem, *Histoire des Berbères*, no date, p. 306 (reference in Graham 1902, 307 n.1).
18 Lepelley 1979, 33.
19 Victor of Vita 1992, 3.
20 Salv. *Gub. Dei* 6.12.

The olive tree is well adapted to dry regions: it does not require much water or fertile land, only space for its roots to spread out; thus olive trees were planted c. 10 m. apart. Though it takes ten years to bear fruit, it requires little upkeep, and thanks to the Pax Romana, long-term planning was possible. Olive trees could support a large population, but not a concentrated one. The enormous amphitheatre at Thysdrus (now El Djem), which could accommodate 60,000 people, is a good example: its size is quite out of proportion with the small surrounding town, but the theatre came into its own on market days or days on which games were presented, when thousands of the inhabitants of the hamlets and peasant villages in the vicinity came and filled the amphitheatre.

In a penetrating archaeological article, Mattingly & Hitchner bring to light that the scale of the olive presses and their overall density in certain regions in North Africa are well in excess of what is found in other regions of the Roman world, and that the olive culture was without doubt the major contributor to the African economy.[21]

Other products

Pliny the Elder (23–79 CE), who was in the late sixties or early seventies procurator in North Africa, made the following remark about this country: 'Nature gave Africa over entirely to cereal, though not depriving it altogether from oil and wine.'[22] Viticulture does not seem to have been a great success – wine was but a minor export product.

Ceramic production, though, constituted quite a part of Africa's economy: there was an abundance of red-glazed pottery, the so-called African Red Slipware, all around the Mediterranean; in fact, from the second century CE these semi-luxury ceramics (for instance, lamps and vases) dominated western Mediterranean markets.[23] African lamps and *amphorae* still reached numerous destinations in the Mediterranean, even through the seventh century, despite the economic decline in other parts of the Roman world.[24]

The forests of Mauretania were stripped bare for citrus wood, of which the most exquisite tables were made – Cicero had one imported for him from Africa at the exorbitant price of half a million sesterces.[25]

21 Mattingly & Hitchner 1995, 190. See also Shaw 1980, 28–60.
22 Plin. *N. H.* 15.8.
23 Lepelley 2001, 88.
24 Mattingly & Hitchner 1995, 200.
25 Plin. *N. H.* 13.2.9

Figure 1.8 Mosaic portraying tigers and lions, favourites in the arena

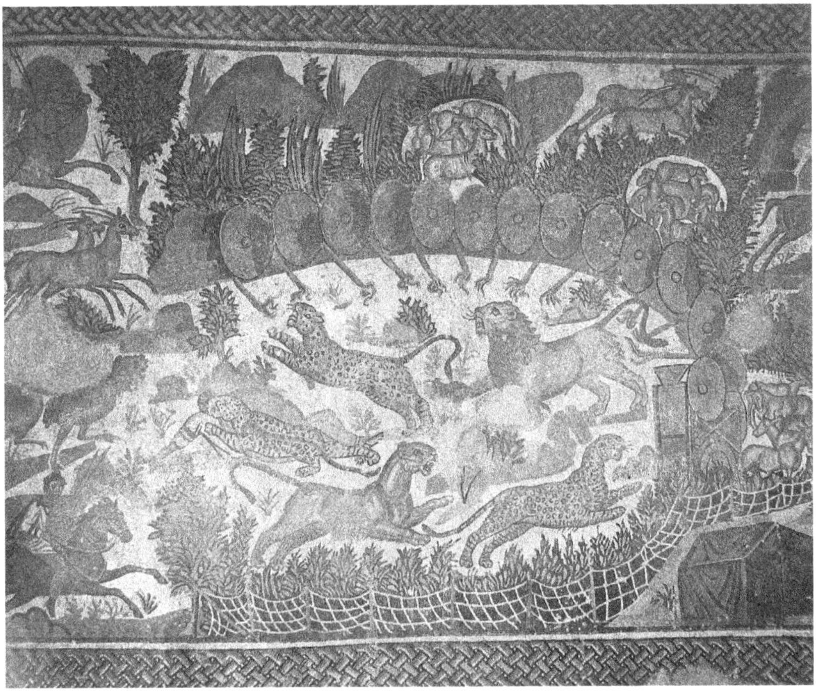

Marble for building projects was also very popular – at Smitthus, quarries were worked for the very striking yellow marble with red veins, which was used for decoration – for instance, in the Pantheon in Rome.

Another luxury product was the costly purple dye secreted by a certain species of sea snail – we read of an imperial purple factory on the island of Meninx (now Djerba) in the time of the emperor Claudius.[26]

Numidian horses, figuring prominently in racing inscriptions in Rome, were famous throughout the Roman world and were highly praised by the first century BCE geographer Strabo.[27] Wild animals like panthers, lions, elephants (extinct by the fourth century), bears and Barbary apes, to be used in the amphitheatre in Rome and for their fur, were ever popular exports.[28]

26 Plin. *N. H.* 9.65.

27 Str. 17.3.19. See also the inscriptions in *CIL* VI.10047, 10053 (reference in Frank 1975, 52).

28 Frank 1975, 24.

Among edible products and exports, figs figure prominently – it was an important element in the diet of the poor in Africa.[29] There is a famous anecdote told by Pliny about the paranoid senator Cato, who, in the time before the Third Punic War, harboured a mortal hatred of Carthage, *inter alia,* because of his fear for the safety of his descendants; he is said to have brought into the senate house a ripe fig from Africa, and, showing it to the senators, asked them when they thought it had been plucked. They all agreed that it was fresh. So Cato said: 'Well, it was picked the day before yesterday at Carthage – so near is the enemy to our walls!'[30] We also read about pears, dates, honey, pomegranates, salt and fish products (for instance, the salty sauce called *garum*) as export products.

Most of the products that were exported were processed in Africa beforehand. However, it has been pointed out that manufacturers had a low social status and that manufacturing was not a major source of wealth.[31] Romans were not supposed to work with their hands (doctors and architects, for instance, were not highly rated socially); wealth came from investment in land or mining. The ancients were thus not interested in technological progress or greater efficiency.

The cities

Development and demise

When Rome started colonizing North Africa in the first century BCE, there were already many towns –as the geographer Strabo mentions[32] – most of which were Punic in origin, but farther inland, Berber (consisting of Libyans, Numidians or Mauri/Moors, with some Hellenistic overlay). Many of the cities were well developed, especially those on the coast, which were cosmopolitan after many centuries of trading. Due to the well-established African culture in these areas, their assimilation to Roman culture took place slowly – in fact, there were few visible traces of Roman influence until the beginning of the second century CE. Then, during the reigns of Trajan and Hadrian, the two second-century emperors who showed an unusual interest in the provinces, the province experienced great prosperity thanks

29 Plin. *N. H.* 15.82.

30 Plin. *N. H.* 15.74.

31 MacKendrick 1980, 324–325.

32 Str. 17.3.15.

to the export of oil, which led to a boom in urban construction, as can be seen in all the monuments and buildings in Roman style.[33] The crisis of the third century – 50 years of civil war – which greatly affected the rest of the Roman world, left North Africa largely unscathed. But changes became visible in the late third and fourth centuries: the pace of building slackened, and the priorities for public buildings changed: 'walls replaced theatres, baths and temples [...] [radiating] the message of a calculated intention to survive'.[34]

Yet the fourth century, the century of Constantine (r. 307–337), started with new vigour. There were 500 small cities in North Africa in that century; only Carthage had c. 100,000 inhabitants; Lepcis Magna had c. 80,000 while smaller cities like Utica and Hippo Regius had c. 20,000 to 40,000.[35] A reasonably high standard of living was kept up until the late fourth and early fifth centuries CE, contrary to the orthodox views of earlier scholars like Mommsen and Rostovtzeff who, disregarding archaeological evidence, believed that the cities were in full decline by the fourth century.[36] The period of anarchy in the third century had little impact on North Africa; in fact, the large estates of the senatorial class continued to flourish for most of the century.[37] And contrary to Rostovtzeff's view, the landed aristocracy did not withdraw into their estates in the countryside like the feudal lords of the Middle Ages – excavations have shown that their villas were within easy distance of the towns.[38]

The Vandal incursion in the fifth century led to radical changes. Mattingly & Hitchner, evaluating the situation from an archaeological point of view, state that the most visible breaks in the Vandal period with the past period of prosperity were buildings that fell into disrepair or were used for more utilitarian purposes.[39] Temples, for instance, were used for Christian basilicas, large peristyle houses were split up into multiple dwellings and workshops, and city walls arose. Carthage in particular suffered heavily:

33 The not-inexpensive mosaics that covered the floors of private houses and public buildings are another sign of the wealth of the inhabitants. Thousands of these visual reflections of everyday life, which greatly enhance our knowledge of North Africa, have been excavated. See especially in this regard Wood & Wheeler (1966).

34 Brown 2012, 11.

35 Brown 2012, 4. Most of these small cities had a population of no more than two to five thousand inhabitants, and though they were close to each other (c. 16 km), they were 'enormously diverse' – some relatively prosperous, others very poor. Brown 2012, 6, 8–9.

36 Rostovtzeff 1957, 535–541.

37 Cameron 2012, 92.

38 Brown 2012, 20–21.

39 Mattingly & Hitchner 1995, 209–211.

wealthy aristocrats were evicted from their homes and often even exiled to make place for Vandal lords. In these dark days, Quodvultdeus, bishop of Carthage, bemoaned the situation: 'Where is Africa,' he lamented, 'which was like a garden of delights for the whole world? [...] Where are those great and most splendid cities?[40]

The Byzantines found a much impoverished country. Smaller towns in the countryside also showed changes: the layout of towns was regrouped around churches and fortresses, no longer around forums, temples and bath complexes.[41] The church came to take the place of the classical city; leadership was now in the hands of bishops, no longer the town council. One must, however, remember that Romanization and urbanization only took place in the eastern Maghreb, that is, the northern and central part of the province (now Tunisia) and in eastern Numidia (now Algeria).[42] Elsewhere it was limited: 'Roman cities were enclaves in the still-foreign world of the Berbers.' This regional differentiation was a serious defect, as became apparent in the course of the sixth century when indigenous tribes attacked the province. The real decline, however, came at the end of the seventh century: Carthage was reduced to ruins during the Arab invasion, and then abandoned by the new conquerors. Kairouan, a new Muslim city, replaced Carthage as capital in North Africa.

As Lepelley details, however, 'archaeological phasing frequently does not coincide with conventional historical periodization, and in compartmentalizing urban activity into periods (Punic, Roman, Vandal, Byzantine, and so on) we are promoting historical over archaeological interpretation of the data. Urban life was a continuum in Africa from the first millennium BCE, in some cases evolving and developing after the Arab invasions of the seventh century.'[43]

In order to complete the picture of the social and economic achievements of the empire, it is enlightening to look briefly at the remains of some individual cities/towns.

40 Quodvultdeus, *Sermo II de tempore barbarico* ('Sermon II on the era of the barbarians') 5.4 (reference in Lepelley 2001, 87).

41 Lepelley 2001, 99.

42 Lepelley 2001, 96.

43 Mattingly & Hitchner 1995, 186.

The environment in North Africa in the fourth and fifth centuries: Some of the cities

Only Carthage will be discussed in some detail, since this was the capital of Africa Proconsularis and was thus the city in which, for instance, Vindicianus as proconsul would have had his residence (see Chapter 5). Many of the physicians mentioned in the following chapters would also have had their consulting rooms there. However, a few other noteworthy cities will also be highlighted to illustrate the environment in which the events in the following chapters took place.[44]

Carthage

Of the North African cities, Carthage was, due to its strategic location and good harbours, one of the oldest. Its turbulent history, with, *inter alia,* three wars against the Romans, has been discussed. The ban on habitation in the area of the destroyed city after the Third Punic War was lifted by Julius Caesar – it was too valuable a site to leave uncultivated and uninhabited. Augustus sent some colonists in 29 BCE, but it took nearly two centuries before the city took shape again. It flourished during the second to fourth centuries; Heather believes that the city fully qualifies to be described as 'a teeming Roman metropolis'.[45] The author of the *Expositio totius mundi* ('The description of the entire world') remarked with admiration on its beauty: the excellent location, the trees that lined the paved streets, the safety of the harbour.[46] During the high Empire, Carthage was the third largest city in the Mediterranean after Rome and Alexandria.[47] The African writer and orator Apuleius (second century CE) left a description of several buildings, such as the Hadrianic theatre, the Severan Odeon (a music hall), the amphitheatre and the circus for chariot-racing, which housed 70,000 spectators.[48] There was also the Antonine Baths, one of the most sumptuous bath complexes in the empire, supplied with water from a new aqueduct bringing water from Zaghouan, 132 km away.

44 The information gleaned from archaeologically based books like that of Wood and Wheeler (1966), Frank (1975), Lepelley (1979 and 2001) and MacKendrick (1980) have proved to be very useful in this section.

45 Heather (2005, 279, 280) states that at its peak Carthage was home to about 100,000 inhabitants, 'a figure exceeded in the fourth century only by Rome and Constantinople, both of whose populations were artificially swollen by subsidized food supplies'.

46 *The description of the entire world* 1966, 200–203 (reference in Lepelley 1981, 24).

47 Lepelley 1979, 49.

48 Apu. *Flor.* 18.

The schools, especially those for higher education, were highly regarded throughout the Roman world – Augustine studied rhetoric and philosophy in Carthage. Apuleius enthusiastically praises Carthage, 'where all the citizens are scholars, where every branch of learning is assimilated by schoolboys, displayed by the young, taught by the old. […] Carthage, heavenly Muse of Africa, Carthage, inspiration of those who wear the toga.'[49] Salvian, a Christian writer of Gaul (early fifth century) also speaks with great admiration of the quality of the schools in Carthage before the Vandal invasion; according to him they taught the liberal arts, Greek and Latin literature and philosophy.[50]

The Vandal arrival disturbed Africa as seat of culture but did not permanently shake it. Even a Vandal poet, Florentinus, praised the city: *Carthago studiis, Carthago ornata magistris* ('Carthage is fit for learning, Carthage is fit for teachers').[51] The schools survived the Vandal conquest. Romans and Vandals alike were taught in the same classroom.[52] In 534, just after the reconquest by the Byzantines, the emperor Justinian provided for the public appointment of two teachers for primary and two for higher education.[53] The survival of the schools is reflected in the literature of the Vandal and early Byzantine eras. All of the writers must have been trained in this educational system.

The passion for the arena and horseracing that so often features in mosaics in Carthage is corroborated by literary evidence: the bishop of Carthage, Quodvultdeus, complained that when the Vandals were at the gates of the city, a great many of the population were still watching events in the arena.[54] Salvian, the monk from Marseilles, writing in 440, stated that the Vandal invasion of the 'African Babylon' was a just chastisement for their vices.[55] The fall of Carthage to the Vandals in 439 was a dramatic event that shook the Roman world. Its impact is comparable to that of the sack of Rome by the Goths under Alaric in 410.

The city suffered greatly during the Vandal occupation when the wealthy aristocrats were dispossessed and even exiled; rural domains were also confiscated. Yet, thanks to the momentum of two previous centuries of prosperity, the city survived during the Vandal occupation and even through

49 Hays 2004, 120.
50 Salv. *Gub. Dei* 7.16, 180 (reference in Lepelley 1981, 25).
51 *Anthologia Latina*, R 376 (reference in George 2004, 134).
52 Hays 2004, 120.
53 *Codex Justiniani* 1.27.1.42
54 Quodvultdeus, *Sermo II de tempore barbarico* 1.1 (reference in Lepelley 1979, 110).
55 Salv. *Gub. Dei* 7.13–17 (reference in Lepelley 1979, 33).

Figure 1.9 Temple of Iuno Caelestis in Thugga

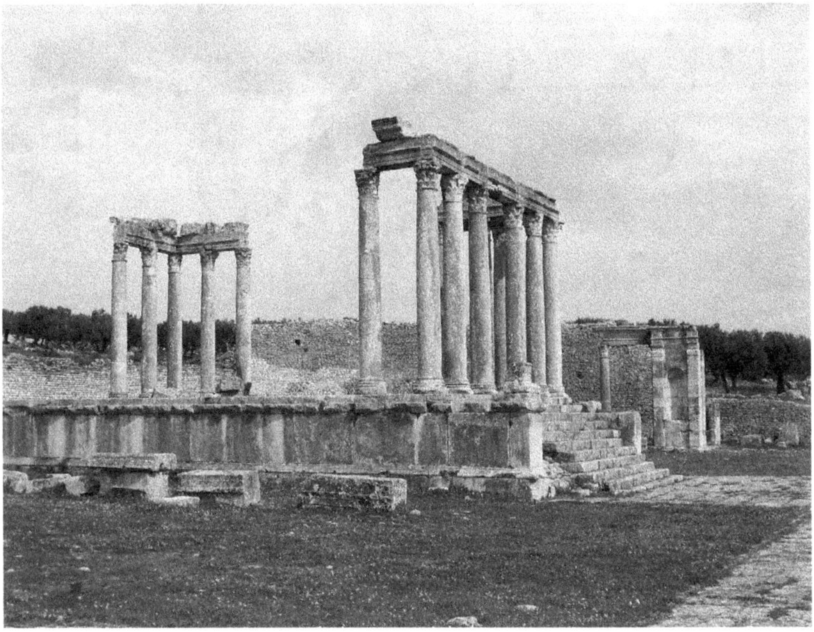

Byzantine times. In fact, Carthage experienced a brief period of prosperity under the Byzantines: the city wall was rebuilt, streets were repaired and the basilica on the Byrsa Hill was converted into a Christian church.

Unfortunately, disappointingly little remains of Roman Carthage today, since it was built over with summer resort villas after World War II, and the remains of ancient monuments were used for buildings in modern Tunis and towns in the vicinity. However, in 1992 there was a report that international salvage operations sponsored by UNESCO have begun to reveal many facts about the ancient city.[56]

Thugga (now Dougga)

Lying off the main road, this little local metropolis had most of the amenities of a big city. It had more, and more varied, cults and religious buildings than any other city in the province, among which the Capitolium, dedicated to Jupiter, Juno and Minerva, and, close by, the well-preserved temple of the Carthaginian goddess Juno Caelestis. There was also a theatre that could accommodate 3500 spectators, and the Licinian Baths, the size of Carthage's Antonine Baths.

56 Ennabli 1992.

Figure 1.10 Mosaic portraying the charioteer Eros and his horses

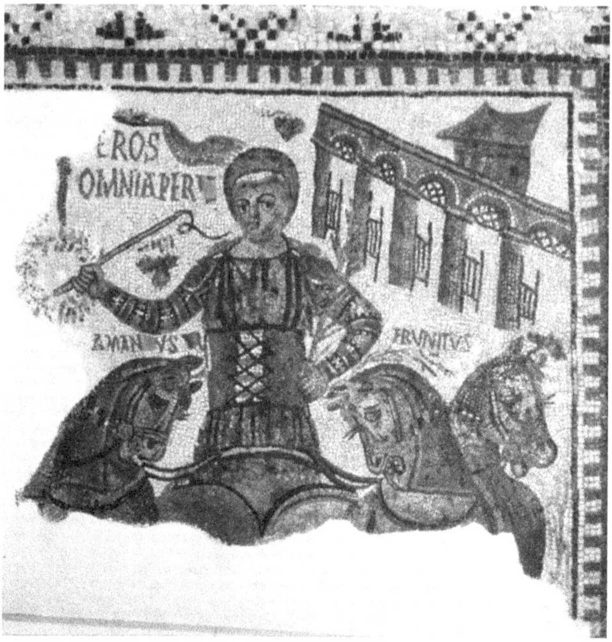

Figure 1.11 Mosaic portraying Vergil seated between Calliope (Muse of poetry) and Melpomene (Muse of tragedy)

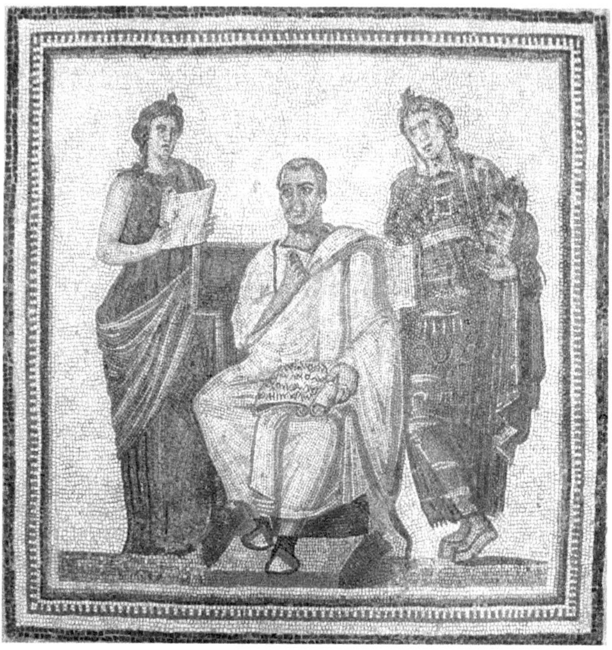

Figure 1.12 Mosaic portraying gladiatorial combats in Zliten

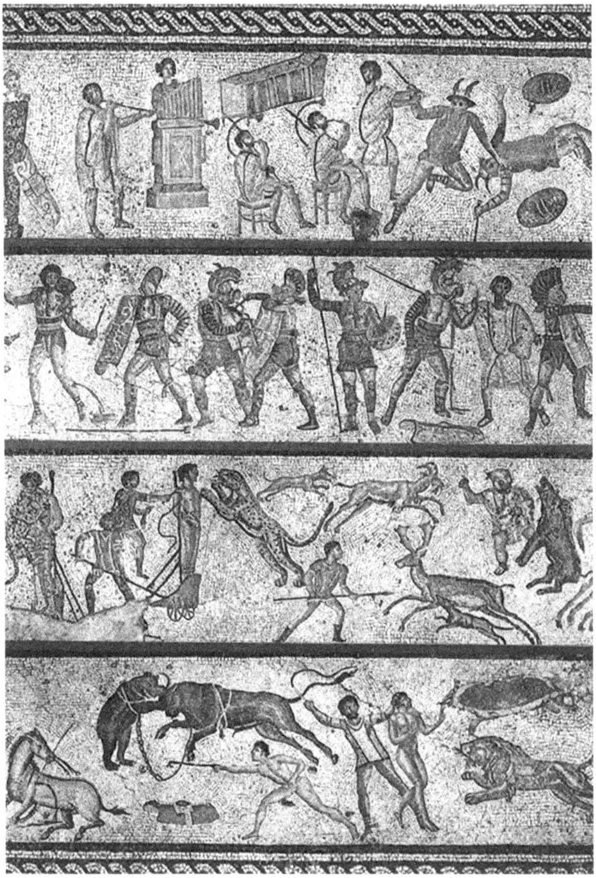

Hadrumetum (now Sousse)
Hadrumetum was the chief seaport on the eastern coast. It was one of the most prosperous cities in the province; more than 250 mosaics were found in private houses and public buildings, among which the famous mosaic portraying Vergil with the Muses Melpomene and Calliope next to him (now in the Bardo Museum in Carthage), and many mosaics portraying horses competing in events in the arena.

Thysdrus (now El Djem)
Reference has already been made to Thysdrus, the small town in the middle of nowhere with the huge amphitheatre which, thanks to olive production, was filled on feast days (especially when gladiator fights were staged) by thousands of farmers coming from farms and hamlets in the vicinity.

Figure 1.13 Hippo Regius

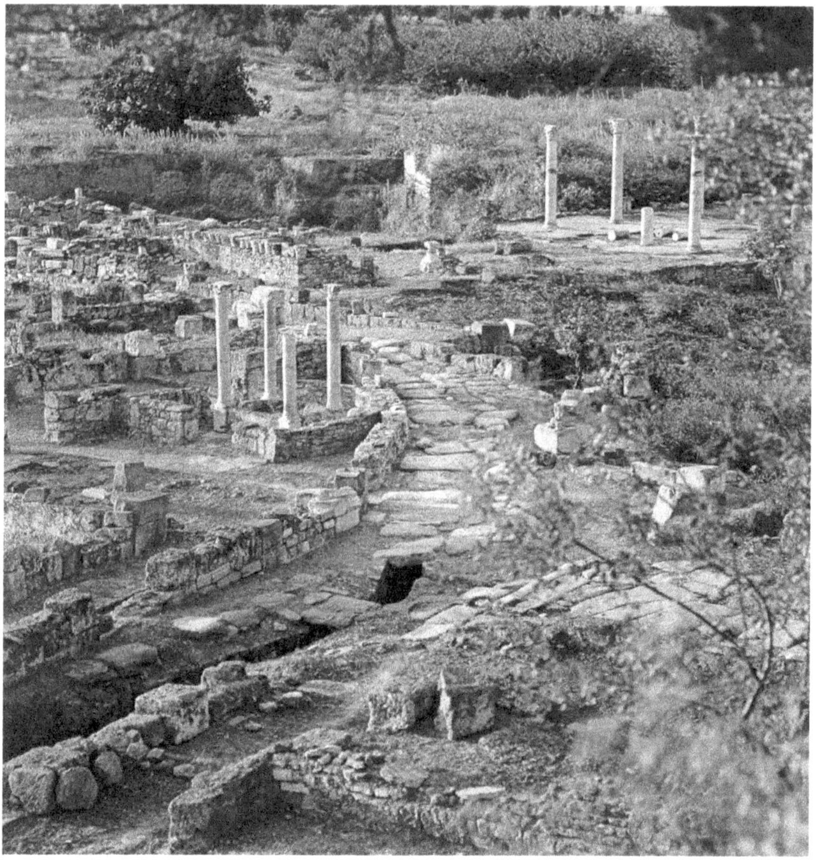

Hippo Regius (now Bône)

This town was, due to its sheltered harbour on an otherwise inhospitable coast, one of the earliest Phoenician foundations. Because of its strategic position, it was soon a regular trading post. The city is in Numidia, but was incorporated into Africa Proconsularis by Augustus. Its pre-Roman origin can be seen in the casual, un-Roman, winding street plan. The famous Numidian horses were bred here. The great Christian bishop St. Augustine had his see here and spent most of his life in this city.

Lambaesis

Lambaesis housed the only Roman garrison in Roman North Africa, the Legio III Augusta. It consisted of three army camps some distance from each other, and is famous because of its *praetorium,* which was a huge four-way

Figure 1.14 Fourway arch in military camp, Lambaesis

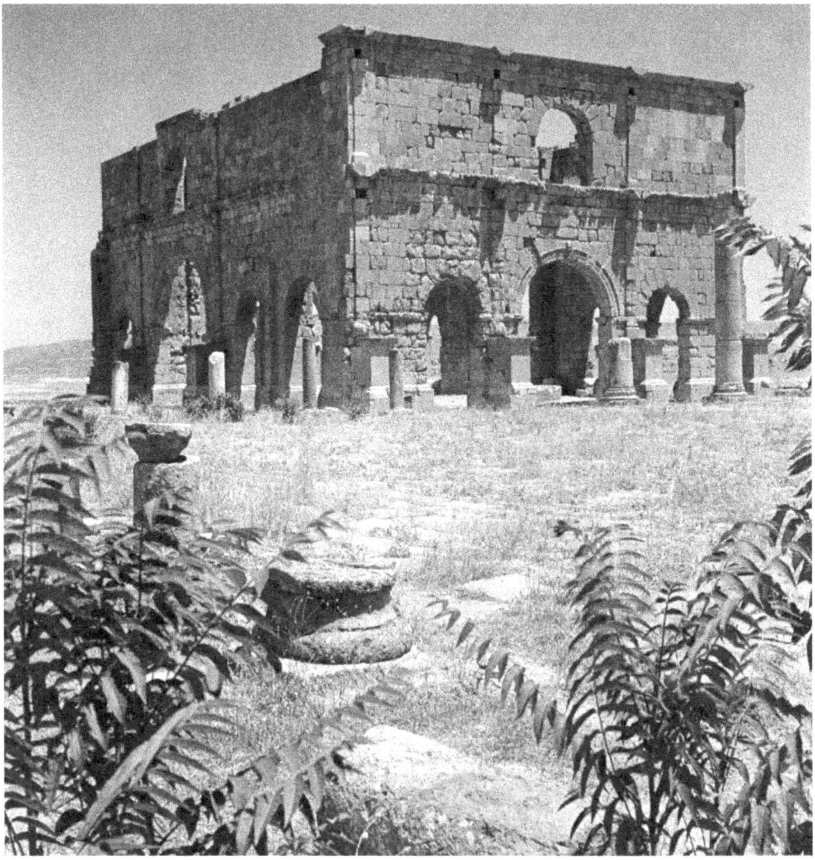

arch with a tile roof and various workshops inside; the building was initially stuccoed bright yellow with the joins in the stonework painted red. The largest camp had baths and a prison; in the nearby town there was a market, amphitheatre, a capitolium and an Aesculapium, or 'hospital' for the sick.

The population

According to the fifth century BCE Greek historian Herodotus, Libya was inhabited by four nations, of which two are indigenous: Libyans living in the north, and Ethiopians living in the south.[57] The Phoenicians and

57 Hdt. 2.53.

Greeks came later. This statement needs qualification: the Greeks used the term 'Libyans' to describe the inhabitants of the whole of North Africa; the Romans later referred to the indigenous people of Roman North Africa as 'Berbers' or Mauri ('Moors'). Apart from them, the peoples the Romans encountered when they first set foot in North Africa were the Phoenicians and the Greeks.

The Berbers

It is believed that Berbers inhabited North Africa from at least 10,000 BCE.[58] From the earliest times they formed the basis of the population in North Africa, and the situation remained thus despite the waves of conquerors that swept over the country. They were a Hamitic people who came from the east across Egypt and spread all over North Africa, even to the Sahara, where they drove the local peoples farther south.[59] They settled in the Maghreb. The ancient Berbers are described as 'long-headed, brown-skinned, black-haired'.[60] They were traditionally nomads, but by the second century BCE gradually settled down to farming; town life later developed. They lived mainly in the Atlas Mountains close to the Mediterranean coast or were oasis dwellers; those living in the Sahara remained nomads. A subsistence economy comprised pastoralism, agriculture and herds.[61] The ancient Berbers were organized in various loosely administered nations, the most important of which were the Maurousioi, or Moors, and the Numidians.[62] There is evidence of trade between Carthage and the Berbers, and of Berbers serving in the Carthaginian army. The Berber elite spoke more than one language: the early stages of the Berber languages that are spoken now, Punic, and occasionally Greek, or later, Latin.[63] Berber civilization reached its peak in the early second century BCE during the reign of King Masinissa

58 See Brett & Fentress (1996) for an excellent summary of Berber history.

59 'Hamitic' denotes a hypothetical language family including Berber and ancient Egyptian. *South African Concise Oxford Dictionary* (1999, 1065).

60 Dennis (1970, 16). He adds further information gleaned from several ancient sources: 'They were lean and squalid. There were blonds as in modern times, but the population was for the most part dark. They [...] plaited their hair, trimmed their beards, cleaned their teeth, and pared their finger nails. They were very healthy and long-lived [...]. Their dwellings were stuffy huts and their couch the ground; their clothing was rough and meagre, often only the skins of beasts which served also for bedding.'

61 Fentress 2006, 20.

62 See Raven (1993, 7): 'for neither Carthaginians nor Romans, Vandals or Arabs invaded in sufficient numbers to alter the ethnic inheritance'.

63 Fentress 2006, 9.

(238–148 BCE), who, during his reign, greatly extended Numidian territory. After his death, however, his sons and grandsons alternately made treaties and war against Rome until Numidia was eventually annexed as a Roman province.

Ancient sources have a negative view of the Berbers, like many scholars of the previous century.[64] In the last few decades, however, scholars have repudiated as Eurocentric the view that the prosperity of North Africa was due to Rome, arguing that 'Rome happily exploited pre-existing social and agricultural systems'.[65]

Famous Berbers in later times included Apuleius, St. Augustine and Pope Victor I (who served during the reign of Septimius Severus).[66] Today there are some 25 to 30 million Berber speakers in North Africa, and the number of ethnic Berbers, mostly living in Algeria and Morocco, is far greater.[67]

The Ethiopians[68]

Herodotus' remark about the Ethiopians 'who lived in the south' would refer to the people from deeper Africa, south of the Atlas Mountains, of whom a small number may here and there have seeped into North Africa, perhaps via the Nile Valley or by trans-Sahara trade routes, though it seems that they did not settle in the Maghreb. A small number of fair-haired, blue-eyed immigrants may have come from the north, but would have been absorbed by the local Berber population.[69]

The Phoenicians

The Phoenicians were an ancient Semitic civilization that inhabited the western coastal part of what is now Lebanon, Syria and northern Israel, and flourished between c. 1500 and 200 BCE. Their origin has been traced back to the third millennium BCE. They are first mentioned in Egyptian

64 In Procopius we also read that the Berbers were noted for their perfidy, that they were superstitious, that women were treated as slaves, and that polygamy was practiced.

65 Merrills 2004b, 14.

66 *Encyclopedia Americana* 2005, III. 569.

67 Wikipedia s.v. Berber people.

68 The name 'Ethiopia' was applied by the Greeks to any region in the far south of Africa. The Greek word *aithops* is related to the word *aithos,* which means 'burning heat', thus the people of 'Aithiopia' were described as 'burnt–faced', i.e., sun–burnt, dark–complexioned, black. An ethnic connotation is already found in Homer (*Od.* 2.22).

69 Wood & Wheeler 1966, 11.

texts from the eighteenth century BCE, and in the ninth century BCE it was Hiram of Tyre who provided cedar wood and artisans for the building of King David's palace and later for Solomon's temple in Jerusalem.[70]

The country inhabited by the Phoenicians in Biblical times was known as Canaan, the land to which Moses led the Israelites and which Joshua conquered.[71] It is widely thought that the Phoenicians originated from the earlier Canaanite inhabitants of the region, which was named 'Phoenicia' by the Greeks; it consisted of port towns on the coast, organized as separate city states.[72] The collection of city states was eventually referred to as 'Sidonia' or 'Tyria'.

The Phoenicians were from earliest times a great maritime people due to the fact that they were hemmed in by a narrow strip of land next to the sea. They were famous for shipbuilding: there are several references in Homer's *Odyssey* to their ships.[73] The Phoenicians were thus great traders, and sold, bought and transported especially luxury goods to overseas markets: wine to Egypt in exchange for papyrus and Nubian gold, silver from the Iberian peninsula, tin from England (which they smelted with copper from Cyprus to make the valuable metal alloy bronze). They also established commercial outposts throughout the Mediterranean, of which the most important, of course, was Carthage.

Their skill in manufacturing articles was also commented on by various authors.[74] In 2 *Chronicles* 2:14 we read about Huram-Abi (the person associated with the building of the temple in Jerusalem) whose father was 'a man of Tyre, skilful to work in gold, silver, brass, iron, stone, timber, royal purple, blue and in crimson fabrics, and fine linens.' But it was especially for the production of purple dye that the Phoenicians were famous. The reddish-purple dye was derived from the secretion of Murex snails, which in early times were profusely available in the eastern Mediterranean Sea but later became extinct due to local exploitation. The dye was probably

70 2 *Sam.* 5:11; 1 *Reg.* 5:1–12 and 7:13–47.

71 In the Amarna tablets of the fourteenth century BCE the inhabitants of this region referred to themselves as 'Kenaani'. The Amarna clay tablets, written in Babylonian cuneiform script and excavated in the late nineteenth century, comprised correspondence between the pharaoh Amenhotep IV, also known as Akhenaten, and his subjects (Hansen 2005, 1336).

72 The word 'Phoenicia' is derived from the Greek word *phoinike*, which meams 'blood-red' or 'purple', and refers to the purple dye of the Murex snail for which the Phoenicians were famous. In Latin it became *Poeni*, *Poenicus* and later *Punicus*.

73 Hom. *Od.* 13.272; 14.295; 15.215 ('men famous for their ships'). See also Ezechiel (26:17): 'o city [...] mighty on the sea'.

74 See Plin. *N. H.* 36.65 par. 191 for the production of glass.

first used by the Phoenicians in the fifteenth century BCE and was highly valued in ancient times because it was colour-fast.[75]

However, the most enduring legacy of the Phoenicians is probably the alphabet, which they transmitted to the Ionian Greeks along the west coast of Asia Minor, whence it spread to Greece and from there to southern Italy, where it was used by the Etruscans before it finally reached Rome.[76]

Some ancient sources also reflect negatively on the Phoenicians. In the eighth century BCE, in Homer's *Odyssey* 14.288, the hero is deceived by a Phoenician, who was on the point of selling him; Zeus saved him by causing a shipwreck, which Odysseus survived. In Roman times, *Punica fides*, or Carthaginian perfidy, became proverbial in the Roman vocabulary, as the historians Sallust and Livy attest.[77] Although undoubtedly biased, the Romans portrayed the Carthaginians as cruel, ferocious and despotic; their chief trait was that of deceit, shown especially in the flagrant breaking of treaties.[78]

The Greeks

The ancient Greeks were from earliest times a seafaring people, seeking opportunities for trade as early as the ninth century BCE and founding new trading stations on coastal sites across the Mediterranean Sea. Greek goods such as pottery, bronze, silver and gold vessels, olive oil, wine and textiles were exchanged for luxury items and exotic raw materials that were then worked by Greek craftsmen.[79] In the eighth and seventh centuries many Greeks emigrated – fleeing famine, drought, the pressure of an increasing population or to expand their trading influence – and formed colonies in southern Italy and Sicily.

The emigration of the Greeks to the western Mediterranean Sea led to a long series of conflicts from 600 to 265 BCE between the Greek cities of Sicily and the Carthaginians (see pp. 15-16). The beginning of the Second Punic War, when the Carthaginians had to use their forces to fight the Romans, put an end to these hostilities.

The Greek traders who visited North Africa left no influence on the Libyan and Phoenician mixture of the population. There is nothing of the

75 A modern researcher reckoned that 12,000 Murex snails yielded about 1.4 gr of pure dye, 'enough to colour only the trim of a single garment'. See also Edwards 2000 on Tyrian or imperial purple and the mystery of the imperial dyes.

76 For more information on the development of the alphabet see Coulmas 2014.

77 Sall. *J.* 108.3; Liv. 21.4.9; 22.6.12; 30.30.27; 42.47.7.

78 Gruen 2006, 469.

79 Hemingway 2000.

quarrelsome gaiety of the Greeks in the Phoenicians, who tended instead to display gloom and hardness, as ascribed to them by ancient authors.[80] And, in any case, the number of Greeks was never very large; only the commercial activities of Hadrumetum and Carthage drew a substantial number.[81] Yet an all-pervading Greek influence was felt and played an important role in North African cultural development.

The Vandals

Although the Vandals were latecomers, they formed an integral part of the population of North Africa after their invasion in the early fourth century, and deserve a closer look. The origin of the Vandals can be traced back to the Carpathian region, in what is today the Czech Republic and western Slovakia.[82] In 406/407 CE a significant number of people, consisting of a loose federation of Vandals, Alans and Suebi, crossed the Rhine and forced their way into the empire. Procopius gives hunger as the reason, but pressure due to the migration of the Huns who settled in the Carpathian region is more likely.[83] The Vandals moved through Gaul, raiding and devastating cities.[84] They eventually settled in Hispania; the Hasding royal house from which Geiseric descended received a very modest and barren piece of land in the northwest, yet they soon spread south, where they made their presence felt. Having reached the coast of Spain, they went farther, plundering the Balearic Islands. At that stage, their leader, Gunderic, died (428) and was succeeded by Geiseric. Jordanes, a sixth century historian, described Geiseric as 'taciturn [...] of violent temperament, extraordinarily resourceful and far-sighted, and prepared to sow the seeds of discord and hatred in order to stir people up against one another.'[85]

Geiseric's name is inscribed in history books because he was the leader who in May 429 led 80,000 Vandals and Alans across the Straits of Gibraltar,[86] but also because he was the most successful of the Vandal kings and lived the longest.[87] After going ashore they marched westward along the coast to

80 Wood & Wheeler 1966, 19.

81 Frank 1975, 108–109.

82 Pohl 2004, 34 and 36.

83 Procop. *Vand.* 1.3.

84 Jerome, in far-off Palestine but well-informed about the course of events in the West, lamented the devastation of the cities (*Ep.* 23).

85 Jordanes, *Getica* 33,168 (reference and translation Pohl 2004, 38).

86 Victor of Vita 1992, 1.2.

87 Pohl 2004, 38.

Hippo Regius, which they besiege for fourteen months. This was the episcopal see of the bishop St. Augustine. The *Comes Africae*, Bonifacius, under whose protection the city was, led an army against the Vandals, but was defeated. The western emperor thus had to conclude a treaty with them, conceding a part of the African diocese to the Vandals. Breaking the treaty, Geiseric took Carthage in 439. The emperor had no option but to renew the treaty, which meant a further allocation of land to the Vandals.[88]

Geiseric had in the meantime acquired a sizeable fleet and soon occupied Sardinia, Corsica and the Balearic Islands; in 455 he broke the treaty for a third time and attacked and plundered Rome for two weeks, 'more thoroughly than Alaric and his Goths'.[89] In 468 the eastern emperor sent a huge fleet to North Africa, but the aged Geiseric had good luck on his side with favourable winds and defeated the Byzantine army. He died in 477 and was succeeded by various kings, until in 530 his grandson Gelimer came to the throne. In 533 Gelimer was attacked and defeated by Belisarius, who occupied Carthage without even a fight and immediately ordered the dilapidated defences to be repaired. Gelimer fled and entrenched himself in a fort in the Atlas Mountains but capitulated in the end; he walked in Belisarius' triumphal procession and then received an honourable exile in Asia Minor.

The Vandal occupation of the country brought great disruption and losses to the upper strata of society, and senators who went into exile lost their possessions. The lands and estates that had been confiscated were donated by the Vandal king to his family and followers, but it seems that the complaints of Victor of Vita and Procopius are exaggerated.[90] It was to the advantage of the Vandals to maintain the municipal systems uninterrupted, and some Romans still reached high positions. The excavations in Carthage show a decline, as elsewhere, but there is no indication of a break in urban development. This brings one to conclude, as George has, that 'the destruction of the Roman cities and imperial buildings of North Africa was not the work of the Vandals, but of their Byzantine conquerors and the African tribes during the expulsion of the Vandals in 534, and by the Arabs in later centuries'.[91]

88 Lee (2013, 117) states that 'the Vandal occupation of the north African provinces as far east as Carthage was a blow of incalculable importance to the western empire, for the provinces in question included the wealthiest in the western Mediterranean, based on their production of grain, olive oil and wine' and meant 'the loss of significant revenues for the government, with all that it implied for its ability to maintain the army'.

89 Pohl 2004, 38.

90 Pohl 2004, 42.

91 George 2004, 134.

It should also be pointed out that learning and culture did not come to an abrupt end with the Vandal invasion, but that it was followed by 'a transitional period of cultural adaptation'.[92] There is even evidence of a small circle of *literati* in the late Vandal and early Byzantine era with Vandal poets like Fabius Planciades Fulgentius, Martianus Capella and Dracontius. These poets shared a common social and educational background and were mostly Christians. Their poems reflect the Vandal interest in and enthusiasm for Roman pastimes and amusements. There was a vigorous cultural life under the Vandals: just over 70 years after the Vandal invasion, their king, Thrasamund, surrounded himself with theologians, rhetoricians and writers.

Language

The history of North Africa makes it clear that the country was in the course of time subject to many cultural changes caused by the successive conquests. The language and culture of the Berbers were replaced by the Punic language and culture, which in turn was replaced by Greek and later Latin and their respective cultures. Latin remained the official language under Vandal rule, but Greek, the language of the Byzantine court in Constantinople, became official during the Byzantine occupation.[93] However, neither Greek nor Latin left a mark in North Africa, since many of the educated people fled to Europe after the Vandal invasion. All of these languages vanished like mist before the sun after the Arab conquest, leaving no language native to North Africa, apart from (modern) Berber. But the contribution of Roman North Africa was the fact that during the 'Golden Age' of the country, the second to the fourth centuries, the culture of the Greeks and Romans had, as it were, merged, and it was a Greco-Roman heritage that was transferred to the provinces in the north: Spain, Gaul and later Germany and even Britain.[94] When the Arabs came, North Africa turned its back to the north, faced east and became part of a new world.

The most important languages in North Africa before the Arab conquest, besides Greek and Latin, were early Libyan and Punic. Early Libyan was the

92 Hays 2004, 111; George 2004, 135,143,142.

93 By the time of the so-called 'last Roman emperor', Justinian (r. 527–565), who was based in Constantinople, Greek (a *koinê* form) had become the official language in the eastern (Byzantine) Empire – Justinian had to publish his famous law code, the *Corpus Iuris Civilis*, in both Greek and Latin (Ostler 2007). However, the inhabitants of provinces in the eastern empire still regarded themselves as 'Romans'.

94 See Chapter 10 on the transmission of the texts.

language spoken by the Berbers, the original inhabitants. At an early stage, merchants and soldiers brought new languages to the coastal cities, but early Libyan continued to be spoken in the countryside. According to ancient sources it sounded 'harsh and barbarous' and could only be pronounced properly by mother-tongue speakers.[95] It was used at the time of the Punic Wars and even during Roman rule, but probably mostly in the countryside (especially in Numidia) – it was the language of the lower and less literate classes. According to some scholars (modern) Libyan is still used today in the rural areas in Libya.[96]

The Phoenician colonists brought with them their language, Phoenician or Punic, when they founded Carthage in c. 800 BCE. It became the official language at that early stage and was the language of the upper classes; it was spoken until the Arab invasion. In the fifth century CE St. Augustine stated that the debased Punic spoken around him was the cultural mark of what was specifically African: *Punica, id est Afra*[97] ('Punic, that is to say African'). It was at that stage on the same level as Latin, the language of the Christians in Africa. However, the difficulty experienced by St. Augustine in finding, for a remote village, a priest who could speak the native tongue gives the impression that there was not a widespread knowledge of Punic among the clergy. One should point out, however, that when St. Augustine died in 430, Punic had been spoken for over 1000 years – it had outlived the Vandals, and was probably still spoken in Byzantine times.[98]

Although the Phoenicians would have become acquainted with Greek merchants and colonists who visited the North African coastal towns from the earliest times, it was during the long and bitter battles between the Carthaginians and the Greeks in the fifth and fourth centuries BCE that the latter left their mark. Greek gradually came into use as the language of culture, even in Carthaginian times;[99] by the second century CE Greek was taught at schools and was greatly in favour among the aristocracy. The emperor Marcus Aurelius, for instance, wrote his *Meditations* in Greek. The influence of Hellenic culture was pervasive in higher circles. But the settlement of numerous Roman colonies in North Africa from the first century onward led to an increasing use of Latin, so that by the end of the fourth century, Greek, though still taught in schools and understood by

95 Sil. 3.305 (reference and translation Dennis 1970, 46).

96 Dennis 1970, 18.

97 *Tractatus in Epistulam Ioannis* 2.3 (reference in Lancel 1995, 437).

98 Lancel 1995, 438.

99 Nep. *Hann.* 13.2 (reference in Dennis 1970, 47).

scholars, was no longer used or understood by the natives in the western part of the empire.

In the second century CE, Greek and Latin were the predominant languages in North Africa. But when a law was passed in 212 by the emperor Caracalla to increase the income of the *fiscus* by making all citizens subject to inheritance tax, Latin was suddenly thrust upon the stage as the world language. This law, the *Constitutio Antoniniana*, conferred Roman citizenship on all free residents of the empire.[100] The advantages of having Roman citizenship at this stage were minimal, but the implication was that Roman law was now to be used in every province of the empire; local laws no longer applied. Lawyers, prosecutors and plaintiffs now all had to know and understand Latin when appearing in court. This led to a great increase in the number of people with knowledge of Latin: thousands of citizens all over the empire were frantically learning it.

The situation in the early Empire can thus be summarized as follows: Latin became the official language of the law and civil service (and eventually also of the Church), while Greek for a long period remained the language of cultural intercourse, and Punic the medium of middle-class exchange. In the background, among the humble Berbers, lurked Libyan and other native dialects.

Cultural life

The wealth and prosperity of Roman North Africa during its 'Golden Age', from the second to the fourth centuries CE, had an advantageous influence on cultural life. Many families had enough money to send their children to school, even in far-off towns or abroad, and authors of all genres had time to devote themselves to writing. Apart from the schools in Carthage already mentioned, there were also centres of learning in Cirta (now Constantine) and Theveste (now Tebessa). Learning started early: local schools in the smallest towns provided an excellent basic education. Although knowledge of Greek was declining across the western empire by the third century, there is testimony that it was still being taught at a small provincial town in North Africa: St. Augustine tells us that he was taught Greek in primary school in the small town of Thagaste (now Souk Ahras). George concludes that 'North Africa challenged, if it did not surpass, Rome, as a centre of culture and learning; the home, in particular of celebrated grammarians, rhetoricians,

100 Boak & Sinnigen 1977, 328.

advocates and theologians'.[101] It is noteworthy that St. Augustine, one of the greatest intellects in Antiquity, spent the greatest part of his life in Hippo Regius – the resources of North Africa and his network of contacts in other intellectual centres such as Rome, Milan and the East appear to have been sufficient to keep him informed of intellectual life and theological developments in the Roman world.[102] A few of these outstanding figures in Roman North Africa in the fourth and fifth centuries will be discussed, starting with the famous author Apuleius.

Apuleius was born (c. 125) in Madauros in Africa Proconsularis in a newly rich family.[103] He received his schooling in Carthage and then used his family inheritance to study Greek and Platonic philosophy in Athens, where he was also indoctrinated in the mysteries of the goddess Isis. Thereafter, to refine his knowledge of Latin, he went to Rome, where, in the second century, there already was an influential group of Africans, including Fronto and Salvius Julianus (see below). He soon squandered his inheritance and returned to Africa. In Oea (now Tripoli) he met an ex-student of his from Athens, who asked Apuleius to stay there for a year and marry his mother to protect the family fortune. Since she was a rich widow, much older than Apuleius, her relatives suspected dubious motives, and took him to court, accusing him of using magic to induce the lady to marry him. He conducted his own defence (later published as the *Apologia*) and was acquitted. He settled in Carthage as a public speaker, where he wrote a brilliant satirical novel, *The Golden Ass*, the only Latin novel that has survived as a whole.

Roman North Africa produced some of the finest lawyers in the history of the Roman Empire. In the late first century CE the satirist Juvenal already referred to Africa as 'the foster mother of lawyers'.[104]

Salvius Iulianus, born in Hadrumetum early in the second century, was one of the most important lawyers to come from Africa. The emperor Hadrian, who had a great appreciation of Iulianus' legal skill, appointed him to edit the praetor's edict. He became consul in 148, and thereafter governor of Lower Germany, then of Nearer Spain, and in 167/168 of Northern Africa. In the codification of law in the sixth century, the emperor Justinian honoured him as the most eminent of Roman lawyers and the precursor of his own codification which became known as the Corpus Iuris Civilis.[105]

101 George 2004, 134.
102 Several letters were exchanged between St. Augustine and St. Jerome in Jerusalem.
103 Harrison s.v. Apuleius in Hornblower & Spawforth 1996, 131–132.
104 Juv. 7.147ff.: 'nutricula causadicorum Africa'.
105 Honoré 1996, 778.

Although not a lawyer – but keenly interested in the administration of justice – a noteworthy person who came from Africa was **Lucius Septimius Severus**, the first African emperor (r. 193–211). He was born in Lepcis Magna of an equestrian family of Punic origin and of considerable local prestige. He was probably a person of colour, as were many of the Phoenician people in Libya. His mother tongue was Punic, but he also spoke Greek and learned Latin at a later stage, both of which he spoke with an African accent. He studied jurisprudence in Rome and followed the normal *cursus honorum* before becoming a commander of legions. After various civil wars he was proclaimed emperor by his legions in 193. He paid much attention to the provinces, and in 202/203 the whole imperial family visited Africa. He made use of the opportunity to visit his home town, which he showered with privileges and buildings. Numerous statues, monuments and triumphal arches erected in his honour attest to his popularity in North Africa.[106]

A great admirer of Severus was **Sextus Aurelius Victor**, the author of the *De Vita Caesarum*, a biography of the emperors from Augustus to Constantius II (360 CE).[107] He came from a humble background, but was not so humble when he stated that he owed his social advancement to his brilliant studies; he remarked that the African background he shared with Severus was clearly capable of carrying the brave to the highest point. Like many other young men of North Africa, he tried to escape what he regarded as the mediocrity of his African background by going abroad. Victor was fortunate enough to meet the pagan emperor Julian (r. 361–363), who favoured pagan intellectuals, at Sirmium, and was honoured by him with a bronze statue and the governorship of Pannonia in 361. This was followed in 389 by his appointment as *Praefectus Urbi* in Rome.[108]

Marcus Cornelius Fronto was born c. 100 in Cirta (now Constantine), studied in Carthage and then went to Rome, where he achieved the consulship in 143 and, at the request of the emperor Antoninus Pius, became the tutor of the emperor's two sons, Lucius Verus and Marcus Aurelius, adopted to secure the succession. Fronto's surviving correspondence with the future philosopher-emperor Marcus Aurelius throws an interesting light on daily life in Rome in the middle and late second century CE. Essentially an orator, he was forever looking for exactly the right word in a sentence. He left no

106 Birley 1996, 1390–1391.

107 Victor states that 'as regards Severus, nobody in the Empire is more celebrated than he' (*De vita Caesarum* 20.6).

108 MacDonald 1996, 222.

work of consequence; it is said that 'he was more interested in how he said a thing than what he said'.[109]

Carthaginian-born **Sulpicius Apollinaris** studied in his home town and went to Rome during the reign of Antoninus Pius (r. 138–161). He too was interested in the meanings of words and in obscure points of etymology; he wrote important commentaries on Terence and Vergil.

Looking back, it becomes clear that Africa was the motherland of Christian literature in Latin. Starting with Tertullian in the second/third century, numerous works were written in the third/fourth centuries in defense of the Christian faith, such as those of **Gaius Marius Victorinus**.

After completing his studies in Africa he became a teacher of rhetoric in Rome in the time of Constantius II (r. 337–340). St. Augustine (who was introduced by Victorinus to Neoplatonism at a critical stage in his life) relates the story of his conversion: a staunch adversary of Christianity, he gradually felt a growing sympathy for the religion; it took him a long time to take the final step because he did not want to cause sorrow to his pagan friends. On the day he was to make his public confession of faith, the clergy offered to read it to him behind closed doors to save him embarrassment, but he bravely came forward and pronounced the formula of faith in front of the congregation; he did it with such conviction that the congregation 'gave him a place in the deepest recesses of their hearts'.[110] He wrote various works defending the Christian faith. He did not have a great mind; his contribution lay in his influence on great minds.[111]

Arnobius was a teacher of rhetoric in Sicca Veneria in Numidia (now Le Kef) in the late third century. Arnobius believed that human reason is powerless to discover the truth on its own: man must not exhaust his frail reason in vain speculation, but give himself entirely to God. In his *Ad nationes* he attacked opponents who state that since Christianity has been on earth, the world has gone to ruin, and used pagan legends to make his point. It has been said that Arnobius knew little of Scripture, made little use of it, and misunderstood some of its leading ideas; he thus 'enjoyed in Christian Antiquity only a very mediocre prestige'. His writings are likewise regarded as suspect from a doctrinal point of view.[112]

Another Christian apologetist was **Minucius Felix** (fl. 200–240 CE); he probably came from Africa, but acted as an advocate in Rome. He states

109 Ogilvie 1980, 270.
110 Aug. *Conf.* 8.2.
111 De Labriolle 1968, 262.
112 De Labriolle 1968, 198.

that he had been a pagan for a long time before converting to Christianity. His famous work, *Octavius*, a dialogue between a Christian, Octavius, and a pagan, Caecilius Natalis, was praised by Lactantius and St. Jerome as one of the finest defences of Christianity.[113]

From Numidia came Lucius Caecilius Firmianus, also known as **Lactantius** (c. 240–c. 320), who became famous as a teacher of rhetoric in Sicca Veneria (now Le Kef). He was summoned by the emperor Diocletian (r. 284–305) to teach rhetoric at his palace in Nicomedia in Bithynia. He did not, however, have success there, since it was a Greek world; furthermore, he lost his position after his conversion to Christianity. In his old age, when he had fallen into extreme poverty, he was called to Gaul by the emperor Constantine (r. 307–337) to become the teacher of his son Crispus. Although Lactantius shows knowledge of the Latin poets and especially Cicero, he has little of importance to say on Christian doctrine. In the Renaissance, Lactantius was, due to the purity of his style, regarded as 'the most classical of all early Christians' and became known as 'the Christian Cicero'.[114]

Tertullian (Q. Septimius Tertullianus, 160–240) was born in Carthage in c. 160 from a pagan family. His conversion to Christianity came late in his life after a wild youth, frequenting public shows and committing adultery. At some stage after his conversion he joined the Montanists, a sect that believed that the Paraclete was incarnate in the person of Montanus; Montanism did however not alter his ideas radically.[115] There are references to Tertullian's 'intense African temperament' and his tendency to fanaticism and rigidness, which is clear from his works.[116] He was still an exponent of the bilingual culture: he wrote in Latin but Greek idioms figure strongly in his works. He left an immense number of works and brought an honest (if undiplomatic) judgment to bear on many of the uncertainties of the growing Christian faith. His *Apologeticum* contains a fiery defence of the morals and beliefs of the Christians against the slander in Rome. His doctrinal works, among which the *De carne Christi* ('On the body of Christ'), *De resurrectione Christi* ('On the resurrection of Christ'), *De anima* ('On the soul') and *De pudicitia* ('On chastity'), were directed against the dualistic view that body and spirit are not one. Tertullian had a great and abiding influence on Christian theology in the West. He is also known for the difficulty of his epigrammatic Latin style.

113 Becker 1967, 952ff.
114 Stevenson 1996, 811.
115 De Labriollle 1968, 60–102.
116 Thieling 1911, 171.

St. Cyprian (Thascius Caecilius Cyprianus, c. 200–258) became a teacher of rhetoric in Carthage and received a classical education. He was a great admirer of Tertullian. However, he broke with his classical background after he became converted to Christianity, and was shortly thereafter ordained as Bishop of Carthage. His works were all in relation to his office as bishop. Most of them provide important information on the persecution by the emperor Decius in 248/249, dealing with the problem of the Christ after the persecution, especially with the problem of the so-called *lapsi* (Christians who had succumbed during the persecution and now wished to re-enter the church). During Valerian's persecution in 257, Cyprian was banished when he refused to sacrifice to the pagan gods. He was recalled the next year, only to become the first African bishop to die a martyr's death. It is said that at his beheading in 258, the authorities treated him with the respect due to his class. He left an immense literary output, among which the most important was *On the Unity of the Catholic Church.*[117]

Medical literature

Medical literature, which will be discussed in detail in the following chapters, flourished in the late fourth and fifth centuries. Whereas Greek had been the language used since the beginning of written medicine, it was the North African writers who in the fourth century started to translate, adapt and summarize Greek medical works into Latin. In making the works of the old masters available to the lay public who no longer understood Greek, these authors played an important role. **Gargilius Martialis** (220–270) was probably the first, writing on agricultural and veterinary science (*Medicina ex holeribus et pomis,* 'Medicines from greens and fruits'). Then the eminent physician and proconsul (in 379 or 380) **Helvius Vindicianus** (c. 330–410) translated and adapted various Greek works into Latin, and also sent a medical treatise highlighting his own expertise, to the emperor Valentian I; in this treatise he styles himself as *Comes Archiatrorum*, which implies a high position (see Chapter 5 on Vindicianus). Vindicianus' pupil, **Theodorus Priscianus** (b. 364?), probably associated with the royal house in the western empire, was well known for his three books of *Euporista* ('Easily available medicaments'), of which the third book, the *Gynecology*, was famous even in the Middle Ages.

117 Matthews 1996, 419.

In the fifth century we find **Caelius Aurelianus** (425–460) from Sicca Veneria (now Le Kef), who translated into Latin the (now lost) books *On acute diseases* and *On chronic diseases*, as well as the *Gynecology*, written by the second-century physician and gynecologist Soranus (greatly abridged and adapted). In this time span too, there was the eminent physician **Cassius Felix** (c. 400–450), probably from Cirta (now Constantine), a respected *archiater*/civic doctor at Carthage, whose *On medicine* was dedicated to the two consuls of the year 447.

The careers of the authors discussed above, who all had contacts in Rome or were in Rome at some stage, reveal the gradual integration of provincials (especially those from North Africa) into the cultural, political and social life of Rome in the third, fourth and early fifth centuries. But after the Vandal conquest the gates closed, as it were, to North Africa. North Africans who used to go to Europe thereafter went as refugees fleeing their native country, no longer as young students or scholars seeking further education or wealth and honour.

2. Health facilities in the cities of Roman North Africa

Dionysius of Halicarnassus, a first-century-CE Greek historian, made the following remark in his book *Roman Antiquities*: 'The extraordinary greatness of the Roman Empire manifests itself above all in three things: the aqueducts, the paved roads, and the construction of drains.'[1] These may seem very mundane aspects to eulogize, but had it not been for the infrastructure provided by aqueducts, bath complexes and sewers, many of Rome's achievements, among them the provision of health care, would not have been possible. The necessary infrastructure was made possible by the amazing level of architectural and technological knowledge of Roman engineers and their expertise in implementing the building plans.

Aqueducts

Aqueducts are, arguably, one of the most distinctive features of Roman civilization. In his famous book, *The decline and fall of the Roman Empire*, the eighteenth-century historian Edward Gibbon described aqueducts as 'the noblest monuments of Roman genius and power'. Not only were they a symbol for everything Rome represented, they were also 'conducive to the health [...] of the meanest citizen'.[2] This was already emphasized in the first century CE by the Roman Water Commissioner, Frontinus, when he compared the vital Roman aqueduct network with the 'useless pyramids and the good-for-nothing tourist attractions of the Greeks'.[3]

However, before proceeding to discuss these technological masterpieces, the bubble must be pricked to deflate some of the glory of the aqueducts. Archaeological excavations in North Africa during the past few decades have brought to light the fact that not many cities had aqueducts,[4] yet thrived on water from traditional sources, such as wells, cisterns, reservoirs, rainwater tanks, and also from water drawn from the *quanat*, a characteristically

1 Cited by Quilici 2008, 552.

2 Gibbon 1974, Vol. I. 52.

3 Front. *Aquaed.* 1.16.

4 As discussed by Shaw (1995, VII.90). See also Hodge (1992, 5): 'Nearly all Roman cities grew up depending for their water on wells or cisterns in individual houses, and some cities (such as London) got through their entire history without ever having had an aqueduct.'

Figure 2.1 The Pont du Gard is part of a 50 km aqueduct built in the first century CE, carrying water from its spring to Nîmes in southern France; it is the highest of all elevated aqueducts and the best preserved

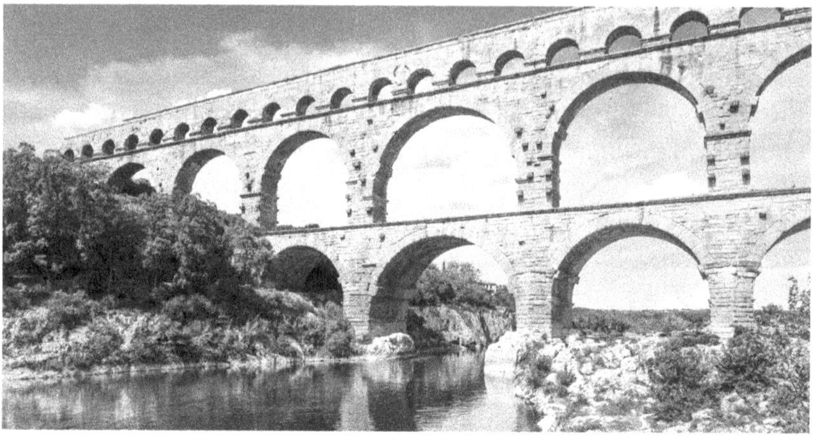

Middle Eastern way of supplying water.[5] Furthermore, little of the aqueduct water reached the ordinary citizen for domestic purposes: pipes from the aqueduct served only a restricted section of the urban centre, since water was mainly used for luxury consumption in prestige projects such as public baths, ornate fountains and the houses of the rich. Aqueducts, contrary to the *quanat*, were not necessary precursors to town development, but were mostly built belatedly after the city had already been established, as an indication of civic pride and an urbane Roman lifestyle (aqueduct building was ruinously expensive). In short, aqueducts were not built to fill a basic human need.

Nor were the Romans the first to build aqueducts. In c. 700 BCE the Assyrian king Sennacherib had a structure built after the fashion of what was later to become a Roman aqueduct, to bring water to his city, Nineveh, from a distance of about 65 km; it is said that parts of it are still visible in Northern Iraq.[6] Roman engineers would also have been familiar with the water management of the Etruscans, their predecessors in Italy.[7]

5 Hodge (1992, 20) describes a *quanat* as 'a tunnel driven into a hillside to tap an aquiferous stratum deep inside it. The tunnel has just enough of a downwards slope for the water tapped to run down it and into the open air by gravity, and is punctuated at intervals [...] by vertical shafts to the surface.'

6 Forbes 1955, 1.156–158.

7 Hodge 1992, 45–47.

In Rome the first aqueduct, the Aqua Appia, was commissioned by the consul Appius Claudius Caecus in 312 BCE. Before that, the citizens of Rome drew their water directly from the Tiber, a method that was practical enough, but dubious from a sanitary point of view, since much of the sewage ended up in the river (see below).[8] Elsewhere water was acquired from streams, springs, publicly owned wells or rainwater tanks.[9] As the city grew, more aqueducts were added, so that by the early Empire there were nine, and by 226 CE eleven aqueducts, supplying water to a city of over a million inhabitants. Hundreds of similar aqueducts were erected in provincial cities and towns throughout the empire. Many municipalities found sponsors to commission the construction of aqueducts, emulating the Roman model; it became an object of civic pride, 'an expensive yet necessary luxury to which all could, and did, aspire'.[10]

In Rome, as in the rest of the empire, only a little of the water brought by the aqueducts served private houses. A private supply could be obtained by imperial grant on payment of a fee, which meant that only wealthy citizens would have been able to acquire private water; others had to employ slaves to fetch water from basins or street fountains.[11] The Romans did not consider the possibility of having pipes laid directly to the kitchen – thanks to many servants, 'that kind of labour-saving device never occurred to the Romans'.[12]

Aqueducts were of course not used in cities only; smaller conduits also provided water for agricultural purposes in rural areas (such as for irrigation), and for industrial purposes (as for water mills and mining operations).[13] In this chapter, though, only the use of water in cities and towns will be discussed.

Since the low rainfall and the uneven distribution of rain in North Africa put a premium on water, it is surprising that archaeological excavations in Volubilis in North Africa brought to light that in this city water was used for purely ornamental purposes. In a wealthy area of the city it was found that many private houses had pipes providing water not for domestic purposes, but exclusively for pools and fountains; these pools were decorated with mosaics showing fish or aquatic scenes, and apparently also served as ponds which would have contained rare fish to be served as delicacies for

8 Front. *Aquaed.* 1.4.

9 See Van Tilburg 2015b, 1-30, on Greek and Roman ideas about healthy drinking water in theory and practice.

10 Gagarin 2010, 1.145.

11 Front. *Aquaed.* 1.103, 105, 118; Vitr. 8.6.2. This would also have been the practice in the provinces where authorization would have been granted by the municipalities.

12 Raven 1993, 118.

13 Hodge 1992, 246–260.

Figure 2.2 Diagram of an aqueduct

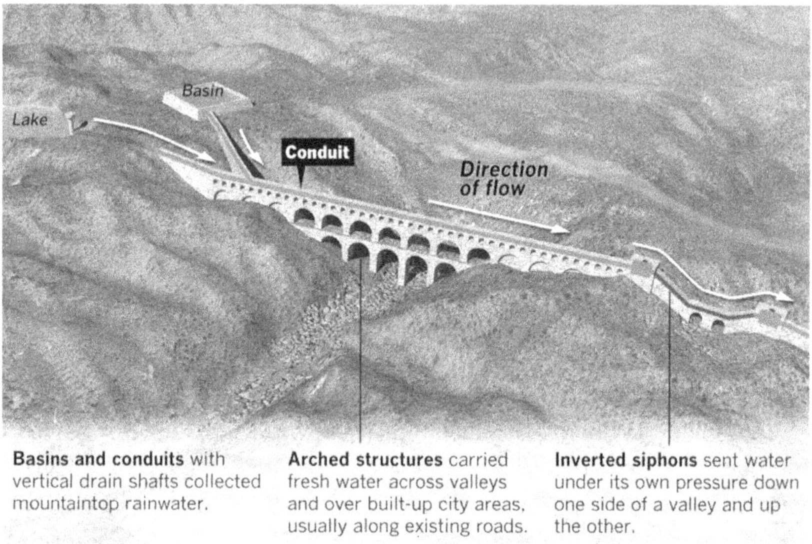

the table.[14] Since the fountains and basins were placed directly opposite the entrance to the house, it seems that running water in Volubilis in c. 60–80 CE was used primarily for the ostentatious display of wealth as a symbol of social status. There is no evidence that the piped water was also intended for domestic purposes; it is, however, of course possible that the water was not potable and thus only fit for decorative purposes or for watering a garden.

Aqueducts were constructed with a slight downward gradient, so that the water moved by gravity alone. The typical aqueduct was a surface channel, but to protect it, it was very often buried some 50 cm to one meter beneath the ground. Those above ground followed the contours of the country, circumventing hills or tunnelling through them, or, where necessary, were carried on bridges over low-lying valleys or syphoned across to deposit the water into water-storage facilities called *castella*. From here it would be distributed to various localities, such as the public baths or fountains or private houses. Aqueducts had ventilation holes, sluices and also sedimentation tanks, allowing impurities to settle on the bottom. The conduits were made of lead, ceramic or stone, but due to knowledge of the health hazard caused by lead pipes, ceramic pipes were preferred.[15]

14 Andrew Wilson 1995, 52–57.

15 Vitruvius (*Architecture* 8.6.1) stated: 'it seems that water should not at all be conveyed in lead pipes if we wish it to be salubrious'. However, Hodge (1992, 308) points out that the calcium

Describing the aqueducts and their working in one paragraph is one thing, but building them was quite another. It is clear that a high level of skill was necessary. Hydraulic engineers were only found in the army[16] – it is therefore no wonder that Lambaesis, the only military camp in North Africa, had an aqueduct. Incidents of failed attempts to build an aqueduct by inexperienced teams due to lack of knowledge are recorded.[17] Vitruvius in his book on architecture left valuable information about the methods of aqueduct building: he described the surveying and mapping of the country to ensure that the water would run at an acceptable gradient for the entire distance, and also the actual construction of the aqueduct. Once the aqueduct had been built, the water had to be kept flowing – a never-ending job. The management and maintenance of the water works were described by the high-ranking ex-consul Julius Frontinus, appointed Water Commissioner by the emperor at the end of the first century CE. In his authoritative book on aqueducts he systematized the maintenance and regular inspection of the aqueducts by appointing gangs of trained workmen; he also investigated the uses and abuses of the water supply, and tried to separate the supply of water so that the best quality went to the fountains for drinking and domestic purposes, while the poorer quality went to the public baths, fountains (their overflow helped to clean the streets), irrigation on farms, mining

carbonate deposit that formed inside the pipes effectively insulated the water from the lead; apart from that, the water was constantly running so that even if it was inside a particular section of the pipe for a few minutes, it was too short a time to become contaminated. An article on lead poisoning from a medical perspective by Retief & Cilliers (2000b, 167–184) confirms this view: they found that the average lead percentage of the Roman population peaked at a level only 41–47 percent of modern Europeans, and classic chronic lead poisoning was first described in the seventh century CE.

16 In peace time, the army participated in many 'community projects', such as the building of roads, aqueducts, sewers, and so on; every major military camp had at least one permanent hydraulic engineer (Raven 1993, 66; Shaw 1995, 69).

17 Shaw (1995, 69–70) mentions two cases, one which was in Mauretania Caesariensis in North Africa, where the governor wanted to build an aqueduct. An expert hydraulic engineer, Nonius Datus, was lent by the army in the neighbouring province, who came and presented a blueprint for the construction of the aqueduct. However, after his departure the construction of the 21-km-long aqueduct soon fell into a morass of difficulties; after twelve years of struggling the governor asked that Nonius be sent again to help with the problems. The work after his departure apparently proceeded for some time, until the laborers encountered a problem when they were tunneling from opposite sides through a mountain; the governor was compelled to ask his neighbour again to send Nonius (by now a retired veteran). When he inspected the work, he saw that the two teams who had started digging from opposite sides had not kept to the line initially established by him. The problem was solved and the aqueduct was completed, two decades after it was begun.

Figure 2.3 The Zaghouan aqueduct in northern Tunisia, part of a 132 km aqueduct (the longest in the Roman Empire), which was built in c. 160 CE and functioned as the main supplier of the city of Carthage

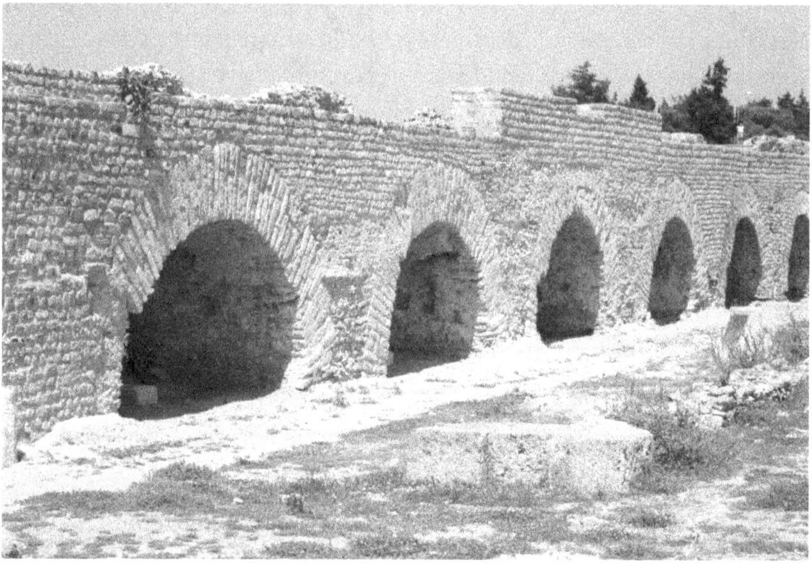

operations, milling, and so on This system was for many centuries followed in all provincial cities and towns.

Excavations of pre-Roman Carthage reveal various water-collection and storage techniques, such as cisterns beneath houses that were built as early as the third century BCE. Some evidence even suggests that there may have been an aqueduct or at least a water pipeline in pre-Roman Carthage.[18] During the Roman occupation, the population increased and new storage and distribution facilities were built. It is reported that in about the first century CE three groups of cisterns and an aqueduct were erected in different areas around the city, including the La Malga cistern complex, one of the largest in the ancient world.[19] Another group of cisterns, the Bordj Djedid cisterns, fed the Antonine Baths. The Zaghouan aqueduct, constructed c. 160 CE, was the main supplier of the city of Carthage during the empire.[20] Its source, a fountain in the Djebel Zaghouan, a mountain range some 60 km south of Carthage, had a splendid colonnaded monu-

18 Wilson 1998, 68.
19 Wilson 1998, 76.
20 Wilson 1998, 80.

Figure 2.4 Nymphaeum built over the spring of the Zaghouan aqueduct

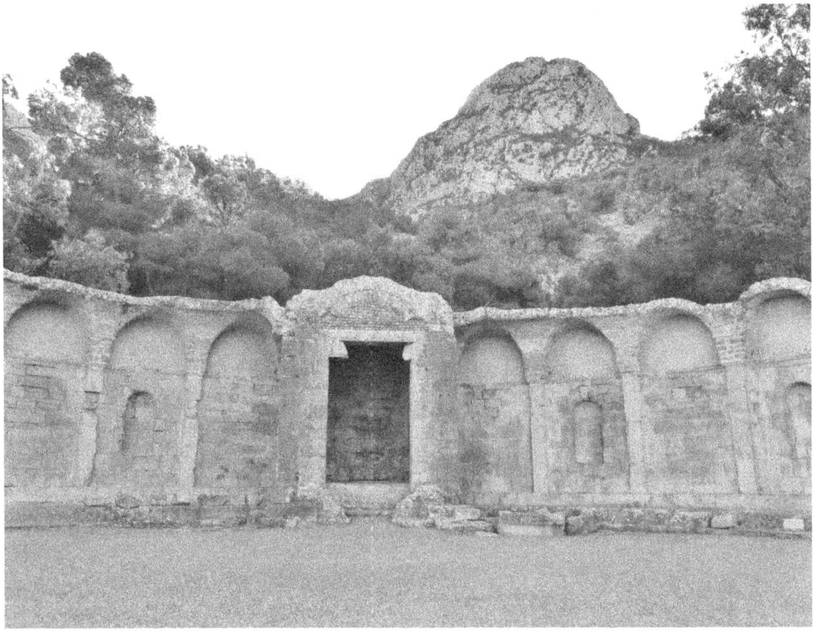

ment surrounding it.[21] It flowed 132 km to the city, making it one of the longest aqueducts in the Roman Empire. This aqueduct is a masterpiece of engineering, considering that the water travel this enormous distance by force of gravity alone.

The Zaghouan aqueduct was destroyed on three occasions: during the Vandal destruction of Carthage in 439, during the Byzantine invasion in the sixth century, and again during the Arab conquest of the city in 698 – but was restored each time. In the sixteenth century it had deteriorated to the point where it was used as a stone quarry. In the nineteenth century the French again restored it, and it is reported that it is still in use today. Aqueducts elsewhere in the Roman world also deteriorated and fell into disuse with time; this occurred in Rome after the emperor Constantine moved the capital to Constantinople in the fourth century CE. There are, however, some aqueducts still standing and said to be in working order, including the Pont du Gard in France, the Aqueduct of Segovia in Spain and the aqueduct supplying the Trevi Fountain in Rome.

21 Water in North Africa was treated with reverence, thus the springs from which the water was tapped often had a marble monument on it – for instance, at Timgad (Raven 1993, 118).

Figure 2.5 The aqueduct at Segovia in Spain, built c. 100 CE

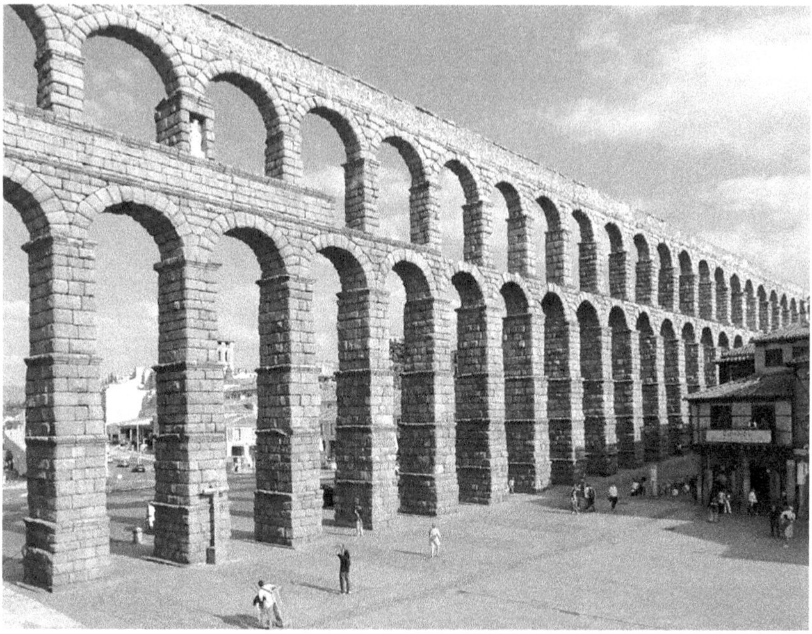

Public Baths/*Thermae*

The Romans set a high premium on health – *mens sana in corpore sano* ('a healthy mind in a healthy body'), wrote the satirist Juvenal.[22] The most conspicuous proof of this view are the innumerable public bath complexes all over the Roman Empire, the ruins of many still with us today. Every town and city worth its name had its own public bath – Thamugadi (now Timgad) even had thirteen![23] The most famous bath complexes or *thermae* in North Africa were the Licinian Baths in Thugga (now Dougga),[24] the Hadrianic Baths at Lepcis Magna,[25] and the Antonine Baths in Carthage.[26]

22 Juv. 10.356.

23 MacKendrick 1980, 232. Hodge (1992, 49) adds that all military forts had baths as standard equipment, as was the case in, for instance, the forts in Hadrian's Wall in England.

24 Dated 250–275, also symmetrical like the Antonine Baths in Carthage.

25 Among the largest in the Roman world, half the size of the Baths of Caracalla in Rome. Also symmetrical, providing bathing for both sexes.

26 Fourth in size among the baths in the Roman Empire, the others being those of Diocletian, Caracalla and Nero in Rome; the Antonine Baths were erected in 145, finished in 162. They were symmetrical, with similar baths for women.

Figure 2.6 Ruins of the Antonine Baths in Carthage, among the largest Bath complexes in the Roman world

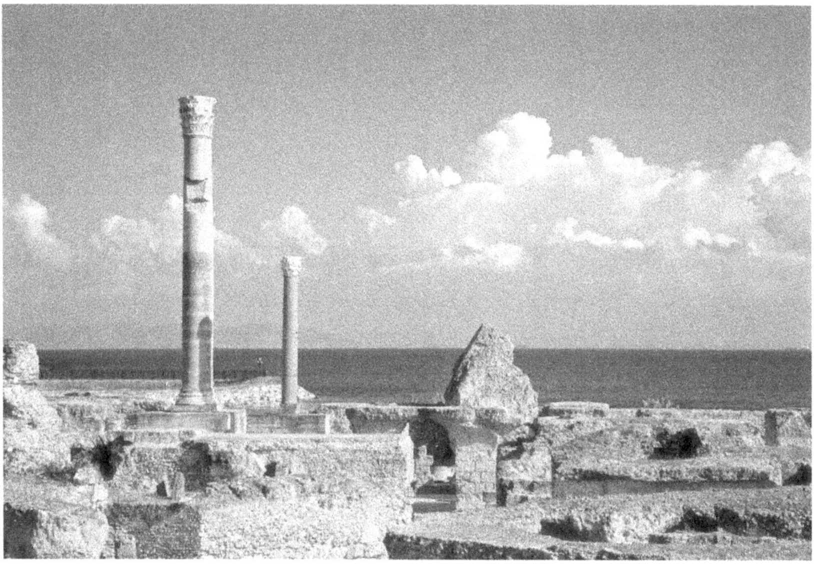

The latter complex was the most impressive surviving Roman building in Carthage; it was unusual in that it faced the sea, so that the front rooms took full advantage of the magnificent view. They were used up to the end of the Byzantine rule in the sixth century CE, but had by then lost much of their grandeur.

It can be argued, from a modern point of view, that it was a great waste to have used so much water for the public baths, that it was consumption for mere luxury purposes – but any tourist who has visited Tunis and its environs in summer will disagree. The unbearable heat and the stifling humidity make it understandable that the Romans, with their practical bent of mind, would endeavour, by all means possible, to make living conditions bearable for the ordinary citizen. Their solution was the building of structures such as bath complexes, public fountains in the forum and *nymphaea*[27] in strategic places.[28] But unlike the Greeks, who were interested in the outside of a

27 Water basins with a fountain and statues, often sheltered by a marble portico. A beautiful three-story *nymphaeum* in the form of a grotto with a fountain and statues between the columns of the portico survives in Lepcis Magna (MacKendrick 1980, 163).

28 Mumford (1973, 273) states that during its heyday, Rome had approximately 500 fountains, 30 public parks, 8 grassy commons and many gardens and libraries.

Figure 2.7 Ruins of the Antonine Baths in Carthage, built c. 150 CE

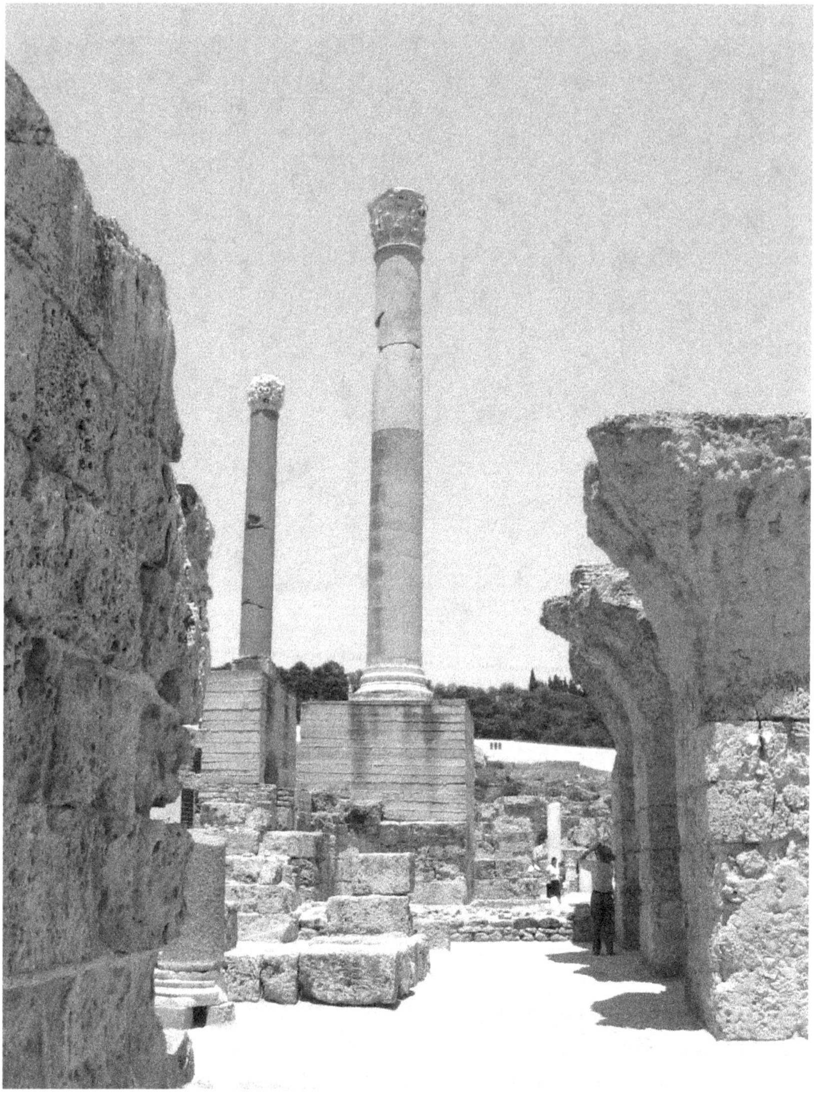

building – consider the beauty of the Parthenon in Athens – the Romans were not motivated to beautify the exterior of buildings,[29] but instead designed interiors: the beautiful inside of Roman bath complexes with their

29 Consider the unattractive outside of the Pantheon in Rome, and the so-called Hunting Baths just outside Lepcis Magna (Wood & Wheeler 1966, 70 plate 15), which look like giant versions of the modest barrel-vaulted houses seen all over North Africa.

vast vaulted ceilings reminds one of a typical medieval cathedral.[30] Most of the *thermae* were furthermore crammed with statues and decorated with beautiful mosaic floors.

The *thermae* were built around three principal rooms:

- the *caldarium* (the room for the hot bath provided with basins, and in large complexes, with a swimming pool),
- the *tepidarium* (a transit room which acclimatized bathers to the difference in temperature between the hot and cold baths; bathers would here be anointed with oil by slaves, and the excess oil would be removed by a *strigil*, a metal scraper),
- the *frigidarium* (the room for the cold bath, smaller and darker).

Rooms for various other functions were added, such as

- the *apodyterium* (a room for undressing before entering the baths; clothes would be taken by slaves, who were notorious for their dishonesty (attested in the *Digesta* 47.17) thus many clients brought their own slaves to carry and guard the clothes, towel and oil),[31]
- the *laconicum* (a dry sweating room, much like the modern sauna),
- the *sudarium* (a moist steam bath).

Many *thermae* also contained a *palaestra* where men could take part in various ball games and exercises, and the wealthy complexes also had a library and *popinae* or shops to buy food and drink.[32] The baths thus served many purposes, and were above all a place to socialize, invite friends to dinner, canvass for an election, discuss business deals, and so on.[33]

The *thermae* opened at noon when the underground furnaces were lit, and closed at dusk.[34] The usual routine was, after undressing in the *apodyterium*, to have oneself anointed in the *unctarium*, followed by a workout in the

30 Raven 1993, 115.

31 The bather's slave also helped his master during the bath, massaged him, plucked the hair from his armpits, and so on (Paoli 1963, 225).

32 Paoli 1963, 223.

33 A comment on the Internet states that the baths were 'the modern equivalent of a combination of a library, art gallery, mall, restaurant, gym and spa' (http://www.wikipedia.org/wiki/thermae).

34 Paoli (1963, 226) explains the methods of heating the water in the baths: 'A furnace (*hypocausis*) fed with charcoal was used for heating the water for the baths and for spreading hot air into the cavities between small brick columns under the floor where the hot air could circulate freely under the floor and in the double walls.' Three bronze tanks were placed above the furnace, one above the other, the cold one on top to be refilled continually, then the tepid one underneath, then the hot one under that, directly on the furnace. They were linked with

Figure 2.8 The Baths of Diocletian in Rome, built c. 300 CE and used until the invasion of the Ostrogoths in the sixth century (outside)

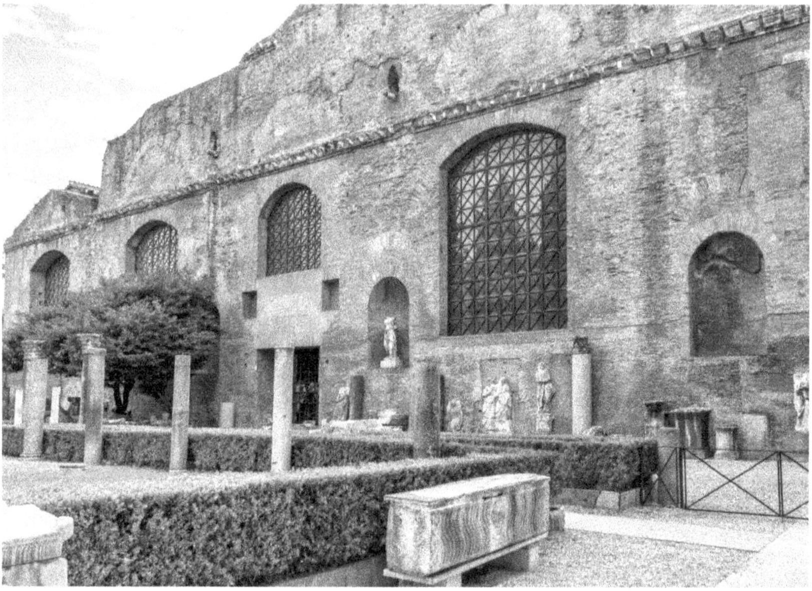

palaestra, scraping oneself down and then enjoying dry heat in the *laconicum* or the sauna in the *sudarium*, then a plunge in the warm pool, then in the cold pool, thereafter again in the warm pool. This lengthy routine was so popular that it was sometimes found necessary to throw darnel seed in the braziers to smoke the patrons out![35]

The *thermae* thus provided physical relaxation for all, even women: most baths were symmetrical, having separate identical but smaller sections for women; otherwise there were different times for bathing for men and women and the very poor (the entrance fee was modest[36]). According to the first-century-CE philosopher-statesman Seneca, the ancient Romans washed their arms and legs, which would naturally have become dirty after working, every day, but they washed completely every nine days.[37] However, during

the different baths by means of pipes. This was the invention of central heating, attributed to C. Sergius Orata in the first century BCE (Valerius Maximus 9.1.1).

35 MacKendrick 1980, 62.

36 *Quadrante lavatum* (one can 'bathe for a *quadrans*', a very small coin), Hor. *Sat.* 1.3.137. Entrance was sometimes free when a rich citizen would arrange a free day to gain favour with the populace.

37 Sen. *Ep.* 86.12.

Figure 2.9 The Baths of Diocletian (inside). In 1560 the Pope ordered Michelangelo to build a church commemorating Christians who, according to legend, died during its initial construction – hence the name: Basilica of St. Mary of the Angels and the Martyrs. View of the *frigidarium*

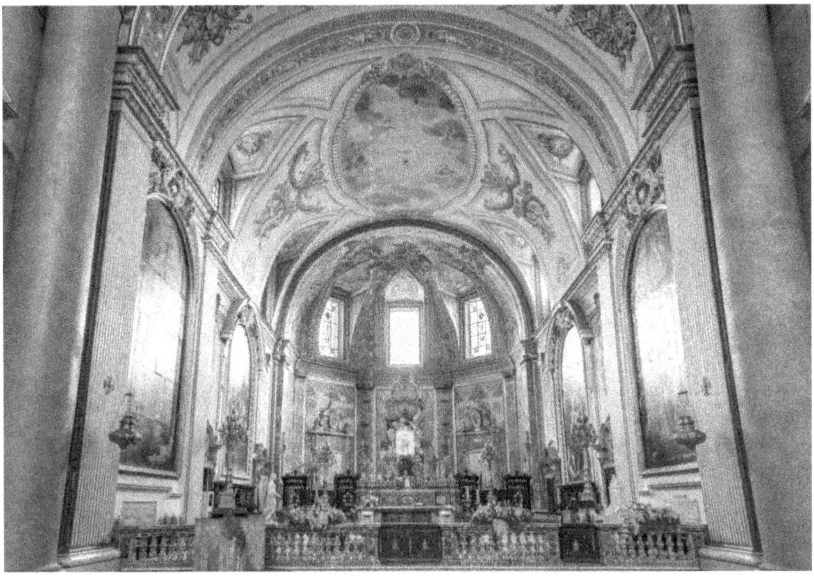

the empire a daily hot bath became the custom.[38] Since the second century BCE some private houses also had a bathroom (*balneum*) in the house.

At Sidi Ghrib, near Carthage, a private bath complex was found in 1983, built by a husband and wife for themselves and their circle of friends.[39] In the cool, high-domed *frigidarium*, the owner advertised his achievement with an inscription: 'I have built more than my income allowed, but never as much as I would have liked.'[40]

Roman society thus seems to have been remarkably clean, and, one would have liked to add, healthy.[41] The flip side of the coin reveals a different picture, however. It has been noted that the first-century-CE medical

38 When asked by a foreigner why he bathed once a day, a Roman emperor is said to have replied, 'Because I do not have the time to bathe twice a day' (http:// www.pbs.org/wgbh/nova/lostempires/roman/day.html. Retrieved 2015-06-03). See also Paoli 1963, 221.

39 Brown 2012, 200.

40 See also Leone (2007), who had made a study of public baths in Africa.

41 *Ancient Roman Baths. Explore Italian Culture* (http://www.explore–italian–culture.com/ancient-roman-baths.html. Retrieved 5 January 2016).

writer, Celsus, on numerous occasions advises patients suffering from a broad range of ailments and diseases to go to the baths as part of their treatment.[42] Some of the many illnesses he mentions for treatment in the baths are fevers (possibly associated with typhoid or malaria, *On medicine* 2.17.4), cholera (4.18.5), dysentery (4.23.3) and diarrhoea (4.26.2). There was thus a real possibility that patrons visiting the baths could become infected with a wide range of infectious and contagious diseases.

The emperor Hadrian (second century CE) made a ruling that the sick have the exclusive right of the baths until the eighth hour (2 o'clock), possibly to protect the healthy from the unhealthy, but it is not certain whether the Romans realized that diseases such as cholera and dysentery could also be transmitted by water.[43] And there is no indication that the Romans used disinfectants in the pools, nor do we know how often the pools were drained and cleaned, but then the water flowed in and out of the pools quite quickly. Nevertheless, *thermae* lingered on in the West until the sixteenth century, when a combination of church preaching and syphilis led to their demise.[44]

Apart from the baths visited mainly for recreational purposes, there was another category of baths: baths 'served by hot springs or water with some mineral content', and visited because of the medicinal quality of the water.[45] This was the equivalent of a spa, which would be frequented by those who wanted to 'take the waters', as it was later expressed.[46] The proconsul-physician Vindicianus did in fact mention the benefits of visiting such a spa to a patient whose excessive eating and drinking led to fever and constipation.[47] The following medicinal baths in North Africa are mentioned: Aquae Calidae (Hamman Righa on the coast), Aquae Flavianae (Aïn el-Hammam near Lambaesis, whose warm swimming pools are still in use), and Aqua Septimiana Felix, in a sanctuary in Timgad, modern Algeria, which had a sacred and therapeutic spring possibly visited by the emperor Septimius Severus himself.[48] Hamman Lif near modern Tunis, where Apuleius is said to have taken the waters, is a spa still used today.[49]

42 Scobie 1986, 425.

43 Scobie 1986, 425.

44 Scobie 1986, 427.

45 Discussed by Hodge 1992, 261.

46 The word 'spa' is derived from Latin: *Sanus Per Aquam* (http://www.explore-italian-culture.com/ancient-roman-baths.html. Retrieved 5 January 2016).

47 Vindicianus' letter to the emperor Valentinian 1, par. 7. In: Niedermann & Lichtenhan 1968, 46–53.

48 MacKendrick 1980, 205, 218, 236.

49 Raven 1993, 116.

The sewers

Among the wonders of the city of Rome, Pliny the Elder (first century CE) mentioned the sewers, which he described as 'the most noteworthy achievement of all', considering their size (one could travel in them by boat) and their solidity (buildings which collapsed in the streets above them did not damage them).[50] And indeed, the Cloaca Maxima, originally constructed by the last Etruscan king in the seventh century BCE to drain the marsh where the Roman forum was later situated, became a landmark in the field of public hygiene. It later acquired all the functions of a modern sewer, and was so solidly built that it is still used for that purpose today, 2700 years and many millions of litres later!

And yet – despite the valuable contributions to public health care made by the aqueducts and baths in Rome and the provinces discussed above – there were deficiencies. In an informative article, Scobie investigates the state of the sanitation in Roman cities and towns. Though he concentrates on Rome and Pompeii, the situation would have been the same (or worse) in the provinces.[51] One of the problems that emerges is the deficiency of the disposal of human and animal waste.[52] Roman lawyers seem to have been more concerned about preventing the burial of the dead within the city walls than about the disposal of human and animal waste within the city.[53]

Very few houses in the Roman world had a built-in latrine. Scobie describes the setup in the houses that did have one: the latrine (built over a cesspit) was situated either in or partly separated from the kitchen, in a small doorless, windowless room.[54] The location had the advantage that the open cesspit could also be used for kitchen waste, but apart from offensive smells, it was a constant source of infection and there was the real risk of food poisoning. The contents of such cesspit toilets would accumulate until a local manure merchant was called, who would cart it away for resale as fertilizer to farmers; the fluid content was used by fullers for industrial use.

50 Plin. *N. H.* 36.24.

51 Scobie 1986, 399–433.

52 See Van Tilburg 2015a, 103-117 on the excrement problem in ancient Greece.

53 'A dead man shall not be buried or burned within the city' (*Twelve Tables* 10.1, *Remains of old Latin* 1969, 496–497). See Cilliers & Retief (2006, 48–49) for information on the burial practices of the Romans.

54 Scobie (1986, 415) notes that 'evidence for the existence of private latrines at Rome is all but non-existent', thus one can conclude that the same would have applied in cities and towns in the provinces. It is, however, amazing to read that 'almost every house in Pompeii had a latrine' (Scobie 1986, 409).

Figure 2.10 The Cloaca Maxima

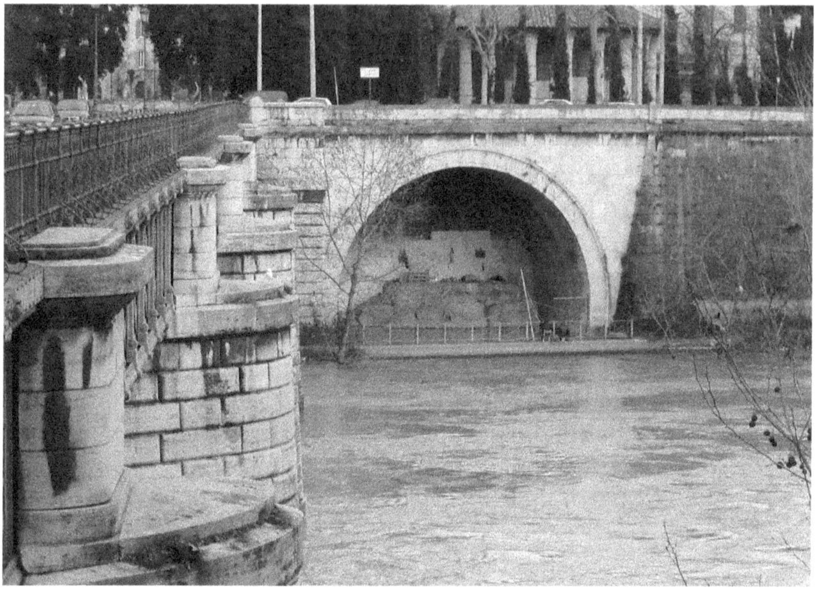

Although a connection with the street sewers could be acquired, house owners for various reasons preferred internal cesspits.[55]

In multi-storey apartments, upper floors had no running water, but sometimes the building would have had a communal latrine on the ground floor.[56] If not, the tenants had to use the public toilets in the vicinity, or pots put on the front doorstep of businesses for possible contributions (fullers in particular needed urine for industrial purposes), or a chamber pot, which would simply be emptied onto the street out of an upper-storey window.[57] The satirist Juvenal (first century CE), when relating the perils facing those walking in the streets of Rome at night, notes that passers-by could count themselves lucky if it was only the contents of the chamber pot that fell on their head and not the vessel itself![58]

55 Scobie (1986, 413) mentions as possible reasons that (i) flushing a toilet down a connecting pipe was wasteful of water, which would have been an important consideration in North Africa where water was so precious, (ii) the manure was very useful as a fertilizer in a pre-industrial society, and (iii) the removal of the manure provided work for unskilled labourers.

56 Hodge 1992, 337.

57 Instances are mentioned by, *inter alia*, two first-century-CE satirists, Petronius (*Cena Trimalchionis* c. 27) and Martial (*Epigram* 6.89).

58 Juv. 3.269–277. There was in fact a law (Ulpian in the *Digesta*, 9.3.5.1–2) on the legal responsibility of the upper-floor tenant if there were an injury in such a case.

Figure 2.11 A typical Roman toilet

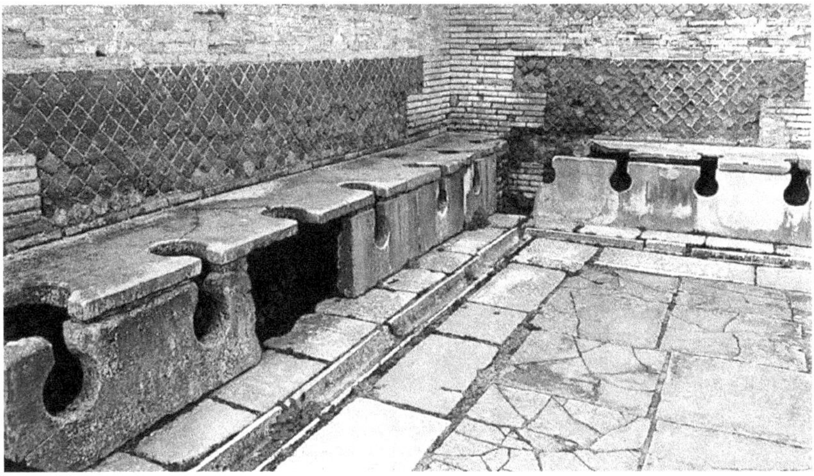

Due to the lack of private toilets or *foricae,* public toilets were well frequented. Some of them were attached to *thermae* but accessible to all members of the public, or else situated at strategic positions – next to the forum, for instance. It seems that the Romans felt no embarrassment in sharing the toilets – on the contrary, it was a place to consort with friends, make business deals or invite one another to dinner.[59] The toilets consisted of a large open room with beautiful architectural embellishments and, along three sides, a row of seats, sometimes as many as twenty per side. The seats were made of wood or marble, and sometimes even had armrests. They were mounted over a constantly flowing stream of water that carried off the sewage; in front of the seats was a small gutter with flowing water in which tenants could wash their hands.

One of the less pleasant tasks of the *aediles*, officials who were in charge of the sanitation of Rome and the Romanized cities and towns in the empire, was oversight of the cleanliness of the streets, which could present a real health hazard.[60] Sewers for the conveyance of domestic human waste were only found in cities where the density of the population justified it; elsewhere, drains functioned for the disposal of surplus water (rainwater and the overflow of the fountains) as well as for sewers.[61] The continuous

59 See Martial's ditty on Vacerra spending a day in the toilets waiting for an invitation to dinner (Mart. 11.66).

60 *Dig.* 43.11.1.1.

61 Hodge 1992, 332.

Figure 2.12 Stepping stones to cross a street in Pompeii

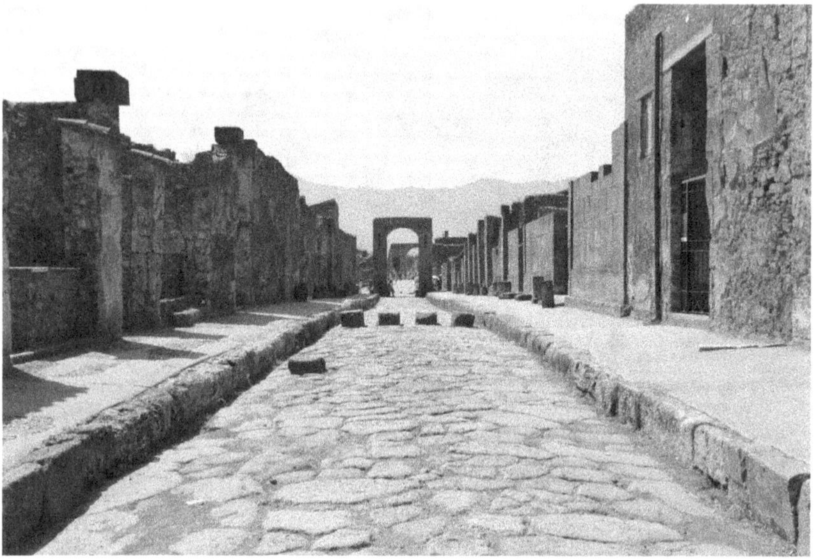

overflow of the street fountains (automatically fed by the aqueducts which could not be 'turned off') thus greatly helped to keep the streets clean.[62] The drain water was then discharged into a large central collector (the equivalent of the Cloaca Maxima) or in a nearby river or the sea, or left to soak away in a nearby field – there is no record of sewage treatment, although it would at this stage have been greatly diluted by the fountains' overflow.

Despite a law prohibiting the throwing of excrement and corpses onto the street, or contaminating the water, or covering anyone with dung or filth, it did happen.[63] The biographer Suetonius (first century CE) reports that the emperor Caligula ordered Vespasian (a future emperor) to be covered with filth when as city *aedilis* he had failed to keep the streets clean.[64] Dogs and carrion birds such as vultures must have played a useful role in the disposal of street refuse, but of course fouled the street with their faeces.[65] It is clear that inadequate street cleaning posed a real health hazard: not only from the pollution of the water basins in the streets with carrion and filth, but also from the pollution of food sold at open-air shops (most probably infested

62 Hodge 1992, 306–307.

63 *Dig.* 43.10.1.5.

64 Suet. *Vesp.* 5.3.

65 Suetonius records that on one occasion, while Vespasian was having lunch (he was emperor by then), a dog brought in a human hand and deposited it under the table (*Vesp.* 5.4).

with flies), through direct or indirect contact with human and animal faecal matter. Diseases that could result from such environmental conditions included cholera, dysentery, gastroenteritis and typhoid.[66]

Hospitals

Hospitals as a feature of public health service are taken for granted today. But the hospital as we know it, an institution where a patient is treated by a physician over a period of time, only came into being in late Antiquity. Some scholars believe that the temples of Asclepius in Greece to which ill people flocked may be regarded as the first hospitals. But there is no evidence that priests regularly treated patients there; they went to the Asklepieia because of dreams in which, they believed, the god revealed to them what treatment they ought to follow.[67] Neither can the *iatreion* or the *taberna* – consulting room of the Greek and Roman physicians, respectively – be regarded as a kind of hospital, since there is no evidence that provision was made for nursing patients over a period of time in either of the two. The question may then be asked where the ill were treated in Antiquity. It seems that the poorer patients were brought to the doctor's consulting room, where they received treatment and then returned home, while the rich were visited at home by the doctor.[68] Hospitals only came into being in the fourth century CE under the influence of Christianity. Hospices, originally called *xenodochia*, initially built to shelter pilgrims and messengers between various bishops (mainly in the eastern empire), eventually also housed disadvantaged and diseased people, and in the course of time developed into hospitals. By the fourth century *xenodochia* had become well-known institutions in the west as well, among other reasons because the emperor Julian the Apostate (r. 361–363), in his attempt to revive paganism, tried to attract converts by establishing *xenodochia* in emulation of the Christians.[69]

With the rapid rise of Christian monasticism, it was logical that charitable endeavours would emanate from monasteries. Infirmaries originated as

66 Scobie 1986, 421.

67 Cilliers & Retief 2013, 69–92.

68 Galen states that on a usual working day he first visited patients and met social obligations and then took a bath (Gal. *San. Tu.* 6.7 and 412 K., reference in Horstmanshoff 1995, 84). That rich patients were treated at home is also confirmed by Celsus (*Med.* 1.65), Cato (*R. R.* 1.1) and Columella (*R. R.* 11.1.18).

69 Jul. *Ep.* 49. On the rise of hospitals see Cilliers & Retief (2002, 60–66), and also Stegers (2004) and Israelowich (2015).

health care facilities inside monasteries, designed for care of the monks. In time civilian patients were also admitted, and later treatments supplied by the monks themselves were supplemented by help from physicians from outside.

Various well-known hospitals in the empire became established in the fourth century – among them, the celebrated St. Basil of Caesarea in the 370s (which apparently had as many wards as there were diseases), soon to be followed by others, such as the one built by the wealthy penitent widow Fabiola in Rome, and two other wealthy ladies, Pulcheria and Pauline in Constantinople and Jerusalem, respectively.[70] The empress Eudoxia also ordered the building of a hospital in Jerusalem.[71] In North Africa there were three hospitals in the fourth and fifth centuries: one at Calama, the others in Carthage where two churches were transformed into hospitals; we know of a third hospital, or, as it was called, a *xenodochium*, in Hippo Regius, because St. Augustine mentions it in a sermon.[72]

Military hospitals, or *valetudinaria*, on the other hand, can be traced back to the first century CE, the first probably built at Carnuntum (near Vienna). They were established after the creation of a professional army when, with the extension of the empire, it was no longer possible to send soldiers home for treatment. *Valetudinaria* were thus established, especially near the frontiers, where wounded and ill soldiers could be treated. Normally the *medici* in charge (the number and experience of the medical staff would have depended on the size and prestige of the unit) would have been competent to deal with a broad spectrum of injuries and diseases, but since they were not equipped for long-term convalescence, seriously ill or wounded soldiers would be sent home or to a nearby spa.[73]

Similar arrangements, though on a much smaller and less satisfactory scale, would have been made for slaves on big estates or *latifundia* – landowners realized the necessity of keeping their labour force healthy in order to ensure that they could fulfil their function.[74]

70 Hier. *Ep.* 77.

71 Allan 1990, 447–450.

72 Aug. *Serm.* 356 par. 10. In this moving sermon St. Augustine explains how he ordered the priest Leporius to build a *xenodochium*; initially the latter had to use the funds intended for the church, but when the congregation saw the building rise, they started to contribute, each in accordance with their situation (http://www.augustinus.it/latino/discorsi/discorso_519_testo.htm. Retrieved 6/01/2016). St. Augustine elsewhere refers to the presence of one or two doctors in the monastery at Hippo (*The literal meaning of Genesis* 12.17). Reference in Benseddik 1988, 672 n. 72.

73 Jackson 1988, 134–135.

74 Jackson 1988, 65.

The province of North Africa was in a unique position since, thanks to the peaceful condition during the early empire, only one legion was allotted to it. The Legio III Augusta was housed at Lambaesis in Numidia, and consisted of three camps. The main camp is famous for its huge *praetorium* or guardhouse (mistaken for an elephant stable by an early excavator!) – basically a huge tile-roofed four-way arch, one of the most impressive surviving structures in North Africa.[75] To the north of the *praetorium* were barracks and possibly a hospital, which Benseddik believes could, among other uses, have accommodated pilgrims who received what we would today call psychosomatic treatment.[76] A civilian town grew up east of the main camp, in which excavations uncovered *thermae*, and also an Aesculapium complex complete with therapeutic baths as part of the health regime prescribed by Asclepius, to which patients with chronic ailments would have gone.[77]

The lack of clear evidence of a military hospital in Lambaesis can probably be ascribed to the fact that in view of the peaceful situation the authorities did not think large-scale provisions for wounded soldiers were necessary. Still, some arrangement would have been made by the medical staff for treatment of the soldiers and sick civilians (who in other parts of the empire went to military forts for treatment). Yet hospitals in the pre-antisepsis era were at best a mixed blessing, given the dismal recovery rate of patients after operations.

Conclusion

Despite all the health facilities by means of which the Romans tried to promote good health among citizens, it cannot be denied that ordinary people in the cities and towns of the Roman Empire lived in a highly unsanitary environment. One must, however, keep in mind that health facilities and laws alone could not achieve much – the main problem in the Roman Empire at large was a lack of knowledge. Only centuries later – after the discoveries of people like Louis Pasteur, with his germ theory of infection, and Joseph Lister, who invented an antiseptic that reduced post-operative mortality – could there be an improvement in health services.

75 MacKendrick 1980, 221–226.

76 Benseddik 1988, 678.

77 MacKendrick (1980, 225) mentions that some 1400 inscriptions of grateful patients who were healed by Asclepius, the god of medicine, were found there, in one of which it is stated *bonus intra, melior exi* ('go in good, come out better')!

One should furthermore not criticize the Roman government overmuch, since the situation in Rome was in many respects similar to that in large European cities till shortly after 1842, when Edwin Chadwick's 'Sanitary Report' was published in London, drawing attention for the first time to the 'appalling consequences of inadequate waste disposal in cities'.[78] Then only was a series of laws passed in England to improve sanitation, living conditions among the poor, and public health services in general. This example was eventually followed by improvements instigated by public heath pioneers in Europe and the United States.

78 Reference in Scobie 1986, 417 n. 138.

3. Greek, Roman and Christian views on the causes of infectious epidemic diseases[1]

In 251 CE a devastating epidemic struck the Roman Empire. A description of the situation in Carthage, capital of North Africa, one of the empire's most prosperous provinces, has survived:

> There broke out a dreadful plague, and excessive destruction of a hateful disease invaded every house of the trembling populace in succession, carrying off day by day with abrupt attack numberless people, everyone from his own house. All were shuddering, fleeing, shunning the contagion, impiously exposing their own friends, as if with the exclusion of the person who was sure to die of the plague, one could exclude death itself also. There lay about meanwhile, over the whole city, no longer bodies, but the carcasses of many, and, by contemplation of a lot which in their turn would be theirs, demanded the pity of the passers-by for themselves.[2]

Some gory details of the symptoms of the disease are mentioned by Cyprian, bishop of Carthage at the time of the epidemic:

> The bowels, relaxed into a constant flux, discharge the bodily strength [...] a fire originates in the marrow, ferments into wounds of the fauces [...] the intestines are shaken with a continual vomiting [...] the eyes are on fire with the injected blood [...] in some cases the feet or parts of the limbs are taken off by the contagion of the disease's putrefaction.[3]

It was said that the epidemic, which lasted about fifteen years, carried off 5000 people a day in Rome, and struck everybody, irrespective of age, gender, status (even the emperor Claudius Gothicus died) or nationality – so many

1 For an overview of the etiology of diseases in Greece and Rome, see Oser-Grote s.v. Ätiologie in Leven 2005, 17-19.

2 Pontius the Deacon, *The life and passion of Cyprian*. Bascome (1851/2–13, 12–13) surmises that about 800,000 persons died in Numidia, and on the coast of Carthage, 200,000.

3 Cypr. *De mortalitate* cc. 15–20.

of the Goths, against whom the Romans were waging war, died that the emperor did not even bother to continue the hostilities.

Under such circumstances it is understandable that the epidemic was seen as apocalyptic, as a sign of the passing away of the world. At times like this numerous questions would have beset the minds of the panic-stricken victims; the most insistent would have been what the cause of the disease was and where it came from. Horrific as the situation might have been, it was by far neither the first nor the last epidemic to ravage the Greco-Roman world. Although the severity of the disease and the resulting death toll might have differed, the question of the cause of the disease would recur. This lack of knowledge about the cause of the disease led to a feeling of complete helplessness and contributed greatly to the terror experienced during the epidemic.

Greco-Roman views on the causes of diseases underwent many changes through the centuries. In prehistoric times it was believed that divine intervention caused diseases. But even before the fifth century BCE it seems that some knowledge of infection was prevalent among the followers of Asclepius, the god of healing – his temples were mostly built in pleasant, healthy sites outside towns, and early laws prohibited the burying of the dead near his temples.[4] In the fifth century BCE, the Hippocratic era, diseases were ascribed to rational, physiological causes – namely, an imbalance of the bodily humours. Thereafter, *miasmata* or potentially harmful powers in the air became the culprit, linked to the theory of 'seeds of disease' in the air or in man, making him susceptible to the disease. During the great pestilence that struck Athens in the late fifth century BCE, the concept of contagion appears in the work of the Greek historian Thucydides, later picked up by a few Roman authors but, for reasons which will be discussed in the course of the chapter, never developed to prevent the spread of an epidemic.

In the early Roman Empire, when Christianity became established, theories that epidemics were caused by natural phenomena were influenced by superstition and religious beliefs, and diseases were again ascribed to divine displeasure and intervention, as in prehistoric times. Nearly two millennia had to pass before the development of the science of bacteriology brought a new insight into the origin of disease. In this chapter the various phases in the views on the causes of diseases will be discussed.

4 Retief & Cilliers 2011, Art. #26.

The religious phase: diseases caused by supernatural agents

An explanation of the presence of evil, sorrow and diseases in the world was first given by the seventh-century-BCE Greek poet Hesiod. In his epic *Works and Days*, a beautiful woman, Pandora, is given by the Olympian gods to Epimetheus as a wedding gift. She brings with her a jar; out of curiosity, not knowing what its content is, she lifts the lid, and a myriad of plagues and evils fly out, which will forever wander among men. When she hastily replaces the lid, only Hope is trapped inside.[5] Some scholars explain this by saying that only Hope, for good or harm, remains within man's control.

In this misogynistic myth the blame for man's suffering is attributed to the gods: Zeus punishes Prometheus (Epimetheus' brother) for stealing fire and giving it to mankind; the punishment is the creation of a woman, the greatest of all evils, and giving the first of the species to the scatter-brained Epimetheus as a wedding gift.

In Homer too we find the view that disease is caused by divine intervention. In his epic *The Iliad* (seventh century BCE), the enraged god Apollo fires arrows at the Greek army that cause a pestilence; this was the god's vengeance because he was insulted by Agamemnon, leader of the army, who had taken as mistress the daughter of Apollo's priest, given to him as part of the war booty.[6] There is no mention of guilt; Agamemnon exonerates himself by ascribing his behavior to *atê*, an irrational impulse caused by a divine agency. It is therefore not a physician who gives advice on how to end the pestilence, but the priest Chryses, who has to appease the god and announce the punishment. The restitution of the priest's daughter and prayers and sacrifices to the god end the pestilence.[7]

It is interesting to note that the whole army suffers because one man has angered a god. It was a cruel world portrayed in the Archaic Age – men were at the mercy of capricious gods who were quick to feel slighted, and punished mercilessly, often by way of disease.

5 Hes. *Op.* 90–100.

6 Hom. *Il.* 1.43–53.

7 For further examples of gods as the cause of disease in Greek epics, see Homer, *Iliad* 21. 483–4; 24.605–7; *Odyssey* 9.407–411, 11.171; Hesiod, *Works and Days* 100–104, 238–245.

The emergence of guilt

The concept of individual guilt emerges in the Greek tragedies of the fifth century BCE, even though the plots represent events that took place during the Archaic Age. Disasters and pestilences were seen as punishment for *hybris* (excessive pride or presumption towards the gods), and the supernatural at this point acquires a moral dimension. Pollution could also, as in the epics, be brought on a whole community by one man who had angered the gods, and was regarded as hereditary (in Aeschylus' trilogy the *Oresteia*, the curse on the house of Atreus extends over three generations).[8]

In Sophocles' tragedy *King Oedipus*, a pestilence has struck the town of Thebes, sent by Apollo as punishment because Oedipus has unwittingly, in fulfillment of a curse, killed his father and married his mother. In contrast with Agamemnon, who exonerates himself of all guilt, Oedipus is devastated when he discovers that he, the very man chosen by the people as ruler and priest-figure, is the cause of the pollution. He accepts responsibility and blinds himself. But the pestilence will only come to an end when the pollution has been cast out of the city by the banishing of Oedipus.

The fifth century BCE: an age of enlightenment

The fifth century was an era of great development in all fields in Greece. In fact, the period of approximately 50 years between the end of the Persian Wars (479 BCE) and the outbreak of the Peloponnesian War (431) is called the *Pentakontaetia*, referring to Fifty (Golden) Years during which there was peace, and all forms of art, literature and philosophy reached unsurpassed heights. The outbreak of the 30-year-long Peloponnesian War between Athens and Sparta and the devastating epidemic that struck Athens in 429 brought a rough end to this era.

The epidemic was described in detail by the fifth-century-BCE Greek historian Thucydides.[9] He was well equipped for such a description, since he was a victim of the plague himself (though he survived). It was most probably smallpox, and killed at least one quarter of the population.[10] Thucydides gives

8 The concept of hereditary guilt and deferred punishment was of course well known among the Israelites, as appears in *Exodus* 20:5: 'For I the Lord am a jealous God, visiting the iniquity of the fathers upon the children unto the third and fourth generation of them that hate me.'

9 Th. 2.47–55.

10 Retief & Cilliers 1998, 50–53.

a meticulous description of the symptoms and the course of the disease, but does not speculate about its cause.[11] It is, however, clear that he ascribed it to natural causes, thereby challenging the widely held belief that plagues were caused by divine intervention. By his account, the epidemic originated in Ethiopia[12] and reached Athens via the sea. Initially the Athenians thought that it was due to the poisoning of their water supply by the Peloponnesians, but this was ruled out. It was exacerbated by the hot pestilential atmosphere in the city (it was summer), which was overcrowded due to Pericles' policy of removing all those living in the countryside and settling them within the Long Walls that connected Athens with the harbour, for protection during the war against the Spartans.[13] This would of course have heightened the possibility of contagion. With grim realism Thucydides describes the fate of the dying victims, staggering about in the streets in search of a fountain to quench their terrible thirst; he tells how the dead are heaped one on top of the other in wagons.

Contagion was a phenomenon not yet recognized in the ancient world. Yet it is implicit in Thucydides' remark that the highest incidence of the disease was among the doctors 'who came most frequently in contact with the sick'.[14] He also mentions that the same patient never got the disease a second time (the first mention in the history of medicine of acquired immunity). He was thus the first person to notice and record the phenomenon of contagion – an advanced perception for the fifth century BCE. There was, however, at that stage, no specific term with which the phenomenon could be described adequately. Nutton mentions that words such as 'sharing' and 'receiving' were used to indicate that proximity to the sick played a role, but the particular manner of transmission was not discussed.[15]

The perception that those who cared for the sick would also contract the disease was mentioned again by the Greek orator Isocrates when defending a claim to inheritance.[16] He argued that his client, who had cared for

11 Thucydides did not have a 'medical' purpose in mind when writing his report, but rather a political, even a moral aim. More than 200 articles have been published during the past 500 years in which authors have speculated about the cause of the epidemic, and the debate is still continuing. Apart from the problem of diagnosing a disease 2500 years after its occurrence, Zinsser (1935, 120) points out that there is seldom a 'pure epidemic', a single malady. The circumstances that favour the spread of one epidemic create opportunities for the transmission of others.

12 Th. 2. c. 5. There was an ancient and traditional belief that all diseases originated in Ethiopia.

13 Th. 2.17.2 and 2.52.1.

14 This remark was first picked up by Crawford in 1914 (*Plague and pestilence in literature and art*), and thereafter elaborated by various authors in the twentieth century.

15 Nutton 2000, 137–162, here 138.

16 Isoc. *Aegineticus* 390b29 ff.

Thrasylochus, a sufferer from phthisis (probably consumption) despite the warnings of friends that those who cared for the sick were themselves killed by it, deserves the legacy bequeathed to him rather than the sister who did not even pay the patient a brief visit. The danger of proximity was thus known in Greece.

Later Latin authors like Livy, Diodorus Siculus and Procopius also mention the phenomenon of contagion in their description of contemporary epidemics, but did not understand why proximity to the sick caused others to contract the disease. It is interesting to note that the Biblical book Leviticus, which was compiled c. 600 BCE, already contains instructions about physical and ritual purification (*Leviticus* 14:8–10), showing that the phenomenon of contagion was known to the Jews, who had developed methods of segregating sick people such as lepers.[17] Only in the sixteenth century was the idea of contagion picked up again by the Italian monk, Girolamo Fracastoro. In his book *On contagion, contagious diseases and their cure* (eventually found to be a summary of earlier writers, especially Galen without acknowledgement), he stated that contagious diseases are spread by the transfer of imperceptible particles from an infected body to another by direct contact. But another three centuries had to pass before technological handicaps could be overcome by the development in the nineteenth century of the new science of bacteriology.

The Hippocratic era: the emergence of a rational approach

Despite the persistence of superstition and magical-religious views – which will probably never be eradicated – great progress was made in the fifth century BCE by the Hippocratic authors with their rational approach to diseases, which is in many respects analogous to our own. An example of this new approach is the Hippocratic treatise *On the sacred disease*, written about 400 BCE. The author explains that the so-called sacred disease (epilepsy) does not have a divine origin, but has a natural cause just like any other disease: it is due to an excessive phlegmatic discharge from the brain, he states, which blocks the blood-vessels supplying the brain with air, resulting in the loss of voice, choking, foaming of the mouth, clenching of the teeth, convulsive movements and eventually unconsciousness. Even though this is not a correct diagnosis judged by modern standards, the explanation that

17 See also Sigerist 1967, 446–447.

the disease is caused by natural factors is a great step forward: personal intervention by the gods in the origin of diseases has now been ruled out.

There were various classifications of diseases, and the Hippocratic doctors had different views on their causes. The main cause of external diseases (which affect many people at the same time in a given place) was putrid air. The Hippocratic treatise *On the nature of man* 6.9 observes that 'plainly the air must be harmful because of some secretion that it contains'.[18] Airborne infections have thus been recognized, but the view was not developed because the ancient physicians were not able to see the microorganisms. This was the beginning of the *miasma* theory, 'bad air' emanating from rotting organic matter.[19] This theory was accepted until the nineteenth century, when it was displaced by the discovery of germs and the germ theory.

Related to this theory is the connection that the Hippocratic physicians saw between the climate, seasons, weather and diseases. In the treatise *Aphorisms* 6.1.20, we read that in the springtime, madness, melancholy, epilepsy, hemorrhages, sore throats, catarrhs, hoarseness, coughs and leprosy are very frequent. The theory that the weather, winds, seasons and floods cause epidemic diseases remained popular until the nineteenth century.

In the 429 BCE Athenian epidemic mentioned above, the populace believed that poisoned drinking water had caused the pestilence. In the Hippocratic treatise *Air, waters, places* 11.7–8, the writer recommends that water should be boiled or that rainwater should be used to prevent certain illnesses. Though water can be healthgiving and salubrious, it was from earliest times realized that it is not always potable.

Then there were internal diseases. The most obvious cause of disease was to be found in one's way of life, or one's regimen. Regimen is a comprehensive term, including diet, exercise, sleeping – in short, one's lifestyle. From the earliest times, balance in all aspects of one's way of life was emphasized, especially in one's diet: the quantity and quality of foods taken in could lead to indigestion causing gas, which in turn leads to certain diseases.[20]

Then there was the humoural theory, the cornerstone of Hippocratic teaching.[21] The word 'humour' is derived from the Latin translation (*humor*, fluid) of the Greek term *chymos*, which means 'juice' or 'fluid' of whatever kind. The four most important humours in the body are blood (which comes

18 See Goodall (1933, 533) for more detail.

19 *Miasma*, Greek for 'pollution', 'defilement' (Liddell, Scott & Jones, *A Greek–English Lexicon*, 1953). This is the modern definition of *miasma*, as given by Last, 2007, *A dictionary of public health*. The word 'malaria' is derived from *mal* (bad) + *aer* (air).

20 Hp. *Alim.* 11.2. Discussed by Mudry 2006b, 483–489.

21 Jouanna 1999, 57 and 62.

from the heart), phlegm (which comes from the head), and yellow and black bile (which come from the gall bladder). Disease results when there is an imbalance in the relationship between the humours, which can be caused by, for instance, a change in locality or the weather (in winter when it is cold, there is too much phlegm and one has a runny nose or sneezes), or too much black bile, which may cause depression. The theory of the four humours was in later times linked to the four elementary qualities (hot, cold, dry, wet) and to the four seasons (summer, fall, winter, spring). It had a prolonged influence on medicine; though outdated now, some terms have survived – for instance, a phlegmatic person is one who has a cold, slow temperament, and a sanguine person is one who is supposed to have a ruddy complexion and is cheerful and optimistic.

It should be noted that the Hippocratic physicians had a physiological and not an ontological approach to disease – a disease was not regarded as a specific entity with an existence of its own, but as the result of a deviation of the normal condition of the patient.[22] It was furthermore believed that each patient had his/her own predisposition that would determine the course and nature of the disease.[23]

'Seeds of disease' as cause of illnesses

In the first decades of the fifth century BCE, the philosopher Anaxagoras mentioned the concept of 'seeds of disease' as a possible cause of illnesses, of course seen with his mind's eye and inferred by logic. It is, however, possible that two of his pre-Socratic contemporaries, Democritus and Leucippus, famous for the atomist philosophy, which links up very well with the seed theory, were the first to suggest this as a possible cause. Nutton remarks that the seed theory is quite apt, since it emphasizes three things: 'the object posited is a living entity, it is in origin very small, and it contains within itself the potentiality for growth.'[24] Epicurus (fourth century BCE), founder of the Epicurean School of philosophy, another proponent of the atomist philosophy, also believed that there are noxious *semina* (seeds) in the air that can on occasion penetrate the human body.[25]

22 Temkin (1977a, 442–448) discusses this in detail.
23 Grmek 1989, 284–304.
24 Nutton 1983, 3.
25 Reference in Grmek 1984, 53–70.

Alexandrian medicine

Contagion was not high up on the list of priorities of the two famous scholars of the Alexandrian period in the fourth century BCE – according to the first-century-CE Roman encyclopedist Celsus, Herophilus stuck to the Hippocratic view of the humoural theory of causation.[26] According to Galen, however, Erasistratus developed a new but short-lived theory that blood seeping into areas of the body where it should not causes inflammation with attendant fever.[27]

Roman views on contagion

During the tyrannical reign of King Ptolemy VIII Euergetes (182–116 BCE), who was hostile to the Alexandrians, many physicians and other members of the intelligentsia fled to Rome, which eventually became the centre of medical activities.[28]

Mirko Grmek made the interesting observation that contagion was often discussed during the late Republic and early Empire by authors as diverse as historians (Diodorus Siculus, Livy, Appian), poets (Lucretius and Vergil), philosophers and encyclopedists (Lucretius, Seneca, Plutarch, Pliny the Elder), authorities in the field of agriculture (Varro, Columella), and veterinary writers (who recorded that one sick animal can quickly infect a whole flock and therefore had the remedy of segregating the sick animal) – but seldom by medical writers.[29] Nutton discusses possible reasons: thanks to a relatively stable disease environment, not many infectious epidemics were spread by contagion in the period discussed in this chapter (c. 700 BCE – c. 600 CE), which caused medical writers to concentrate on diseases of individuals rather than on those of groups.[30] Another possible reason mentioned is that the veterinary practice of segregating infected animals could not be applied to humans: those suffering from a contagious disease could not be locked up or exiled, since

26 Cels. *Prooem.* 14–15.

27 Gal. *Plen.* 7.537-543 K.

28 Hornblower & Spawforth 1996, 1273.

29 Grmek 1984, 53–70.

30 Nutton 2000, 155–158. Nutton (p. 157) mentions four epidemics: the Athenian plague of 430–427 BCE, the Antonine plague of the 160s CE, the plague of Cyprian in North Africa in the mid–third century CE and the plague of Justinian in the sixth century.

medical ethics forbade it.[31] Knowledge of the danger of proximity in the case of certain diseases was thus of limited value, especially given that it was not widely believed.

The first Roman author to pick up the topic of epidemics was the Latin poet **Lucretius** (94–55? BCE). In Book VI of his philosophical poem *On the nature of things,* he again describes the Athenian plague, clearly based on Thucydides' account.[32] He gives a vivid description of the symptoms of the disease – particularly those of intense fever and thirst, and in lines 1182–1207 of Book VI a horrific picture of the signs of death is given. All perished – the brave and selfless ones trying to help the sick, and the cowards who refused to touch them. The only difference was that the latter suffered the shame of dying alone and unmourned. In line 1090 Lucretius tries to explain the cause of the disease – noxious particles or seeds in the air (Lucretius was an adherent of the atomist theory of Democritus; see above) exhaled by the infected bodies of the sick and dead and communicated to those tending or touching them.

Some decades later the theme of the plague was taken up again by the Latin poet **Vergil** (70–19 BCE), whose agricultural poem the *Georgics* shows many verbal, thematic and stylistic similarities to Lucretius' *On the nature of things*. Vergil's poem is, however, about a fictitious plague among animals (who are given human emotions), and the setting is in Noricum, far away from Rome. In agreement with Lucretius, Vergil attributes the plague to polluted air that affects the livestock through food and water supplies.

The Greek historian **Diodorus of Sicily** (first century BCE) also stated in his *Library of History*, a monumental universal history from mythological times up to 60 BCE, that the disease in Athens was transmitted from person to person. He further added that the 'multitude of people in cramped quarters, breathing air which had become polluted' was the reason why great numbers of people succumbed to the disease.[33] It should, however, be noted that this remark in Diodorus and the use of the word 'contagion' in some later Latin authors does not imply that they are referring to the transmission of a disease entity as we understand it today. At most it refers to diseases caused by proximity to the sick and by inhaling the patient's bad breath.

31 See below and Chapter 7 (pp. 177–178) regarding Caelius Aurelianus' view on exiling foreigners when infected with leprosy. Celsus (*On medicine* 1.10.1) advised travelling abroad in case of a pestilence, but that would of course only apply to individuals.
32 The rejection of plagiarism was not a principle valued by the Romans; in fact, *aemulatio*/imitation or direct translation was highly acceptable and widely practiced in Latin literature.
33 D. S. 12.45.

Marcus Terentius **Varro** (116–27 BCE) was a prolific writer on a great number of subjects, but is mainly known for his books *On the Latin language* and *On agriculture.* The latter work, a treatise on farming, deals with agriculture in general, and gives advice to men of his own class. He knew Anaxagoras' seed theory, and warns prospective farmers not to build their houses in the neighbourhood of swamps, 'because there are bred certain minute creatures which cannot be seen by the eyes, which float in the air and enter the body through the mouth and the nose and there cause serious disease.' He also refers to unhealthy *miasmata* and bad air as a cause of diseases and therefore advises that houses should be built on high ground, exposed to healthy winds.[34]

A century later another agriculturalist, **Columella** (4–c. 70 CE), took Varro's invisible minute creatures a step further. In his book *On agriculture* he also warned that a house should not be built in the neighbourhood of a marsh, 'for it breeds animals armed with mischievous stings, which fly upon us in exceeding thick storms'.[35] This is probably the first mention of mosquitoes – malaria was endemic in the low-lying areas around Rome.[36] In various remarks elsewhere Columella emphasizes the importance of wholesome air; in 1.3 and in 1.5, for instance: 'for the surrounding air, when it is corrupted, brings very many causes of hurt and offence to our bodies'.

A different approach is found in the work of **Aretaeus** of Cappadocia, an excellent physician who is credited, among other things, with original descriptions of various major diseases. For some ill-understood reason, however, his work did not get the recognition it deserved. If placed in the first century CE, he was the first to explicitly state that contagion was the cause of disease: he believed that elephas/leprosy spread by direct contact.[37]

A medical author born in North Africa (in Sicca Veneria, now Le Kef in Tunisia), **Caelius Aurelianus** (fourth and fifth centuries CE), made a valuable contribution by adapting and translating into Latin some of the (now lost) works of the famous second-century-CE Greek physician Soranus. In his *On acute diseases* and *On chronic diseases* Caelius states that leprosy,

34 Varr. *R. R.* 1. c. 12.

35 Col. *R. R.* 1 c. 5.

36 Retief & Cilliers 2004, 127–138.

37 Retief & Cilliers (2009, 23–39) place Aretaeus of Cappadocia in the first century CE; Hornblower & Spawforth (1996, 152–153) place him in the second century CE, as a contemporary of Galen. Regarding the cure of elephas, Aretaeus says: 'There is a danger in living or associating with it no less than with the plague, for the infection is thereby communicating by the respiration' (*The extant Works*, s.v. Elephas, in Adam 1856, 494).

incubus and plague are spread by direct contact.[38] In some countries, he notes, leprous people are sent into distant exile to protect the citizens from contact with them, but he rejects this procedure as foreign to the humane spirit of medicine.[39]

The plague of Athens was again referred to by the historian **Ammianus Marcellinus** (c. 325–c. 392 CE), who was born in the Greek-speaking East but wrote his *Roman History* in Latin. When describing the pestilence that struck Amida in Armenia (now Turkey) in 359, he likens it to the Athenian plague of 429 BCE, which, according to him, also originated in Ethiopia and had the same characteristics. He ascribes it to excessive heat aggravated by the great number of people, but adds that, fortunately, on the tenth day after the first attack, the 'dense air was softened by rain and the health of the garrison was restored'.[40] Once again the *miasma* theory was revived.

Another epidemic with symptoms similar to those of smallpox was the pestilence of **Orosius**, which affected North Africa and Italy in 125. Once again it was said to originate in Ethiopia, following a famine caused by a heavy locust invasion.[41]

Galen (129–?199/216), arguably the greatest physician of the Greco-Roman era, was a Roman citizen from Pergamum in Asia, but ethnically and culturally he was a Greek, and his medicine too was basically Greek. He was a prolific writer – the 21 volumes of his work that have survived (about one third of what he wrote) are already twice as much as the whole Hippocratic Corpus – and dominated medicine throughout the Middle Ages up to the beginning of the modern era. He had a great admiration for Hippocrates as well as for the anatomical and physiological works of Herophilus and Erasistratus (see above).

Galen's contribution to the development of views on the etiology of disease is to some extent a combination of views current in the second century CE.[42] He played with the idea of seeds of disease in the atmosphere, but added that the seeds are not the disease itself, but merely trigger a situation that could eventually lead to the actual disease if it enters a body with a predisposition

38 Cael. Aur. *Tard.* 4.1.13; Cael. Aur. *Acut.*1.1.12. However, Nutton (2000, 147) indicates that all six references in which Caelius uses the word '*contagio*' are problematic, and in none of them is there an explanation of the actual process of transmission.

39 See also Chapter 7.

40 Amm. 19.4 1–8.

41 Discussed by Retief & Cilliers 2000a, 271.

42 A more philosophical approach to Galen's view of the cause of disease is given by Van der Eijk (2014, 366–368), who states that there is no evidence that Galen considered divine agency as a factor in bringing about disease; Galen did, however, believe that in our sublunary world there are restrictions on what nature (which often heals diseases by itself) can achieve, and he holds an unhealthy lifestyle responsible for some diseases.

or susceptibility to disease (thus a body with a humoural disorder or some or other malfunction). The strictly humoural theory, ingrained in his way of thinking, was thus rejected in favour of the suitability of an individual to be affected by, for instance, an unwise regimen or a rise in temperature. In this combination of theories, he went outside the ambit of current ideas. This was his explanation of why, in a crowd watching games on a hot day, only a few spectators would develop fever or heat stroke – all are subjected to the heat, but not all have the predisposition to be affected.[43] Elsewhere, when explaining contagion, Galen brings the *miasma* theory into play – he states that plagues are spread by the inhaling of air infected by a 'putrid exhalation', for instance, from swamps in summer, but in this he was merely paraphrasing the Hippocratic treatise *On the nature of man* 6.2.3–4, without any further discussion. Yet he adds that this external cause is not enough by itself; it needs a suitable body to be affected by the putrid air, for instance, one full of residues or with blockages of pores.

Vivian Nutton believes that the theory of the seeds of disease was never fully developed by Galen because for this he needed an ontological approach, whereas he and all the other writers in the Hippocratic tradition had a physiological approach (see above). In any case, it did not fit into his overall scheme of diseases. Nor was it of any use to him or, for that matter, to any contemporary Roman doctor in his daily task of trying to cure patients. 'The hypothesis of causative seeds was a philosophical luxury for the intellectual practitioner.'[44]

During Galen's lifetime, one of the most catastrophic epidemics of all time struck the Roman Empire. It became known as the Antonine Plague because it occurred during the reign of the emperor Marcus Aurelius Antoninus (r. 161–180), or as the Plague of Galen, because he was one of the authors who described it.[45] It was brought back to the Roman Empire by troops who had been engaged in campaigns in the Near East. It was probably smallpox, though there is not enough evidence to be certain, and Galen's report is uncharacteristically incomplete due to his haste to leave Rome at the first signs of the disease.[46] The death toll is estimated at about five million – from a quarter to a third of the population. The social and military impact was

43 Gal. *Caus. Morb.* 7.101–108 K. Emphasized again in his commentary *On Hippocrates' Epidemics* 17.3.7 K.

44 Nutton 1983, 1–34.

45 The volume in Dio Cassius' books *Roman History*, which would have covered the epidemic, is missing, but he describes the later outburst as the greatest he had knowledge of (72.14.3–4).

46 Gal. *MM* 10.1–6 K.

enormous; whole towns were wiped out.[47] Marcus Aurelius' campaign against the Marcomanni (the emperor was on the northern border of the empire for the greatest part of his reign fighting against barbarian invaders) had to be postponed due to lack of manpower. In the chaos, many people turned to magic for protection, but others converted to Christianity in response to the Christians' unstinting assistance to all victims of epidemics.[48]

It is clear that the calamitous epidemics that swept the Greco-Roman world again and again had a profound effect on the availability of manpower and the ability of the Romans to keep the barbarian invaders at bay, and hastened the end of the Roman Empire.

The Christian view

In 251 a severe epidemic (mentioned in the first paragraph of this chapter) struck the empire. To pacify the populace, emperors such as Gallus (r. 251–253) and Valerian (r. 253–260) stepped up the persecution of the Christians, to whom the disease was ascribed. **St. Cyprian**, Bishop of Carthage at the time (he was martyred in 258), left the best-known description of the disease (it thus became known as the Epidemic of St. Cyprian). The epidemic, which, like the others, was said to have originated in Ethiopia, raged through Egypt and North Africa before it reached Europe. It lasted close on fifteen years – it swept over the same regions repeatedly – and was extremely contagious, spreading not only by direct contact but also through clothing.[49] It showed a seasonal incidence, with maximum impact in autumn and winter, which is typical of epidemics spread by the respiratory route, such as smallpox, measles and influenza. The absence of skin lesions suggests influenza, with gangrene of the extremities as an unusual complication. The clinical picture also points to influenza.[50] Mortality was high and terror extreme. What makes this

47 Zinsser 1935, 100.

48 Lucianus, *Alex.* c. 35; Stark 1992, 162. Zinsser (1935, 139) cynically remarks that 'throughout the early Christian period every great calamity – famine, earthquake, and plague – led to mass conversions [...]. Christianity owes a formidable debt to bubonic plague and to smallpox, no less than to earthquakes and volcanic eruptions.'

49 Archaeologists working in Thebes (modern Luxor) in Egypt which was also affected by this epidemic, found charred human remains buried in a mass grave in lime (used as disinfectant in ancient times), and believe that it is evidence that the corpses had to be disposed of in a great hurry due to the disease's extreme contagiousness (http://www.ees.ac.uk/publications/Egyptian-archaeology.html).

50 Retief & Cilliers 2000a, 271.

epidemic remarkable is St. Cyprian's description of the charitable work done by the Christians during the epidemic, even helping the pagans, to the extent that a century later the emperor Julian (r. 361–363), who hated the 'Galileans', launched a campaign to institute pagan charities in an effort to match the Christians.[51] Cyprian tried to console his parishioners by saying that the suffering was a spiritual exercise for all Christians and that they should rejoice, and embrace 'the benefit of the occasion' to give proof of their faith.[52] In fact, it was debated whether trying to avoid epidemic disease was scripturally acceptable, in view of the Church's dogma of the virtue of suffering.[53]

This was also the view of the biblical scholar and Christian historian **Eusebius** (c. 260–339), who, when describing the epidemic of 312/313, probably smallpox of the virulent hemorrhagic kind, again stated that it was a schooling and testing of the Christians' faith.[54] Thus, whereas the other faiths were failing their adherents, only Christianity offered an explanation and comfort, and the promise of a rewarding afterlife. Eusebius also mentions the love and care with which the Christians ministered to the sick, fearlessly, even though they knew that they could contract the disease through contact with the sick or dead. The heathen, in contrast, rebuffed the sick and avoided their dearest friends when sick and dying.

One last major pandemic remains to be described: the disastrous plague bearing the name of **Justinian**, which struck Constantinople and the surrounding countries in 542.[55] The vivid descriptions by various contemporary writers, but especially the sixth-century-CE Greek historian Procopius, of the symptoms, the portents and hallucinations of the sick, and the disposal of the dead, rival Thucydides' description of the Athenian pestilence.[56] But this time it was not smallpox or some other contagious disease, but bubonic plague (*Yersinia pestis*), which is spread by infected fleas on rats, and is not directly contagious (it was also the cause of the medieval 'Black Death'). The cause of the Justinian plague baffled contemporaries – Procopius stated that 'it is impossible to conceive in thought any explanation, except indeed to refer it to God'.[57] The Bishop, John of Ephesus, also believed that it was

51 Nursing the sick was valued highly by Christians, because in showing love (*agapê*) in this way they imitated Jesus (*Matt.* 25:36; *Cor.* 13). Reference in Leven 1995, 393–407.

52 Cypr. *De mortalitate* cc. 15–20.

53 Nutton 1984a, 8.

54 Retief & Cilliers 2000, 271; Eusebius, *Historia Ecclesiastica* 7.22.

55 Retief & Cilliers 2000b, 249–254.

56 Procop. *Pers.* 2.22.2–5.

57 Procop. *Vand.* 22.22.1.

sent by God because of the sins of the world. It is estimated that about one third of the population of the Roman world died; the disposal of the dead in Constantinople was such a problem that when every possible cemetery was full, the dead were piled up into the watch towers of the fortifications, or put on empty boats to be swept out to sea. Famine, inflation, the depopulation of the countryside and a critical shortage of manpower in the army brought Justinian's military attempts to reunite the eastern and western parts of the empire to a premature end.

Later views

Towards the end of the Roman era, after Galen, few writers contributed significantly on the subject of infection. The Spanish encyclopedist **Isidore of Seville** (seventh century) did write on the contagious nature of pestilences, which he ascribed to God's punishment on sin. He also believed in dangerous pestilential seeds in the vicinity of disease, which could cause death.[58]

Various medieval Arab scientists showed interest in the subject of infection, and translated many of the Greek and Roman works on this topic. They tended to replace the concept of seeds of disease with vague descriptions of corrupt air and vapors, thus propagating the *miasma* theory.[59]

In 1546 the monk **Girolamo Fracastoro** published his famous book *On contagion and contagious diseases and their cure,* in which he propounded a theory of airborne seeds. Why and how the contagion occurred depended, according to him, on the composition of the seeds. It was initially regarded as an important contribution to the subject, but in the course of time Fracastoro's book was recognized as not original, but merely an extensive summary of the views of authors from the Greco-Roman era and of Galen in particular (without acknowledgement). The technological handicaps that his – and his predecessors' – theory of seeds faced were only overcome in the nineteenth century when the new science of bacteriology, developed by Robert Koch, brought insight into the mysterious theory of the seeds of disease, by identifying the specific causative agent of some diseases.

58 Isid. *Etym.* 4.16.17.
59 Nutton 2000, 19.

Conclusion

The contribution of the ancient Greeks and Romans to the development of views on the causes of infectious diseases was enormous. This becomes clear if one compares the approach of the Greeks and Romans with modern science: Hippocratic physicians believed that a disequilibrium of body humours leads to disease. Galen took it one step further and stated that a body had to be predisposed by, for instance, a disequilibrium before infection could take place. Today we know that a disease or a malnourished body predisposes the patient to epidemic infection of any kind. And *miasmata* or seeds of disease clearly represent the pathological microorganisms that today we know are responsible for infectious disease. These organisms could travel by air, bad food or water on their way to the patient. And obviously, close contact with the patient diminished the distance infecting organisms had to travel from the infected patient to potential victims.

The Hippocratic notion that some diseases are transmissible by air still guided public health measures in England in the nineteenth century, when it was believed that infection was the result of putrefied air. This theory eventually gave way to the then newly developed science of bacteriology that substituted pathogenic microorganisms for the *miasmata* – a remarkable discovery indeed, but without the intellectual substructure provided by Greco-Roman thought, it is doubtful whether this development would have made such rapid progress in the twentieth century.As to the role of Christianity, mention has been made of the Christians' sympathetic care of the sick, regardless of their own health, even during virulent epidemics. This eventually led to the establishment of hospitals.[60] On the negative side, the veto on dissection because of the view that the body is the temple of God greatly retarded advances in medical science, as did the Christian belief in demonic possession and miracle cures. Nor did admonishments that epidemics and diseases were punishments for sin or that Christians should acquiesce in suffering since it was a preparation for everlasting life stimulate research in medical science.

60 Cilliers & Retief 2002, 60–66.

4. The knowledge and competence of physicians in the late Roman Empire

In 175 CE Galen, then one of the court physicians of the emperor Marcus Aurelius (r. 161–180), gave a public lecture in Rome on the knowledge and competence of contemporary physicians.[1] In the lecture he pointed out some serious problems in this regard and suggested a number of criteria by which the best doctors could be recognized. Although the standard set by this brilliant (but insufferably arrogant) physician was unrealistically high (he took himself as norm), there must have been some truth in his statement, since the information about the (in)competence of doctors described in another later source is equally negative. In a compilation of letters serving as introduction to a collection of medical recipes assembled by Marcellus (end of fourth and early fifth centuries), a Gallic nobleman of Burdigala (now Bordeaux in France), it appears that doctors were found lacking in many respects.[2] In addition to this there is a letter from Vindicianus (late fourth century CE; proconsul of the province of Africa Proconsularis, but also renowned physician) to the emperor Valentinian I, in which Vindicianus fulminates against his colleagues who, because of ignorance, applied the wrong therapy to a seriously ill patient.[3]

The problem

Criticism of doctors can be traced back to the earliest medical manuscripts and occur in practically every literary genre.[4] The problem is that there was no official licensing by the state, or by a body such as a general medical council, to ensure that those presenting themselves as doctors have the

1 Galen's lecture was published shortly thereafter with the title *De optimo medico cognoscendo.* Before the original Greek text got lost, it was translated into Arabic in the ninth century by Hunain ibn Ishaq; the Arabic text was translated into English in 1988 by A.Z. Iskandar, who gave the treatise the English title *On examinations by which the best physicians are recognized.*

2 In Niedermannn & Liechtenhan 1968. The compilation of letters, which were written by various authors between the first and the fourth centuries CE, is discussed by Cilliers 2010, 401–418.

3 See c. 5 on Vindicianus for a discussion of this letter.

4 See Nutton (1988a, 30–58) for an extensive account of the criticism of doctors.

necessary medical knowledge and competence.[5] There was also no consensus about what the training of those aspiring to become doctors should comprise. People with little or no competence could thus practise as doctors, with the result that doctors acquired a bad reputation, as is reflected in the works of, *inter alia*, the satirist Martial, who remarks in one of his epigrams, 'Diaulus was a doctor until recently, now he is an undertaker; what he does now he also did as doctor.'[6] And in the first century CE Pliny the Elder, in his encyclopedic work the *Natural History*, has much to say about the ignorance of doctors that put patients' lives at risk. His remark that only a doctor can commit homicide with complete impunity speaks volumes.[7]

Galen's criticism, mentioned in the first paragraph, touches another aspect as well: the ignorance of lay citizens who would summon a doctor without having any prior knowledge of his competence, and who are too lazy or too busy seeking pleasure to acquire medical knowledge so as to distinguish between good and bad doctors.[8] This criticism must be seen against the background of the time when an educated Roman gentleman was expected to have at least some knowledge of medicine.[9] In one of the anecdotes related by Aulus Gellius (second century CE) in his *Attic Nights* 18.10.1, he states that it is a gross solecism for a man of learning to be so ignorant of medicine as to confuse veins with arteries (this was specialized knowledge in ancient times).[10] In the fourth century Oribasius, personal physician of the emperor Julian (r. 361–363), also stated that it is the duty of educated Romans to learn medicine 'so that they can become good advisors in everything that is related to public safety'.[11] Medical knowledge in the early Empire was thus not limited to physicians – the works of learned authors like the philosopher-politician Seneca (first century CE) and the philosopher-biographer Plutarch (first/second century) are interspersed with medical information, and the learned Galen did not deign it *infra*

5 The term 'healer' could carry different meanings and would easily allow a broad range of styles and statuses (Nutton 1988b, 33).

6 Mart. 1.48.

7 Plin. *N. H.* 29.8–14, 29.18.

8 In *On examinations* c. 8.10, Galen remarks: 'For his own safety, when healthy, a person must diligently test and examine the skill of a physician so that he can rely on him during any illness, and hope to recover at his hands.'

9 Canizares (2010, 87–99) draws attention to the Hippocratic treatise *Affections*, which as early as the fourth century BCE had as aim to transmit the medical knowledge every intelligent layman should possess.

10 See also Apuleius in North Africa, who referred to people who do not have a basic medical knowledge as 'country bumpkins' (*Apologia* 48–52).

11 Orib. *Letter to Eunapius* 3.164.

dignitatem to include – without comment or apology – recipes which he acquired from a barber, a eunuch and a boxer.[12] Galen furthermore raised objections against doctors who attempted to make themselves popular, especially among the rich, by not prescribing treatments conducive to good health, but pleasurable regimens that would keep them as doctors employed and their purses full, but which in the long run led to a deterioration of the patient's health.[13] A serious complaint made by Galen in his speech that one sometimes still hears today is that some would-be doctors never had the earnest desire to cure the sick, but that 'their only aim is to gain money, power and position'.[14]

The role of the state in the maintenance of medical services

In view of the incompetence of doctors discussed above, the question may well arise whether the state could not in some way or other address the problem. The answer is yes, the state did make attempts to address the problem – on numerous occcasions. There is a long list of decrees, starting with Julius Caesar, and continued by the emperors Claudius, Vespasian, Hadrian, Antoninus Pius, Alexander Severus and Diocletian.[15] Other measures, mentioned by the biographer Suetonius, the authors of *The history of the Caesars*, the various legal codes and digests, and other sources, pertain to privileges conferred on teachers of liberal arts, rhetoricians, philosophers and *medici* (whether physicians or teachers of medicine). This usually comprised exemption from certain public duties or from the payment of taxes, or involved a grant of a special salaried chair or a lecture hall.[16] Or there were the edicts of the emperor Domitian (r. 81–96) withdrawing tax privileges previously granted to doctors by Vespasian (r. 69–79), since doctors, in pursuit of wealth rather than the care of patients, were found to teach medicine to slaves, thus increasing the number of uneducated doctors.[17] There was also the attempt to make foreign doctors register before

12 Gal. *Comp. Med. Loc.* 104, 204 and 294, 13 K.

13 Gal. *Opt. Med. Cogn.* 1.5–9. It was easy for Galen to say this because he did not have financial problems. This was not, however, the case with most doctors – while a living could be made from medicine, the average doctors had to gain access to rich patients to make an easy living.

14 Gal. *Opt. Med. Cogn.* 1.10.

15 Drabkin 1944, 246–247.

16 See note 47 below regarding the excavation of *lectoria* in Qumm ad Diqua at Alexandria in Egypt.

17 *Fontes Iuris Romani ante–Iustiniani* 1.77, in Riccobono 1968, 427–478.

granting them citizenship; another curb was the restriction of the grant of financial privileges and tax exemption, and the limitation of the number of doctors in accordance with the status of the town or city they served.[18]

Another measure that one would think should result in the appointment of competent doctors was the selection and appointment of *archiatri* (city physicians) by the local city councils. But most of the members of the city councils consisted of laymen with no medical background, who could easily have been swayed by the eloquence of an applicant who had all the necessary rhetorical skills but very little medical knowledge or a rather mediocre former career. The idealistic pronouncement of the jurist Ulpian in the second century CE, that a doctor must be elected on the basis of his moral probity and his professional skill (in that order!) probably also had very little influence on the election.[19]

In 368 the emperor Valentinian I (r. 364–375) established a College of Physicians in Rome to which fourteen doctors (one for each of the districts in Rome) were elected by their peers on the basis of their competence. But this College was still not a kind of medical board that could regulate appointments and see to it that a reasonable standard was maintained.[20] According to our sources, these doctors, responsible to the emperor only, received a salary from the city and were in return expected to render honourable service to the poor, rather than humiliating obsequiousness to the rich.[21] It seems to have been a lifelong appointment, since a new member would only be elected when one of the members of the College died, resigned or was appointed in another capacity by the emperor after serving for a period, as was the case with Vindicianus (see Chapter 5). The new member was to take the lowest place and would gradually rise in seniority as longer-serving

18 Drabkin 1944, 346–347. This could also be due to putting the interest of finance above that of public health by preventing the number of doctors immune from financial burdens from becoming excessive (Nutton 1971, 52–63).

19 *Dig.* 27.1.6.4 and 50.9.1.

20 *Cod. Theod.* 13.3.8–9 and 13.

21 *Cod. Theod.* 13.3.12 of 379 *De medicis et professoribus*: 'That neither grandeur not financial gain should be sought, nor should they tire themselves to acquire an inheritance. And these also, on whom the office of *comes* (count) has been conferred, should, as custom demands, be satisfied with a low salary.' See also in this regard Nutton (1988d, 19–20). In another article Nutton (1988e, 209) gives the background of this rather astonishing step of Valentinian: the emperor Julian the Apostate (r. 361–363) noted that the charitable acts of the Christians 'extended to all members of society, pagans included, while the poorer pagans lacked assistance even from their own community', and therefore numerous hospices open to all were established. Valentinian in turn 'sought to institutionalize still further the Christian ideal of charity in the very stronghold of paganism'.

archiatri died.[22] It is interesting to note that the *Codex Theodosianus* also looks at matters from a deontological point of view: in 13.3.8.1 doctors are exhorted to keep their pretensions within reasonable limits, such as that 'they may receive from the infirm that which they (sc. the patients) would have been able to offer in a state of good health, but not that which they had offered in a period of ill-health.'

The renowned North African physician Vindicianus, to whom reference has already been made, was elected as *Comes* (Count) of this prestigious College. That such a renowned physician from North Africa was appointed is evidence on the one hand of the high profile of doctors in the fourth and fifth centuries, and on the other hand of the importance of this province in the view of the government in Rome.[23]

Different levels of healers

The subject of this chapter covers many centuries and many countries. It is therefore to be expected that there will be a great variation in the level of medical knowledge, in the standard of the service provided and in the social status of the medical practitioners. Clear evidence of the diverse medical scene is found even in a single period – namely, the late fourth and early fifth centuries. The authors of the letters included in the compilation introducing Marcellus of Bordeaux's recipe collection were of varied origin (Gaul, Rome and Africa), belonged to different levels of society (Marcellus a land owner, Scribonius Largus an army doctor and Vindicianus a proconsul and master physician), practiced medicine on different levels (a layman's advice, a 'country clinic', and a city practice), and had different objectives. [24]

Marcellus was an educated layman from Bordeaux in Gaul (late fourth and early fifth centuries).[25] The recipes are the typical traditional remedies of country folk and remind us of the agricultural recipes of, for instance, the

22 *Cod. Theod.* 13.3.9.

23 Nutton (1988e, 12) remarks: 'The doctor in late antiquity has a much greater public profile beyond the confines of his city and civic life. He becomes a bishop, a church leader, even a saint; an ambassador, a provincial governor, even the Master of Ceremonies.'

24 The letters are the following: (i) Marcellus to his sons; (ii) Largius Designatianus to his sons; (iii) Pseudo-Hippocrates to King Antiochus; (iv) Pseudo-Hippocrates to Maecenas; (v) Pseudo-Pliny the Younger to his friends; (vi) Cornelius Celsus (in reality Scribonius Largus) to C. Julius Callistus; (vii) Pseudo-Cornelius Celsus to Pullius Natalis; (viii) Vindicianus to the emperor Valentinian I.

25 He was probably not a doctor by profession. However, in the absence of certification the dividing line between an educated layman and a doctor would have been thin.

elder Cato (second century BCE) and Pliny the Elder (first century CE).[26] The main objective of such recipe collections was to teach men how to survive without doctors – given their bad reputation – and especially without surgery.[27] The recipes are a sort of do-it-yourself manual, providing readers with the necessary medical information to make them self-sufficient, or serving as first aid for travellers. Marcellus dedicated the book to his sons, requesting that they disseminate the knowledge widely (par. 4).

Vindicianus (a slightly younger contemporary of Marcellus), on the other hand, was a learned, professional master physician from Carthage. His letter to the emperor Valentinian I is written in a florid, rather bombastic style, clearly revealing his rhetorical upbringing. It contains the description of two case studies in which he demonstrates that his fellow-doctors' diagnosis and treatment of both patients are completely wrong (par. 2–4 and 8–9); fortunately, however, he could in both cases save the situation. He too asks that his remarks about remedies should be made public, but leaves it to the emperor to transmit them to future generations (par. 10).

Scribonius Largus was an army doctor in the first century CE. His letter is addressed to Callistus, freedman of the emperor Claudius (r. 41–54). This letter is remarkable in being the only (Latin) plea that practicing physicians should maintain the Hippocratic principle of healing and not harming, and of not using abortifacients or poisons, even if the patient is one's enemy (pars. 4 and 5). The letter also contains a plea that doctors maintain a high standard in their vocation by acquiring a comprehensive knowledge of the totality of medicine, and not specializing in only one disease (pars. 10 and 11).

Then there was another level, that of women, who as female doctors and midwives had, over the centuries, carved out a very specific niche for themselves.[28] Since the fourth century BCE a distinction was made in Greece between the midwife (*maia*) who took care of confinements, and the female doctor (*iatrinê*) who handled gynecological problems in general.[29] In Roman times they were respectively known as *obstetrix* and

26 Cato, *R. R.* 156.1 and 157.12. According to Cato 'cabbage is the most outstanding of vegetables', and is a panacea for most of the common diseases. Pliny was a great advocate of traditional folk remedies, and pleaded for a return to self-help medicaments, of course adapted to accommodate a Roman gentleman (*Natural History, passim*). Oribasius (fourth century) in his *Letter to Eunapius* also supported self-help medicaments.

27 On the horrors of surgery, see Augustine's *City of God* (22.8.106–119), where the anxiousness of a man awaiting surgery is described.

28 See Cilliers & Retief (1999, 47–65) and Laes (2010, 261–287) for more detailed discussions of the role of women in medicine.

29 See Plato's *Theaetetus* (149a1–c2) and *Republic* (V. 454d2ff.), in which it is clear that the occupation of midwife was firmly established and respected by the fourth century BCE, and

Figure 4.1 Birth chair used by midwives. Relief erected in honour of midwife Scribonia Attikê, found in Ostia, 2nd century CE

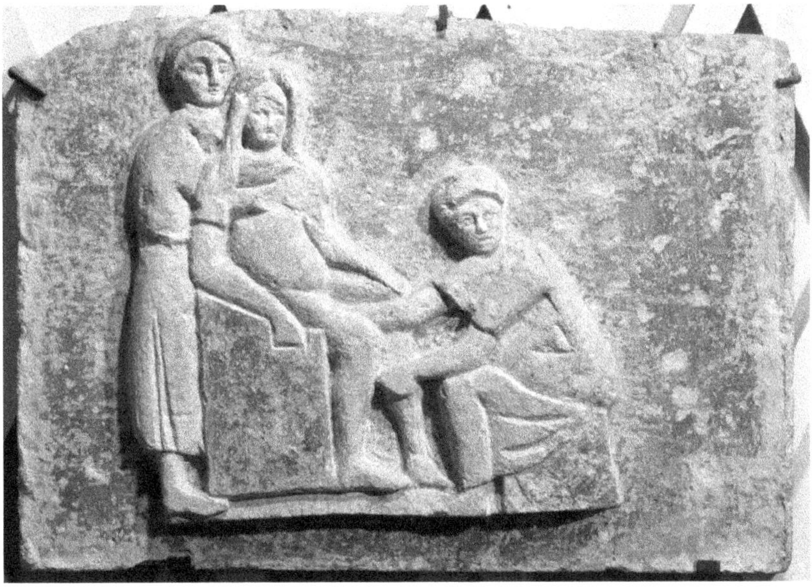

medica, though there would undoubtedly have been overlapping of their tasks in practice. Midwives had little more than a rudimentary practical training obtained from other midwives – knowledge passed on from generation to generation, often tinted with superstition and folklore. About the training of female doctors, we know very little; they could not participate in the lectures given to male would-be doctors, so their training would have been apprenticeship to family members and, since they would probably have been able to read, knowledge gained from books. Apart from the Hippocratic gynecological treatises (fifth and fourth centuries BCE) there were also Herophilus' (now lost) *Maieutikon* ('On midwifery') on obstetrics and gynecology (third century BCE), Soranus' *Gynecology* (first century CE), after its disappearance preserved in Caelius Aurelianus' work by the same name (fourth century CE), which contained a wealth of information on pregnancy and delivery. Galen's treatise on *The construction of the embryo* (dedicated to a midwife) would also have been useful, as well as the North African physician Theodorus Priscianus' *Gynecology* on female problems (fifth century CE), also dedicated to a midwife, and the

also the laudatory inscription of Phanostrate (fourth century BCE) who is called both *maia* and *iatros*, since her services comprised more than assistance at a confinement.

Gynecology of the North African Muscio or Mustio, which had as professed aim the improvement of the midwives' standard of knowledge.

Pliny the Elder also mentions some women who wrote treatises on obstetrics and gynecology – for instance, Sotira, Salpe and Olympias, and Aëtius mentions one Aspasia (second century CE); we also know of Metrodora (second/third century CE) who wrote treatises on diseases of the uterus, sterility and contraception.[30] According to Soranus, midwives varied from the humble wise woman of the town to those better qualified in theoretical aspects of obstetrics and gynecology, and finally to those who could be regarded as the equivalent of doctors, since they had received training in therapy, diets and the preparation of medicaments. Midwives were slaves or freedwomen, while female doctors were mostly free and came from different levels of society, some from high classes. By the sixth century female doctors were recognized as on a par with male doctors.[31]

The training of doctors

Although Galen was in no respect a typical doctor, it will be of interest to follow his career in order to get an idea of the ideal doctor's training – he also happened to be the only doctor to leave extensive information about his career.[32] Born in Pergamum in 129 CE into a wealthy family, he did the normal elementary studies in reading, writing and arithmetic, followed by secondary studies in mathematics, literature and rhetoric, probably from the age of 12. Galen states that he was taught geometry and mathematics mainly by his father, Nikon, who was an architect.[33] Thereafter he attended lectures in philosophy in Pergamum, selected by his father, who also accompanied him. It was as a result of a dream that Nikon had, seemingly sent to him by Asclepius, the god of medicine, that Galen turned to medicine. Nikon's death three years later affected Galen greatly; however, he was left with a substantial income, which enabled him to pursue his medical studies with teachers in various cities in the Mediterranean.

Due to the lack of requirements for starting a medical practice, the length and character of medical studies varied greatly – it not only depended on financing but also on the aptitude and enthusiasm of the pupil, as well as

30 Plin. *N. H.* 28.53 and 54.

31 See the Law of Justinian 530 CE (reference in Kudlien 1970, 35 n. 71).

32 Gal. *Lib. Prop.* 19 K.

33 See Nutton (2004, 216–7) on the profound influence that Nikon had on his son's education.

on the requirements of the teacher, the possibility of specialization and so on. The physician, Thessalus, for instance, attracted hordes of disciples with his claim that he could teach medicine in six months by dispensing with geometry, astronomy, dialectics and music.[34] Galen, at the other end of the spectrum, devoted eleven years to study at various centres of excellence before starting to practice medicine in Rome. We do not know the details of his medical studies apart from the fact that most of his teachers were supporters of Hippocrates and wrote commentaries on the latter's works (hence Galen's great admiration for Hippocrates throughout his life), and emphasized the importance of anatomy. Galen mentions Pelops at Smyrna and Pelops' teacher, Numisianus at Corinth, who unfortunately died young, which caused Galen to visit Alexandria, where he hoped to reconstruct from others some of the teaching of Numisianus.[35] The latter's teacher, Quintus, greatly impressed Galen, who described him as the best doctor of his era, *inter alia* because he had made important anatomical discoveries.[36] Quintus in turn had been the student of the slightly older Marinus (beginning of second century), praised by Galen for bringing anatomy into the foreground again.[37] Also mentioned by Galen among his teachers at Alexandria is Satyrus of Smyrna, apparently one of Quintus' best students.[38]

Alexandria was, in the second century CE, *the* 'university city' (in the broadest sense of the word), where all of Galen's teachers had studied and later taught, so he stayed there for a number of years. It was in his late twenties, in 157, that he got his first job in Pergamum, as surgeon to the troupe of gladiators that the high priest of the city maintained for performances during festivals. This was no mean job: Pergamum had a magnificent amphitheatre carved out against a steep hill, and gladiatorial combats were a very popular form of entertainment all over the empire. During the five years Galen spent at the gladiator school, he would have gained valuable experience as a general practitioner, but especially as a wound specialist. Keeping gladiators was expensive – it was important to keep especially the good ones alive and well. Apart from stitching up their wounds after a performance, Galen would also have had to attend to their diet and general health.

In 162, already in his late thirties, Galen went to Rome, where he remained for most of the rest of his life, serving as one of the court physicians to

34 Galen bitterly criticized Thessalus; see *On the method of healing* (10.1.1 K.).
35 Keyser 2008, 634, 584.
36 Keyser 2008, 717.
37 Keyser 2008, 532.
38 Keyser 2008, 728.

Figure 4.2 Roman theatre in Alexandria, Egypt

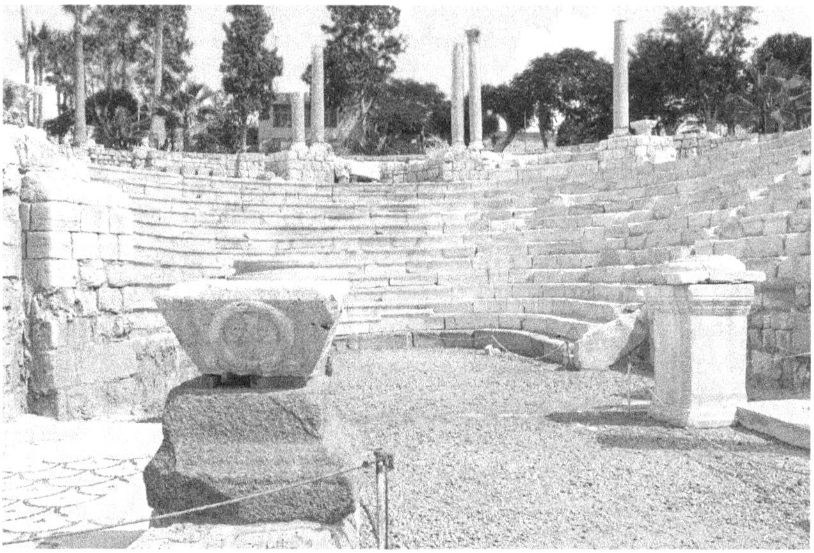

the emperor Marcus Aurelius, as well as doing research (mainly anatomical), lecturing and writing. Nutton, who gives an insightful description of Galen's life and career, mentions the interesting fact that his first important patient in Rome was his old philosophy teacher, Eudemus, who believed that Galen had come to Rome to establish his reputation as a philosopher, not a physician.[39]

There is a great difference between Galen's training as physician and that of the ordinary doctor in the second century CE. The vast book-learning that he displayed was made possible by his wealth, which enabled him to buy or have copies made of every possible medical book, whereas humbler doctors may at best have owned or borrowed only a few short handbooks or digests of earlier doctrines to supplement what they had learned by word of mouth during their apprenticeship or by watching other doctors operate. And then there was Galen's 'educational odyssey', which was 'both longer and geographically more extensive than any other known to us'.[40] It is clear that learning from books and from the masters (local or in another city/country) were the two cornerstones in medical training – theoretical knowledge and practical experience.

39 Nutton 2004, 224. Philosophy was for Galen an integral part of medicine, as is evident from the title of one of his books, *The best doctor is also a philosopher.*

40 Nutton 2004, 218.

Centres of medical education

Alexandria

Higher studies in medicine were throughout the ancient world in the hands of individual teachers (as we have seen in the case of Galen's peregrinations to teachers in various cities) rather than in medical schools or universities as is the case today. However, in certain cities, centres of instruction did develop. Nutton indicates that from the third century BCE the courts in Alexandria, Antioch and, later, Pergamum attracted individuals of all occupations (among them doctors) from all parts of the world.[41] Alexandria, with its magnificent Museum and Library, splendidly furnished by the Ptolemies, soon became the lighthouse of Greek medical knowledge, thanks to the first two enlightened Egyptian rulers in Hellenistic times.[42] During their reign, two physicians, Herophilus and Erasistratus, would make huge strides in the development of anatomy by being able to dissect human cadavers, a practice previously prohibited by religious and other scruples.[43]

In the middle of the second century BCE, however, savage persecution under Ptolemy VIII caused many of the researchers in the Museum and Library in Alexandria to flee the country; they were enthusiastically welcomed elsewhere in the Greek world. Alexandria's reputation suffered but it continued to be a prestige centre to visit. After Rome's conquest of Egypt in 30 BCE, various emperors visited the Museum and even extended the buildings. We have also noted that Galen spent time there with various lecturers; despite his disdainful description of the city (the food, the climate, the natives, the quality of teaching), the fact that he spent six years there speaks for itself.[44]

41 Nutton 2004, 130.

42 The Greek word '*mouseion*' originally referred to a place connected with the Muses or the Arts inspired by the Muses. In Alexandria, the Museum housed the scholars and this was where discussions and symposia were held and research was done. The Library housed practically every manuscript in the Greek world, acquired by fair or foul means: it is said that the Library in Alexandria borrowed the original manuscripts of the Greek tragedians from the library in Pergamum against an enormous sum in collateral, but then told Pergamum that they could keep the money, while they themselves would keep the original manuscripts (http://www.eduscapes.com/history/ancient/200bce.htm). Nutton (1972, 165–176) states that 'the Alexandrian Museum had no connection with the teaching of medicine'; although there were doctors among its members, it was never a teaching institution comparable to a university. The informal relationship between (exceptional) master and student was what 'study in Alexandria' implied.

43 Von Staden 1989, 29.

44 Nutton 2004, 217.

Figure 4.3 A doctor reading in front of his desk with bookrolls and medical instruments

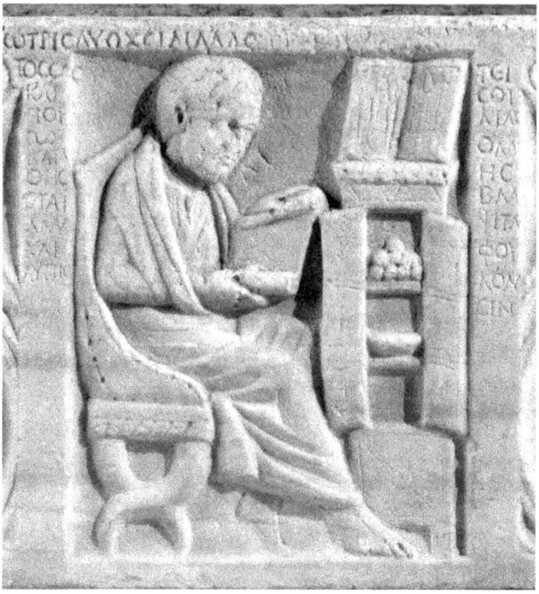

Alexandria was destroyed after its occupation by Zenobia in 272 CE, and the Library with its more than 40,000 priceless scrolls was devastated after the fire of 389 when the Christians, instigated by Cyril, Archbishop of Alexandria, burned the 'pagan material'.[45] The climate was ready for this, since the emperor Theodosius' declaration of Christianity as the state religion and his order that all pagan temples be destroyed followed in 391. Yet Alexandria somehow recovered and even experienced a revival: in the fourth century the historian Ammianus Marcellinus could still state that 'it is enough for a doctor in advertising the merit of his craft to mention that he was educated at Alexandria'.[46] The city survived for another three centuries and was still active during the fifth to the seventh centuries, as is shown by the remains of an amphitheatre, baths and thirteen amphitheatre-lecture halls, which could accommodate as many as 5000 students in total, excavated by a Polish-Egyptian archaeological team in the early 1980s at Qumm ad Diqua.[47] But in 646 the Muslims

45 See El-Abbadi & Fathallah 2008 for details about the destruction of the Library at Alexandria.

46 Amm. 22.16.18. See also Nutton 1972, 165–176.

47 The excavation by a Polish-Egyptian archaeological team revealed thirteen amphitheatre-style *lectoria* in Qumm ad Diqua at Alexandria in Egypt in the 1980s, some of which still had

Figure 4.4 Doctor treating a patient

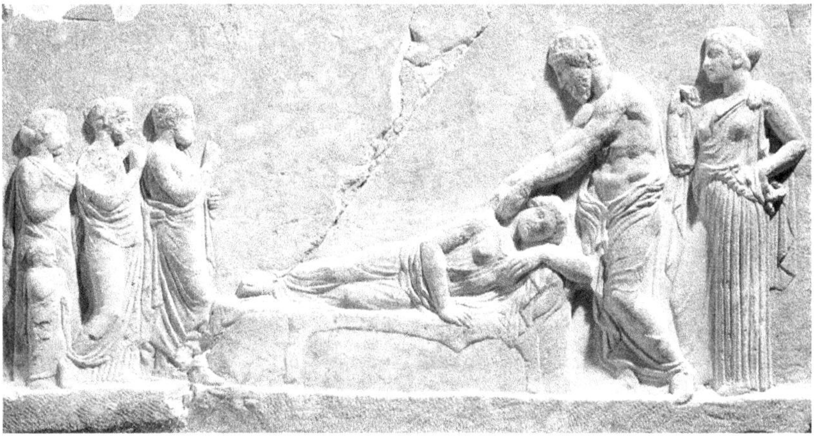

finally burned what was left of the Library, believing that if a book agreed with the Koran, it was superfluous, and if it disagreed, it was heretical. Hereafter, it seems, Alexandria with its Museum and Library slowly slipped into oblivion.

Carthage

In the fourth and early fifth centuries, a time when Rome had been ravaged by civil wars and barbarian invasions and Alexandria had lost much of its former glory, Africa Proconsularis (now Tunisia) with Carthage as its capital, seemed 'to possess the treasure house of the whole world' and excited admiration and envy around the Mediterranean.[48] North Africa was peaceful, since it was not affected by the civil wars, plundering and epidemics of the previous century, and it was rich and prosperous – the export of olive oil, which was in great demand all over the empire, was very lucrative. These favourable circumstances would have enabled scholars to spend time on medical and other studies and to acquire manuscripts by travelling to Alexandria and elsewhere, and could have been a reason for the unusual number of medical texts produced in North Africa in the

a pedestal *in situ* in the middle of the hall for the lecturer. This dates to the seventh century, showing the intellectual vitality of the 'university' of Alexandria until the Arab conquest. (www.freerepublic.com/focus/fr/1137153/ accessed 10 August 2014.) See also in this regard Porman 2010, 425.

48 As stated by the fifth century CE Gallic monk Salvian (*The government of God* 7.13–17).

late Roman Empire.[49] During these years, Vindicianus' *Gynecology* and his *Letter to his nephew Pentadius* appeared,[50] as well as his student Theodorus Priscianus' *Euporiston*, Cassius Felix's *On medicine* and Caelius Aurelianus' *Gynecology* (an adaptation of Soranus' *Gynecology*) and *Medical Responses*. Though not original contributions but rather translations and adaptations of Greek originals, these works were of great importance since the knowledge of Greek in the western part of the empire had by the fourth century declined to the point where the ordinary doctor could no longer read it.[51] Had these translations/adaptations not been done at that stage, the works of the Greek masters of old might have been lost forever.

Two factors can be adduced to explain the density of scientific works. While bilingualism in the West had dropped sharply by the fourth century, even among educated Roman citizens, knowledge of Greek was still regarded as important in certain towns and cities of North Africa. We have evidence in two passages of St. Augustine's *Confessions* where he remarks that he was taught Greek in a primary school in Thagaste (a small provincial town).[52] This bilingual upbringing of the youth would have given them a good basis for eventually becoming scholars who would have been able to translate Greek manuscripts. We also know that Greek was taught at the 'university' of Carthage. Salvian, the monk from Marseilles, spoke with great admiration of the schools in Carthage before the Vandal invasion – according to him, they taught the liberal arts, Greek and Latin literature and philosophy and were second only to Rome.[53]

We know as well that there was contact between Carthage and Alexandria. Augustine, for instance, tells of a retired advocate, Innocentius, who summoned a physician from Alexandria after unsuccessful surgery in Carthage.[54] Furthermore, Vindicianus in the introduction to his *Gynecology* refers to 'experts of earlier times who practised medicine at Alexandria'. Some of the names that he mentions were those of anatomists who belonged to a movement that originated in the second century CE at Alexandria, of which Marinus, Pelops and Quintus were among Galen's teachers (see above).

49 For more information on the situation in North Africa in the fourth and fifth centuries, see Cilliers 2008, 49–63. On Vindicianus, see Chapter 5 and Sabbah 1998, 131–150.

50 On the authenticity of this letter see Chapter 5.

51 Green 1985, 130.

52 Aug. *Conf.* 1.13.20 and 1.14.23.

53 Salv. *Gub. Dei* 7.16. Also transmitted is a letter from St. Augustine to a wealthy Greek who was planning to come and study in Carthage: 'these two large cities, Rome and Carthage, are masters in Latin literature' (*Ep.* 11).

54 Aug. *Civ. Dei* 22.8.3.

Physicians in Carthage were thus in contact with and knowledgeable about trends in medical sciences in Alexandria in the late fourth and early fifth centuries, and one can reasonably expect that would-be doctors in North Africa would have followed basically the same course in their training, even if the curriculum might have differed.

The curriculum

There was a debate in ancient times about whether someone could call himself a *iatros* (physician) if he had read a book or two and happened to know some remedies. Plato (c. 429–347 BCE) and a generation later Aristotle (384–322 BCE) both had the same opinion: that medicine was a craft, and that one could not learn the art of medicine from books.[55] The author of the Hippocratic treatise *Affections* made the qualification that though a literate layman could not become a *iatros* by reading books, he could learn to help himself in diseases and to choose the best physician for his family members and slaves.[56] By the time of the early Roman Empire, however, if we read the treatises of Galen (especially *On my own books*, in which he gives an overview of his studies and skills), it is clear that the theoretical and practical aspects of medical training are equally important.

Apprenticeship with a knowledgeable physician was an indispensable part of the training: observing how the master arrived at a prognosis and requisite therapy when examining the patient (sickrooms were usually full of family, friends, apprentices and curious bystanders) by touching him, taking his pulse, looking at and smelling his urine and asking him or his family members about the history of his illness. Furthermore, looking on while operations were being done and learning about bandages, poultices and various kinds of therapies and medicaments were all part and parcel of the training.[57] The study of anatomy was the key – Galen emphasizes this *ad nauseam*. In *Anatomical Procedures* 2, 220–221 K, he states that 'students need to learn the shape of each bone, not only from books but also by studying them with their own eyes.' For that reason he advised them

55 Pl. *Phdr.* 268c. A thought attributed to Diocles (Fr. 6) was more explicit: 'Books are reminders for those who have learnt, but for the ignorant they are tombstones.' Reference in Totelin 2010, 294 n.35.

56 Hp. *Aff.* 1.6.1–7 and 8.1–8.

57 Craik (2010, 230) states that surgery was not formally taught; the tyro had to look, learn and do likewise.

to go to Alexandria for further study, since they would there still have the opportunity to observe lecturers doing dissections.[58]

Even though most of the ordinary physicians' training would have consisted of a mere apprenticeship with whichever doctor was willing to take him, it is a fact that the more medical information from the writings of the past the would-be doctor absorbed, 'the more likely he was to profit from face-to-face instructions from skilled professionals and to acquire *ta iatrika* (medical knowledge) for himself'.[59]

A useful overview of the subjects studied at Alexandria is given by Marasco, from which the following information has been gleaned.[60] Great importance was attached to philosophy – medicine was associated with philosophy from its earliest origins.[61] We have also noted the emphasis placed by Galen on philosophy, and his view that logic was essential for diagnostics.[62] There was also, of course, the prestige that went with it.

Other, more specifically scientific subjects that were necessary for practical requirements were mathematics, geometry and astronomy. Mathematics was necessary for calculating the course that diseases take and the periods of treatment,[63] geometry to acquire knowledge of the region and of the condition of areas,[64] and astronomy to be able to determine the time of the change of the seasons and of the rising and setting of stars, since when the seasons change the innards of people change correspondingly. Marasco points out that astronomy played a 'vital part' in the determination of the treatment of many diseases, especially epilepsy.[65]

There were a number of subjects that had no direct relation with medicine: grammar, poetry and rhetoric. Knowledge of grammar was regarded as necessary because students learned to write and speak correctly and to

58 Gal. *AA* 2.220 K.

59 Hanson 2010, 188.

60 Marasco 2010, 205–222. An account of the late Alexandrian medical curriculum is given by Iskandar (1976, 235–258); the information is derived from Ibn Ridwan's *Useful book on the quality of medical education* (1060 CE). Basically the same works are studied as in the earlier period, but the course is divided into seven grades, with specific works prescribed for each grade.

61 See, *inter alia*, Edelstein 1967d, 349–366.

62 See above and *The best doctor is also a philosopher* 1.53–63 K. Galen emphasizes that Marcus Aurelius used to call him 'the first among the doctors and the first among philosophers' (*On prognosis* 14.660 K.). For Galen's view on logic, see *The best doctor* 1.3 K.

63 Isid. *Etym.* 4.13.2.

64 This was already emphasized in Hippocratic times, as stated in the Hippocratic treatise *Airs waters places* c.2.

65 See also Temkin 1971. Augustine (*Ep.* 7.6.8) recounted that the proconsul Vindicianus warned him against the science of astrology (telling people's future from the stars).

explain the ancient texts.[66] Poetry might seem a strange requisite, but Marasco explains that it 'contributed to general cultural standing',[67] and we should keep in mind that many physicians in ancient times were well versed in the composition of works of poetry.[68]

These subjects may seem very 'humanistic' to us since they appear to have little bearing on medicine, but Marasco points out that the dichotomy between sciences and humanities only developed in the nineteenth century and that it was unheard of in ancient times.[69] He surmises that knowledge of humanistic subjects might have inspired physicians to adopt a less technical and more humane attitude towards patients.

Rhetoric was a particularly important subject; from Hippocratic times it was regarded as a requirement for practicing medicine. With his rhetorical skills, a doctor could, for instance, persuade a patient of the necessity of cauterization or of some other unpleasant therapy. And would-be doctors could learn how to handle the never-ending arguments about questions of prognosis and therapy with colleagues, or, if they happened to have the confidence that Galen had, display their superior knowledge.[70] But perhaps the most important advantage of being eloquent was in the selection of *archiatri* or city physicians, which was from Hippocratic times up to the early Empire done by the City Council. Making a good impression by being eloquent in such an 'interview' would obviously have been imperative for candidates who wished to start a successful medical career. Rhetorical skills seem to have become an integral aspect of a medical career; in fact, inscriptions found in Ephesus reveal that there was a regular two-day contest in Ephesus during a festival in honor of Asclepius, the god of medicine, where physicians competed in certain categories, trying with their eloquence to convince the jury of their medical skills.[71]

66 Isid. *Etym.* 4.13.1.

67 Marasco 2010, 212.

68 For instance, Andromachus the Elder, master physician of the emperor Nero, who wrote a treatise on theriac in metric verse that was passed on to us by Galen (*On antidotes* 14.34–42 K.), and Eudemus, who wrote down the recipe for theriac for King Antiochus VIII Philometer in verse form. It is also possible that Nicander's *Theriaca* and *Alexipharmaca* were the recipes of King Attalus III of Pergamum in verse form.

69 Marasco 2010, 215.

70 Another example of the use of rhetorical skills is shown by the renowned fourth-century physician Magnus of Nisibis, who was so eloquent that he could convince patients who had been treated by other doctors that they were still ill. Eunapius, *Vitae Sophistarum* 20 (reference in Marasco 2010, 213).

71 Mattern 2008, 69–72, 80–83.

Didactic techniques

The subjects mentioned were taught by way of lectures and/or demonstrations in Alexandria by so-called *iatrosophists* (professors of medicine) who would explain the medical views of, for instance, Hippocrates and Galen in the amphitheatre-style *lectoria* (see above p. 106 n. 47). The original texts of the Hippocratic and later treatises were of course for many centuries already no longer available, but copies had been made of the manuscripts, and along the way also summaries (as still happens among medical students nowadays). More detailed abridgements were also made by scholars, some of which were longer than the original text!

Furthermore, scholars like Galen had written very useful commentaries on a great number of the Hippocratic treatises, explaining them and adding their own opinions.[72]

A favourite way of teaching then (and now) was by way of catechisms (*erotapokriseis*, question-and-answer format), of which many copies have been transmitted.[73] Porman further mentions that the method of division (*diairesis*) and subdivision proved to be a very useful mnemonic device: 'By compartmentalizing the medical knowledge, it becomes easier for the student to remember the material.'[74] Copies of branch diagrams transmitted show that it was also a useful mnemonic technique.

Two very helpful basic texts that would probably have been prescribed are the Pseudo-Galenic *Introduction* and *Medical Definitions*. The latter claims in its preface that especially young students will find it useful, while the *Introduction* contains an overview of the whole of ancient medical history, followed by a section on medical topics, like diseases, body parts, physiology and the like. There were two additional Hippocratic treatises, *Aphorisms* and *Epidemics*, the former stating some principles in a very concise way, and the latter giving valuable examples of views on diseases. Galen also wrote some textbooks specifically for beginners: *On sects for beginners*, *On bones for beginners*, *On the pulse for beginners* and *Therapeutics to Glaucon*. For more advanced students a selection of books of Hippocrates and Galen – of the latter the so-called *Sixteen Books of Galen*, of which different versions have been transmitted, was popular.

72 See Pormann (2010, 419–442) for more information on the teaching techniques and also on textbooks.

73 The question–and–answer technique. See Hanson (2010, 192–197) for more information in this regard.

74 Pormann 2010, 429–431.

In Carthage, Vindicianus' abridgement of anatomy, the *Gynecology*,[75] would certainly have been prescribed, as well some years later Theodorus' *Euporiston* and Soranus' *Gynecology* (or if already lost, then Caelius Aurelianus' Latin version).

Encyclopedias were another genre that developed in the fifth century.[76] Their aim was to give already qualified practitioners 'a well-organized and comprehensive handbook' so that they have easy access to the relevant information.[77] Oribasius of Pergamum's encyclopedia was one of the first (fourth century).

Conclusion

It is, finally, time to return to the problem stated in the first paragraph of this chapter and to take stock of the standard of doctors in the light of what has been discussed above. Where possible, the focus will be on the situation in Roman North Africa in the fourth and early fifth centuries.

The idea of an 'African School' of physicians as proposed by the French scholar Guy Sabbah should of course be understood in the broadest sense of the word, and cannot be compared with the situation in Alexandria, where there has for centuries been a tradition of excellent teachers from whom would-be doctors could receive training. Even though one could not call it a 'School of Medicine', the idea gives a valid evaluation of the vibrant medical activity in Carthage and vicinity in the late fourth and early fifth centuries. Unfortunately, we know very little about the actual training of medical students in North Africa, apart from the two facts that schools in North Africa were highly praised by the French monk Salvian, and that Greek was still taught at primary school level. However – and this is where Carthage's medical contribution shines like a lighthouse in the twilight years of the Roman Empire in the West – while the knowledge of Greek was declining in the West to the stage where the works of Hippocrates and other masters of old would have become totally unknown to ordinary doctors, a number of North African physicians like Vindicianus, who was still bilingual, realized the necessity to pass the treasure of Greek works on

75 On the title – a misnomer – see Chapter 5, and Cilliers (2005, 153–236).

76 A useful custom in the writing of medical treatises from earliest times probably used in these encyclopedias was to order it *a capite ad calcem* (literally from head to heel), which facilitated the consultation of a treatise in a long book roll.

77 Pormann 2010, 423.

by translating them into Latin, a language understood by all at that time. There was now at least the opportunity for would-be doctors to enrich their apprenticeship, and for established physicians to delve more deeply into the knowledge of the human body. Even more importantly, these translations were the texts that scholars fleeing the country after the Vandal invasion in the fifth century took with them to Europe, from where they were further disseminated. Thanks to the erudition of a handful of scholars in fourth- and fifth-century North Africa, priceless Greek medical texts could in the nick of time still be translated and thus preserved for posterity.

5. Vindicianus

Physician, proconsul, mentor

Background

During the twilight years of the late Roman Empire in the West, the province of Africa Proconsularis, with Carthage as its administrative capital and centre, experienced a flowering of scientific and, in particular, medical activity. North Africa had, up to the Vandal invasion in the early fifth century, escaped the disasters that struck the eastern and western empires in the third century. Great parts of the empire had been ravaged by internal civil wars, Persian and Germanic invaders defeated Roman armies and the country experienced a financial crisis that reduced the coinage to almost nothing.[1] In fact, in the late fourth century, the re-founded Carthage was the largest city in the western empire after Rome, and the province was peaceful and prosperous.[2]

The tranquil circumstances in North Africa during the late fourth and early fifth centuries could have been one of the reasons for the amazing number of medical texts coming from this small but vibrant province. The French scholar Guy Sabbah pointed out that in the period from c. 370 to c. 450 CE the greatest number of medical works produced in the Roman world at large were written by four medical writers – Helvius Vindicianus, Theodorus Priscianus, Caelius Aurelianus and Cassius Felix – all of whom lived in or near Carthage.[3] One of the main reasons advanced in the course of his article is North Africa's good school system. The fifth-century-CE Gallic monk Salvian wrote with admiration about the schools in North Africa where Greek, Latin and philosophy were taught.[4] Sabbah even suggested the existence of an 'African School' of physicians and medical writers, but that is perhaps taking it a step too far. Still, that there were highly intellectual circles in Carthage where medical matters such as the urgency of translating Greek works into Latin for ordinary doctors, and the

1 Ward-Perkins 2005, 33.

2 Hornblower & Spawforth 1996, 34.

3 Sabbah 1998, 131–150.

4 Salv. *Gub. Dei* 7.68. See also Lepelley (1981, Vol.II, 23–25 and 31–2), who refers to Carthage as 'une métropole intellectuelle' ('an intellectual metropolis') (p. 31), and the fourth-century-CE Roman poet Ausonius who regarded Carthage as second only to Constantinople (*Order of famous cities*, Bk. 11; Riché 1995, 9–17).

provision of text books for aspiring medical practitioners of whatever level of expertise, were discussed, cannot be denied. In fact, the works by the aforementioned authors give the impression that they were didactic, lecture notes, as it were, written for students who study medicine. Vindicianus' *Gynecology* is a prime example, as will be seen below; his letter to his nephew Pentadius likewise; Theodorus Priscianus' *Gynecology* is written for midwives or people assisting with births (see Chapter 6), Cassius Felix's *On medicine* would also have been useful for students studying medicine (see Chapter 7).

The relative proximity of the medical school of Alexandria, where medical activities were still flourishing despite the disasters of the third and fourth century (see pp. 107–108) would undoubtedly also have contributed to the remarkable interest in medicine in Roman Africa during this period.[5]

The fourth and fifth centuries CE: an era of compilations, adaptations and translations

In Roman North Africa, the late fourth and early fifth centuries CE was an era characterized by a rich medical culture based on extensive knowledge of the long tradition of Greco-Roman medicine. The emphasis, however, was on using existing knowledge rather than on research and original contributions.[6] Most of the works of this period are thus 'second-hand', being translations from Greek into Latin, and adaptations, compilations or condensations of excerpts from earlier medical texts (especially medicinal recipes). Nutton refers to these fourth-to-sixth-century authors as the summarizers, the encyclopedists, 'medical refrigerators of Antiquity' who have been studied not for themselves but for the earlier sources that they happen to encapsulate.[7] Yet he admits that they were not mere copyists, translators or compilers, but that they selected, added fresh material and compressed the old material.

The question arises as to why fourth- and fifth-century medical writers started to translate and compile the earlier medical texts.[8] Vindicianus

5 For further information on Alexandria see Chapter 4, Strootman 2011, 292–310, and Tieleman 2011, 368–376.

6 See Marasco (2000, 166): 'l'érudition avait effacé presque entièrement l'intérêt pour la recherché' (The [emphasis on] knowledge had nearly completely effaced the interest in research).

7 Nutton 1984a, 2–3.

8 See Ensslin/Deichgräber (1961, 36): 'Die Bemühung um Latinisierung des Griechischen ist Hauptzweck seiner Arbeit' ('The endeavour to Latinize the Greek is the main objective of his

himself gives the answer – to disseminate the Greek sources on which his work is based for the benefit of those who could no longer understand Greek. Until the third century CE Latin was still the language of the courts and the forum, and Greek the language of the sciences, philosophy, the Church and medicine. But knowledge of Greek and of Greek literature started to decline in the West after a brief revival of the enthusiasm for Greek culture under Hadrian and the Antonines.[9] By the fourth century a functional knowledge of Greek was unusual even among educated Romans and seems to have become inaccessible to the general medical practitioner.[10] A need for the translation of Greek medical texts arose.[11] Vindicianus was the first to realize it; he was to be followed by his three compatriots in making the works of the old Greek masters available to the masses in Latin – a language they would understand. Regarding Vindicianus' contribution, Langslow remarks: 'His works herald the beginning of what may be seen as a 'Golden Age' of ancient Latin medical compendia, in that a number of relatively stylish, sophisticated and authoritative compilations were produced in Latin by practising doctors in the period c. AD 370–450 in the prosperous and still partly bilingual province of Africa.'[12] The importance of these authors' contributions can hardly be underestimated.

The practical and eclectic approach to Greek sources and their condensation and translation into Latin – of which Vindicianus' *Gynecology* is a prime example – was not, however, a new idea in the fourth century.[13] Cadden refers to the Roman poet Lucretius, who in his poem *On the nature of things* in the first century BCE gave a simplified Latin version of Epicurus' Greek philosophy.[14] And then in the first century CE, Celsus collected

work'). The encyclopedic Latin works of Varro and Celsus were reference books for educated laymen, not the kind of medical texts physicians would use (Green 1985, 133).

9 McGuire & Dressler 1977, 15. Green (1985, 131) remarks that in late Antiquity 'Greek lost its status as the medical *lingua franca* of the Mediterranean world'.

10 Langslow (2000, 39 n. 111) refers to Cassius Felix's 'frequent explanation of Greek medical terms' which assumes a defective knowledge of Greek among his readers.

11 Two centres responded to this need: Ravenna in Northern Italy, where the works of Hippocrates (mostly *Diseases of women* and *Aphorisms*) and Galen were translated from Arabic or Greek into Latin, and Northern Africa, where translations and adaptations of Soranus' Greek works were made (Green 1985, 140–155 and Cadden 1993, 45).

12 Langslow 2000, 63. His catalogue of the extant corpus of Latin medical works (2000, 60–75) reveals that the vast majority of surviving ancient Latin medical texts dates from 300 to 600 CE.

13 See Cadden (1993, 40) who, referring to especially the fourth to the sixth centuries, states that we then find 'a condensation of earlier learning and an emphasis on handy access and on practical or literary utility'.

14 Cadden 1993, 40–42.

and condensed the information on medicine in his encyclopedic eight books from diverse Greek and Latin sources. Also in the first century CE, Pliny the Elder in his *Natural History* had collected and indiscriminately imparted snippets of information about the natural world gathered from any available Greek or Latin source, without any thought about a theoretical basis or consistency – and in keeping with the Romans' practical bent, he added many medicinal recipes. The eclectic approach of the Romans and their inclination towards brevity together with their preference for practicality at the expense of theory are thus obvious. However, this tendency co-existed with a Greek-orientated approach, as exemplified by Galen with his 'theoretical, systematic and even grandiose vision of medicine and natural philosophy'.[15] Authors and translators were thus faced with a choice not only regarding sources, but also regarding models: the brevity of Pliny presenting information only, and the longwinded philosophic-theoretical approach of Galen. These choices were made deliberately and reflect the climate of the period.

Apart from preserving the precious heritage of the past, the translations and adaptations had a secondary advantage: that of making self-help among the laity more widely accessible.[16] Since few if any doctors could be trusted, self-help was of the utmost importance.[17] Fortunately, the emphasis in Roman medicine was on utility; theory and speculation were avoided as far as possible; even the provenance of the material which medical writers incorporated into their works was not mentioned since it was regarded as of secondary importance.

The contribution of these fourth- and fifth-century Latin medical works thus lay in 'transmitting the legacy of the past rather than by inventing a new system of thought', in contrast to the Arabic East, where the ancient inheritance was 'actively manipulated to create an entirely novel entity' – in the West the only manipulation was the condensation and adaptation of existing material.[18]

15 Cadden 1993, 42.

16 Langslow 2000, 63.

17 See Cilliers (2010, 410) on the recipe collection of the fifth-century Marcellus of Bordeaux: 'This recipe book forms part of a long tradition of do-it-yourself books on healing, written in the first place to teach men to do without doctors [...] and to make the reader self-sufficient.' Cilliers also refers to Pliny the Elder's *Natural History*, written 350 years before Marcellus, which pleads for 'a return to the traditional Roman self-help medicine'.

18 Green 1985, 171–172.

Vindicianus' life

This was the intellectual milieu in which Helvius Vindicianus, a person with a truly exceptional career, found himself in the 370s and 380s.[19] He was born in North Africa and probably also educated there – the first datable Western physician and medical writer to have come from Africa.[20] In the 360s and 370s he served as one of the *archiatri sacri palatii* under the emperor Valentinian (r. 364–375 CE) and his son Gratian (r. 367–383 CE) in their court in the Gallic city of Treviri (now Trier).[21] Thanks to meritorious service he was appointed Count of the College of Physicians,[22] established by Valentinian in 368 CE;[23] in that role, he had to guard the privileges and obligations of the other physicians of the College.[24] To become one of the physicians at the imperial court was already a great honour, and then to be appointed the Count was the highest post that a doctor could attain.[25] This board was the first instance of doctors being appointed on merit – a new aspirant to the board was obliged to undergo an examination to determine his suitability before a commission composed of seven senior medical doctors currently in service.[26] The court doctors were salaried to 'relieve' them of obsequious

19 There was some uncertainty regarding the name of Vindicianus. He was erroneously identified with one Avianus Vindicianus, *vicarius* in a diocese in the West and *consularis Campaniae* (*CIL* X.1683), but it was rectified by Beschaouch (1968, 133–135 and 209–210); see also Marasco 1998, 259 n. 46 and Fiorucci 2012, 483.

20 Cassius Felix, in mentioning one of his recipes, calls him 'Vindicianus Afer' (*On medicine* 32.4), Theodorus Priscianus was his pupil, and St. Augustine, who was in Africa at that time, mentions him in various letters. For more information see Fischer 2017, 607.1 and Sabbah 1998, 132–136.

21 Matthews 1975, 72–73; Fiorucci 2012, 485. Treviri was one of the imperial residences of the emperor in the western half of the empire; he often lived in Gaul, or in Illyricum, at Sirmium, and when in Italy normally resided in Milan; the emperor in the West only paid brief ceremonial visits to Rome (Jones 1973, 133).

22 *Comes archiatrorum* (*Cod. Theod.* 13.3.12).

23 *Cod. Theod.* 13.3.8. Although Valentinian I is said to have been a Christian, Nutton (1984, 11) believes this 'less as a gesture of imperial philanthropy than another attempt by Valentinian to reduce senatorial patronage'. It is perhaps no coincidence that the board was established just one year after Valentinian had suffered such a serious illness (Jones 1973, 140) that he promoted his eight-year-old son, Gratian, as Augustus (Amm. 27.6.1 and 4).

24 The *Codex Theodosianus* 13.3.12, promulgated on 14 September 379, is addressed to Vindicianus and states that he, as the Count, should see to it that the court doctors do not tire themselves with obsequious service to the rich for inheritances since they do receive a salary from the state.

25 Nutton (1988, X, 11) explains the title *comes archiatrorum* as '"count of the doctors" to take charge of all the doctors of the city'. According to Korpela (1987, 140) the *comes archiatrorum* had, in the fourth century, the highest position in the inner hierarchy of the privileged group (see *Cod. Theod.* 11.18.1).

26 *Cod. Theod.* 13.3.9.

service to the rich and make them available for honourable service to the poor.[27] Jones states that the court physicians (*archiatri sacri palatii*) were 'the aristocracy of the profession', enjoying special exemption from all the normal burdens of their elevated rank, including the *gleba senatoria* (a tax on land).[28] Vindicianus' appointment as proconsul of an important province after having served in the College, illustrates the tendency in the late Empire that *archiatri*, when transferred by favour of the emperor to an administrative career, could assume a more important role in public life and society, entering the ruling class and as such representing the cultural elite.[29]

While in Treviri, Vindicianus probably met the Greek physician Julius Ausonius, whose son, the famous poet Decimus Ausonius, had great influence at the court, being the tutor of the young emperor Gratian. Decimus could have played a role in the appointment of Vindicianus, then already at a mature age, as proconsul of Africa Proconsularis for 380 to 381.[30] An inscription was found in Mustio, a Roman town in Tunisia, dedicated by Vindicianus to the emperor Theodosius (r. 379–395), in which the former is called a 'v(ir) c(larissimus) ampl(issimus)q(ue) proc(osul) (sic) p(rovinciae) A(fricae) vice sacra iudicans', which Beschaouch translates as a 'proconsul de très haut rang'.[31]

It was in his office as proconsul that Vindicianus, at an advanced age,[32] laid upon the head of a young man the wreath that he had won in a poetry competition.[33] It was Augustine, who later became known as one of the greatest Churchmen in Western history; he was at that time teaching in Carthage (379–383) and had a great admiration for Vindicianus – as physician and as person.[34] In his *Confessions* he left the following testimonial of the mentor of his youth: 'There was at that time a man of deep understanding, who had an excellent reputation for his great skill as a doctor [...] he and I became better acquainted and I listened intently and without fail to what he had to say, for though he was not a gifted speaker, his lively mind gave weight and charm to his words.'[35] It appears, too, that at a critical stage in Augustine's life, when he had developed a leaning towards astrology,

27 *Cod. Theod.* 13.3.8. For more information on this board and the conditions of service of the doctors and the motive for its establishment, see Chapter 4 pp. 100–101.

28 Jones 1973, 1012.

29 Marasco 1998, 282.

30 Fiorucci 2012, 486.

31 Beschaouch 1968, 117–224.

32 Aug. *Conf.* 7.6.8.

33 Aug. *Conf.* 4.3.5.

34 Aug. *Ep.* 138.3.

35 Aug. *Ep.* 138.3.

Vindicianus in a kind and fatherly way advised him not to 'waste further pains upon such rubbish, because there are other more valuable things to be done'.[36] Vindicianus could speak from experience, since he himself had apparently studied astrology as a young man, intending to make a living by it, but had eventually abandoned it and taken up medicine because he found the divinations of the astrologers to be 'utterly deceptive', and, being an honest man, did not want to earn his living by deception (*Conf.* 4.3).

Vindicianus' fame as physician and as person has spread widely. According to his student, Theodorus Priscianus, his fame after his death was even greater that during his lifetime.[37] Somewhat later another African physician, Cassius Felix, refers to Vindicianus as 'vir illustris Vindicianus' when mentioning one of the latter's recipes.[38] Knowledge of this renowned African physician had also spread to Europe, where Marcellus of Bordeaux,[39] a slightly later contemporary of Vindicianus, quotes one of his recipes.[40]

Medical sects in the early Empire[41]

Before carrying on with Vindicianus' contribution, it is necessary to give some background information about the various medical sects[42] or schools of thought that existed in the early Empire, since that will enable us to better understand Vindicianus' views and approach (see below). The three most important sects were the Methodists, the Empiricists and the Dogmatists.[43] The difference between these schools of thought was in essence the way

36 Aug. *Conf.* 4.3.5.

37 Theod. Prisc. *Physica* Praefatio.

38 Cassius Felix, *On medicine* c. 69.

39 In 394–395 Marcellus was the Master of Offices (akin to a Prime Minister) in the court of the emperor, Theodosius I (see Cilliers 2010, 402–404).

40 Marcellus, *De medicamentis* 16.100.

41 The bibliography on the medical sects is vast and confusing, since there was not only opposition between the sects, but also among the members of the sects themselves. In the following discussion I made use of the excellent explications of medical sects in, *inter alia*, Drabkin (1944), Edelstein (1967c), Hanson & Green (1996), Gourevitch (1998), Van der Eijk (2005) and Scarborough (2008).

42 Gourevitch (1998, 105) defines a 'sect' as 'a group that accepted leadership, and followed a set of teachings'. The word 'sect' acquired a pejorative meaning during the growing influence of Christianity, but in medicine still had its initial meaning in the early Empire.

43 These three medical schools were named after their guiding principle rather than their founder, in contrast with numerous other groups, like the Herophileans and Erasistrateans. The principle on which the Dogmatists based their views is derived from the Greek word *dogma* ('theory'), while the Empiricists based their views on experience (*empeiria* in Greek);

in which medical knowledge was acquired, the nature of the knowledge, its origin and its final purpose – all this would determine the treatment.[44] There are numerous references in the works of the medical writer Celsus (first century CE) and Galen (second century CE) to the competition between these sects, 'jostling each other for pride of place at the bedsides of wealthy Romans'.[45]

The **Dogmatic/Rational/Logic sect** was the oldest, tracing their origin back to Hippocrates (fifth and fourth centuries BCE), where the foundation of a 'rational' approach to medicine was laid. They emphasized theoretical principles and believed that by reconciling reason with observation and experimentation, they could infer the existence of the most recondite entities and causes; but in order to be able to do this, the physician needed to study anatomy and physiology.

The **Empiric school**, founded in the third century BCE, had its roots in Sceptical philosophy, rejected unobservable entities and causes and believed that medicine is simply 'an accumulation of knowledge through what were essentially fortuitous observations'.[46] With this negative approach, no doctrine could develop. Since nature was incomprehensible, there was no need to study anatomy and physiology as aid to the treatment of disease.[47] Observation formed the foundation of medicine, and treatment would be determined by the recorded experience of other doctors and similarities amongst various cases that had been observed. As a disease was composed of symptoms, it did not matter what the cause of disease was; it was the cure that was important.[48]

The **Methodists** occupied a middle position between the Dogmatists and the Empiricists.[49] Most of the works of the Methodists survive only as fragments, but fortunately we have in the works of Caelius Aurelianus translations/adaptations of Soranus (first/second century CE), the most important representative of the 'School of the Method'. Like the Dogmatists, they believed that experience was not enough for a physician, but on the

the Methodists believed that treatment consisted in following the path or method (Greek *meta* + *odos*) prescribed by viewing the phenomena (Edelstein 1967c, 187).

44 Van der Eijk 2005, 28.

45 Hanson & Green 1996, 989. This was still the case in the fourth and fifth centuries CE: Theodorus Priscianus (*Faenomenon* 1.2) also complained about the doctors who, instead of being motivated by pity for a dying man, competed with each other as in an Olympic contest. See also pp. 130–131 below.

46 Gourevitch 1998, 109.

47 Drabkin 1950,16.

48 Gourevitch 1991:73.

49 Cels. 26.26.

other hand they opposed the Dogmatists' theory of hidden things and reasoning that leads to the therapy, and also rejected the humoural pathology, so prominent among Dogmatic principles. Like the Empiricists, they emphasized observation of the phenomena presented by the disease, but avoided prescribing a multitude of drugs, characteristic of the Empiricists. Doctors of the School of the Method looked for two universal principal qualities, called 'communalities', in every patient's illness: the state of tension (excessive constriction) and the state of relaxation (excessive fluidity). The third state was a mixed one. Treatment consisted in bringing about the opposite of the pathological state: in relaxing a tense body and in bringing tension to a constricted body (the allopathic principle of *contraria contrariis*). Observable manifestations give the clue to the state. Symptomology and differential diagnosis were thus developed to a high degree of perfection.

The School of the Method developed in the first century CE. Thessalus of Tralles, regarded by some as the founder of the sect, practiced in Rome in the time of the emperor Nero (r. 54–68). Due to the apparent simplicity of its doctrine (Thessalus claimed that he could teach everything a physician has to know in six months), Methodism was very popular in the first century – it did not have rigorous, demanding rules, but prescribed massage, exercises, bathing and the use of wine; in short, a treatment that was quick, safe and pleasant.[50] This appealed to the Romans, who abhorred strenuous and disruptive treatments. References in later works reveal that Thessalus was uncompromisingly opposed to other medical sects and to non-Methodist physicians; in this he differs from later Methodists, who showed a more eclectic approach.

Vindicianus' relationship with predecessors

It has up to now been regarded as impossible to assign Vindicianus, on the basis of his works, to a particular medical sect.[51] However, Gourevitch refers to the existence of an intellectual movement in Alexandria at the beginning of the second century CE (not mentioned by Galen or later medical writers),

50 According to Galen (*On the therapeutic method*, 781 and 927 X K.) who bitterly criticized the Methodists. The pleasant approach can possibly be traced back to Asclepiades of Bithynia (first century CE) or his pupil Themison; the former played an important role in the establishment of Methodism. Yet this approach met with opposition in the second century CE, thus they adapted their doctrine, reinstating, *inter alia*, a study of physiology. Themison, according to Galen, introduced the concept of communalities.

51 Langslow 2000, 65.

which, because it has no name, she calls the 'Anonymous Sect'.[52] Marinus, Quintus and Numisianus were the main exponents of this sect. This group, whose adherents are found as far afield as Pergamum, Corinth, Rome and Macedonia, had as main interests anatomo-physiology, Hippocratic exegesis, clinical medicine, pharmacology, and were known to be excellent teachers. According to Gourevitch they wished to 'reconcile humoural pathology with a location-oriented conception of disease' (which is exactly what Vindicianus tried to do), and to integrate new discoveries regarding the human body into a single system, along with classical Hippocratism, especially the theories in the treatises *On the nature of man* and *Epidemics*, and the clinical theories of nosology and prognosis.

On closer investigation it appears that not only does Vindicianus' approach and his use of sources (in particular Hippocrates' *On the nature of man*) resemble that of this group of medical writers,[53] but that in the foreword of his *Gynecology* he specifically mentions the names of Marinus, Satyrus, Pelops, Lycus and others as famous predecessors who worked in Alexandria,[54] all of whom were Alexandrian anatomist-physicians of the early second century CE. It thus seems that right at the beginning of the treatise Vindicianus is placing himself within a certain medical tradition represented by a group of anatomists that he held in high esteem.

It is, however, strange that the name of Galen is not mentioned in the list of respected predecessors. With his long-winded, discursive style, which did not appeal to the Roman frame of mind, Galen was admittedly not well known or popular in the West. Temkin[55] describes the Romans' approach as disadvantageous to Galen: 'Where only bare facts, shortened and summarized, were admitted, there Galen the systematist, the logician and sophist, could not possibly become a hero.'[56] But the fact that he was a pupil

52 Gourevitch 1998, 117–120.

53 That this group was *de facto* a sect as Gourevitch states (1998, 120) is probably giving it too much of a formal status; at most it seems to have been an intellectual movement. Their teaching, however, had a decisive influence on the system that was later known as Galenism.

54 The manuscripts of the *Gynecology* differ greatly in the set of names transmitted – perhaps to be explained by names written in the margin of manuscripts by copyists that were later interpolated into the text.

55 Temkin 1977a, 176–177.

56 Nutton (1984b, 316) also refers to 'the scarcity of references to Galen by his contemporaries and to the total silence about him and his achievements among the Latin medical writers before Cassius Felix in the fifth century. From this one might justly conclude that Galen never enjoyed as great an authority in the Latin-speaking half of the Roman Empire as he did in the Greek East.' In the East, however, Galen's prolixity was definitely not a disqualification – 128 of his more than 200 works were translated into Arabic, while in the West only four were translated into

of Satyrus and Pelops practically eliminates the possibility that Vindicianus was not aware of Galen's works, since it was probably through the latter's works that Vindicianus came to know Satyrus and Pelops. But there is no direct trace of Galen in the *Gynecology* – the short and very general remarks in c. 17 on the uterus do not show any resemblance to Galen's *On the anatomy of the uterus*, and the latter's two great works on anatomy (*On the utility of parts* and *Anatomical procedures*) would have been much too detailed for Vindicianus' purposes.

An omission that is more difficult to explain is the name of Soranus of Ephesus, whose works on anatomy and gynecology exerted a great influence in the western part of the Roman Empire in late Antiquity, and especially in the Roman province of Africa.[57] Soranus was mentioned with great respect by highly esteemed scholars in North Africa such as St. Augustine,[58] Tertullian[59] and St. Cyprian,[60] and three of the four adaptations of his gynecological works were made by medical authors from North Africa: Theodorus Priscianus (fifth century), Caelius Aurelianus (fourth and fifth centuries) and Muscio (sixth century). The fact that Theodorus Priscianus, who was Vindicianus' student, made an adaptation of Soranus's *Gynecology* in the third book of his *Euporiston* confirms that Soranus' works were available in North Africa during Vindicianus' lifetime. The question of why Soranus' name does not occur in the doxology of any of the manuscripts of the *Gynecology* despite the above-mentioned facts seems unanswerable. It must of course be stated that he had no influence on Vindicianus; in fact, there were some basic differences between their approaches. Apart from the fact that their respective gynecological works were not intended for the same reading public, Soranus' system is characterized by the rejection of certain Hippocratic principles, of which the most important was the Hippocratic theory of the four humours.[61] Although no mention is made of the humoural theory in the *Gynecology*, Vindicianus is evidently a supporter

Latin (Hanson & Green 1994, 1045). Galen's theories gradually filtered through to the West in the early Middle Ages via the works of Oribasius and Paul of Aegina, for instance, who translated some of his works into Latin, but this was many centuries after Vindicianus.

57 Hanson & Green 1996, 1045. In the eastern parts of the Roman Empire, Methodism (Soranus was referred to as the *Methodicorum princeps*) apparently never took a strong hold. Except as a gynecological author, Soranus did not play an important part in Eastern medicine, but the situation was different in the Latin West. Methodist influence remained strong among authors such as Theodorus Priscianus (late fourth and fifth centuries CE).

58 Aug. *Contra Julianum* 5.14.51.

59 Tert. *Anim.* c. 6.

60 Cypr. *Ep.* 69.

61 Green 1985, 25–36.

of this theory, as is clear from his letter to Pentadius, which is based on the Hippocratic humoural theory. Furthermore, the Hippocratic tenet of the polarity of left and right does not find a place in Soranus' works, whereas in Vindicianus the right/left theory, which associates the more favourable right side with a male fetus and the unfavourable left side with a female fetus, is the point of departure for his determination of the sex of the fetus.[62] But, of course, the brevity of the *Gynecology* as well as the fact that we do not have the complete works of Soranus preclude any deductions about possible resemblances between these two authors' gynecological works.

Works

Time has not been kind to Vindicianus – very few of his works have been transmitted. The remainder of this chapter will explore his three most important works.

a. *Epistula Vindiciani comitis archiatrorum ad Valentinianum imperatorem* (*'Letter of Vindicianus, Count of the physicians, to the emperor Valentinian'*)[63]

This letter comprises the introduction to Vindicianus' lost collection of pharmaceutical recipes, *Quae homines docti de expertis remediis prodiderunt* ('Proven recipes transmitted by learned men'), dedicated to the emperor Valentinian.[64] It was written between 371 and 375 while Vindicianus was still in Treviri – his confident tone reflects his superiority as Head of the College of Physicians.[65] It is written in the first person to the emperor personally – the only instance of a physician being so close to the emperor, besides Oribasius, who was the personal physician of the emperor Julian (r. 361–363).[66]

This letter of Vindicianus is unusual – Nutton remarked that medical texts in Antiquity 'have a bias towards theory rather than the realities of day-to-day practice', but here we have a medical text that contains two complete case histories, describing the symptoms, diagnosis, prognosis,

62 Vindicianus, *Gynaecia* c. 21.

63 Text in Niedermann & Liechtenhan 1968, 46–52.

64 Only four recipes were transmitted, found in the works of Marcellus (*On drugs* 16.100: a reference to the 'unparalleled remedy of Vindicianus against the cough') and Cassius Felix (*On medicine* cc. 32, 42 and 69).

65 Fiorucci 2012, 496.

66 Fiorucci 2012, 495.

therapy and the outcome.[67] It resembles the case histories in the Hippocratic *Epidemics*, but is much more detailed; however, it lacks auscultation, the urine test and the critical days often referred to in the Hippocratic case histories.

Though addressed to the emperor Valentinian I and his family, the letter is clearly written with a wider audience in view, in fact for posterity, as Vindicianus himself states in the last paragraph. The important point that he wishes to make is that the authority of renowned doctors of the past should be recognized, and that medications whose efficacy have been verified should be used and not just any remedy that comes to mind; his admonition is of course a gentle reference to his own (effective and tested) recipes that would have followed.

In the letter, Vindicianus shows his superior medical knowledge by describing his handling of two cases. The first is a patient who has developed a fever after having been constipated for twelve days.[68] Vindicianus' colleagues suggested the application of a clyster, but he stepped in and prevented it, for after first observing the appearance of the patient like a good Hippocratic doctor, he deduced from his color that the man was dehydrated and exhausted.[69] His therapy then basically consisted in giving the patient three potions and sending him to the baths to rehydrate his body.[70] The first was a potion of cold water with salt[71] – to the horror of the other doctors, who believed that cold water should not be taken when the patient is feverish.[72] Vindicianus, however, used his common sense – a feverish patient is dehydrated and thirsty and will feel better when drinking cold water. It is reported that the patient did indeed feel better after the

67 Nutton 1988b, VIII.24.

68 Celsus (*On medicine, Introduction* 55) distinguishes between three kinds of diseases: 'one a constriction, another a flux, the third a mixture'. This case would in ancient times have been a classic example of the first: *strictum*, constipation advancing to intestinal obstruction.

69 See Hippocrates (*Prognosis* c. 2): 'In acute diseases the physician must conduct his enquiries in the following way. First he must examine the face of the patient, and see whether it is like the faces of healthy people, and especially whether it is like its usual self.'

70 It is to be noted that the potions, as well as the 'diet' that Vindicianus prescribed when the patient has recovered, do not resemble the typical 'Dreckapotheke' of folk medicine and contained no magical elements, but are the result of pure common sense: salt water and extracts of plant and animal products (see also in this regard Kollesch 1966, 29).

71 If enough salt had been added in the water, it would have had the same effect as magnesium sulphate – namely, to cleanse the bowels; an enema only cleanses the colon, whereas a salty potion will cleanse the small intestine.

72 This view is confirmed by Hippocrates, *Epidemics* 6.3.6 and *Places in Man* c. 27, and even Galen (*On habits* 11–12) stated that 'there was a good chance of healing the patient if he drank nothing cold'. The belief is still going strong today.

drink, and that he then fell asleep, and started to perspire heavily when the fever abated. When he woke up, there was a drastic evacuation of the bowels.

Then follows Vindicianus' diagnosis – excessive eating and drinking – and the prognosis of the (terrible) course the disease would have taken had he not intervened at the right moment.[73]

In the case of the patient who had a continuous flux of tears,[74] Vindicianus permitted the court doctors to try to heal the malady by incising the eyelids, cauterizing the vessels in the temples, shaving the head, making incisions in the veins on the head[75] and putting tinder on the scalp (presumably to cauterize the wounds). The procedures followed by the court doctors were quite in accordance with current medical practice,[76] and were apparently used even up to modern times among the Libyans in Northern Africa.[77]

In this case, Vindicianus did not propose an alternative treatment, but intervened when he saw that the treatment was totally useless and extremely painful, and reprimanded his colleagues for subjecting the patient to such torments, especially when they were about to inflict phlebotomy on the patient, who was already half dead.

A number of enlightening insights come to the fore in this letter about the medical scene in the imperial court, and about Vindicianus as person. It is clear that the treatment of a patient was not entrusted to one doctor only, but that there were a number of doctors working together. It is equally clear that these doctors, who would have belonged to different medical sects, seldom agreed on the therapy, the method of healing and the medication – numerous sources mention the competition and unceasing rivalries among them.[78] Being part of the imperial court, they were in the limelight, and

73 The prognosis was by the Hippocratic authors and even Galen regarded as more important than the diagnosis – if correct, it would greatly enhance the reputation of the doctor and enable him in future to recognize similar diseases and to determine whether the patient would survive or not. Hp. *Prog.* cc. 1–2.

74 In Hippocrates' *Places in Man* (c. 9), there is an explanation of the origin of fluxes: 'Fluxes arise when the tissue is over-chilled, overheated, or when there is an excess of phlegm', and 'the tissues becoming too full are not able to make room for it all, and whatever fluid they are not able to make room for flows wherever it chances to go'. The peccant fluid is then carried down to the eyes by superficial veins and the patient then has a constant flux from the eyes.

75 Referred to as 'arteriotomy' by the Greeks.

76 See Hippocrates' *Places in Man* c. 13: 'when food and medications given to dry the flux did not help, the treatment would be to 'make incisions [...] in order that whatever collects in them will escape more quickly by flowing off through the wounds'. These procedures are also described in the Hippocratic treatise *On sight*: scarification of the eyelids (cc. 2 and 4), incisions in the scalp (cc. 4 and 8) and phlebotomy (cc. 3, 7 and 9) (discussed by Craik 2006).

77 Spencer 1953, III, 354.

78 Marasco 2000, 170–171.

whether their opinions prevailed and proved to be efficacious or not would be important for their reputation. It is thus not surprising that Vindicianus emphasizes his successes in contrast with the erroneous therapies of his rivals because success was the basis of one's prestige and authority.[79] And then, having shown up his colleagues' ignorance, he gives a learned, detailed exposition of the causes of the malady and of the course the malady would have taken had it not been for his intervention.

That these rivalries at the imperial court were quite normal is confirmed by a document of the fifth and sixth centuries, the *Formula comitis archiatrorum* ('Directive of the Count of the physicians'),[80] from the time of the emperor Theoderic.[81] This document, addressed to the court physicians, exhorts them to lay aside their arguments because they have a negative influence when refusing to cooperate and do not seek and accept the best opinion without envy.

Vindicianus' letter to the emperor also gives us some interesting glimpses of the cultural milieu of that era. A characteristic of especially the fourth and fifth centuries was the emphasis on erudition rather than on research.[82] The letter does indeed show Vindicianus' vast but also detailed knowledge of not only the medical tradition as we have seen above, but also of literature and of rhetorical techniques.[83]

Vindicianus' knowledge of literature is revealed by two echoes of ancient authors (clearly showing that he was absolutely competent to judge the literary competition in which he put the crown on Augustine's head). In the first paragraph of the letter in which there is an allusion to the fragility of the condition of man when he neglects the advantages of the medical art, one is reminded of the first line of Sallust's *War with Jugurtha* 1.1, which also contains an ungrounded complaint about the fragility and brevity of man's life when it is ruled by chance rather than virtue.[84] Then also, in this paragraph, Vindicianus cleverly uses the traditional comparison of a helmsman steering his ship through a tempest and man, who is continually

79 See Vindicianus' sarcastic references to the 'great number of renowned colleagues' (par. 2), the 'distinguished' doctors (par. 4), 'eminent' doctors (par. 8), and then straightforwardly their 'ignorance' in their treatment (par. 9).

80 The content of the document is reported by Cassiodorus (*Variae* 6.19.5).

81 King of the Germanic Ostrogoths, reigned in Italy from 493 to 526.

82 See Marasco 2000, 166, and Nutton 1988e, X, 1–4.

83 Information on this section was partly gleaned from the informative article of Marasco 2000, 166–171.

84 'Without reason do mankind complain of their nature, on the ground that it is weak and of short duration and ruled by chance rather than by virtue.'

threatened by ill health, to illustrate his point that knowledge of one's art is indispensable.[85]

A second echo of an ancient author occurs in the second case history, when Vindicianus states that the patient, weeping and groaning of pain, quoted the elder Cato, who stated that one must entrust one's body to a trustworthy doctor,[86] to which Vindicianus added 'And I say, "to an experienced one"'.[87]

Vindicianus furthermore uses his knowledge of the techniques of rhetoric to great effect – the tone of the letter is in a high key and quite dramatic: in the first paragraph the inexperienced helmsman (*rudis gubernator*) who does not know of all the dangers (*incertus periculorum*) is uncertain of his salvation (*dubius salutis*). The first patient is in a critical condition (par. 2), and when Vindicianus gives him cold water to bring down his fever, the other doctors exclaim that he has killed the patient (*occidisti hominem*). When his fever abates and he starts perspiring, it is so abundant that it seemed as if the Nile was flowing out of his body (par. 3). And when he awoke and started evacuating there was such a stench that the doctors believed that his intestines had rotted, and all fled (par. 4).

Vindicianus' discussion of the cause of the disease in both cases and his prognoses are equally dramatic and leaves no doubt that, after the other doctors' drastic treatment, both patients would have died if he had not intervened.

The letter also gives us a glimpse of Vindicianus' personality. In contrast with his colleagues, who employed drastic and painful therapies, his therapies are mild and show respect for his patients' dignity (for instance, he advises against the use of a clyster in the case of the patient with constipation) and compassion for the patient who has already suffered much pain (when preventing phlebotomy). It is also interesting to note that Vindicianus does not suggest an alternative treatment in the second case when the traditional one proved to be ineffective – he knew how far one could go before causing more, probably unnecessary, torment. What angered him about his colleagues was that they did not uphold the Hippocratic principle of helping, or at least not harming, the patient.[88] Furthermore, his diagnoses and prognoses not only reveal his medical knowledge, but also his common sense – for instance, giving a feverish patient a cold drink, against current custom.

85 Used since Plato, and also by Cicero, Quintilian, Seneca and so on. See Marasco 2000, 167 (notes 14–16) for references.

86 Cato, *R. R.* 2.22.2.

87 Letter to the emperor Valentinian, par. 9, Niedermann 1968, 50.

88 Hp. *Epid.* 1.11.

The letter gives no indication of Vindicianus' religious belief, but it is doubtful that he would have held such high positions during the reign of the Christian emperors in the late fourth century if he had not, at least, shown some sympathy for the Christian cause.[89]

b. *Epistula ad Pentadium nepotem suum de quattuor umoribus in corpore humano constitutis ('Letter to his nephew Pentadius on the constitution of the four humours in the body')*[90]

This letter gives a brief account of the theory of the four humours, and is written for Vindicianus' nephew, Pentadius, who had just started his medical studies. It is a didactic letter[91] that purports to be a translation of 'the core of the medical works of Hippocrates',[92] but is in fact a medical treatise in its own right, and gives an account of the theory of the four humours (blood, phlegm, yellow bile[93] and black bile) as it was interpreted in the late fourth century CE. It is stated in the letter that man consists of these four humours and that the characteristics of each correspond with the four seasons. The varying predominance of each of the humours is shown to be linked to a season of the year, and also to specific hours of the day as well as to the stages in the life of man. The letter also mentions its influence on the pulse rate and on man's character: an excess of black bile tends to make men melancholic, blood would make them sanguine, phlegm phlegmatic and red/yellow bile choleric. Finally, the diseases caused by an immoderate increase in one of the humours are mentioned with relevant therapies.

In relating the humours to diseases, Vindicianus follows the Hippocratic principle that health depends on the equilibrium and right mixture of the

89 See Fiorucci (2012) and the discussion in Chapter 9 on the question whether Vindicianus was a Christian or a pagan.

90 Text in Rose 1894, 484–492; Latin text, German translation and discussion in Schoch 1996; also discussed in Cilliers 2014, 122–127.

91 See Schoch (1996, 123), who also regards it as a 'typischer Lehrbrief' (a 'typical didactic letter'). Langslow (2000, 74) points out that letters feature 'quite prominently in the Latin medical corpus', either as prefaces to collections of recipes (for instance, that of Scribonius Largus and Vindicianus) or as theoretical treatises in their own right (as Vindicianus' letter to Pentadius). We know nothing about the addressee of this letter; it could be a fictitious name.

92 Rose 1894, 485.

93 Vindicianus describes it as 'red bile' (*cholera rubea*). Schoch (1996, 82) gives the following explanation: 'Die Farbe der Säfte bleibt in den verschiedenen Jahrenzeiten nicht gleich' ('The colour of the humour does not remain the same in the different seasons'). He adds that it also has to do with the 'Lebensweise' of a person and should thus be regarded as changeable.

four humours.[94] However, during a specific season of the year one of the humours will increase, which can then make man predisposed to diseases associated with this humour: blood increases in spring, red bile in summer, black bile in autumn and phlegm in winter. And when that particular humour has increased immoderately, then disease sets in, which will last long if, according to Vindicianus, an inexperienced or negligent doctor does not recognize from which humour it has originated. Treatment is based on the Hippocratic principle of *contraria contrariis*: a disease of the blood, which is sweet and wet and hot, must be counteracted with a medicament that is cold and bitter and dry.[95]

This letter is the first systematic exposition of the humoural theory in Latin.[96] It was an authoritative work throughout the Middle Ages, and according to Schoch, who traced the development and application of the humoural theory to the modern day, this 'Roman' version of the theory of the four humours played a role until the late nineteenth century with practically no change in content.[97]

One must, however, remember that it is not original work – original scientific research ended with Galen at the end of the second century CE – but rather a translation/adaptation of a Greek text, as Vindicianus himself states. As such, it is part of a long tradition: the theory of the four humours was first written down by Hippocrates' son-in-law, Polybus, in the fifth century BCE in the treatise *On the Nature of Man*. Thereafter it seems that little attention was paid to it during the Hellenistic Age at Alexandria; it was Galen who first pointed out that the theory of the four humours formed the basis of the Hippocratic works.[98] However, Galen did not make much use of the theory himself, since his system was based on the four elementary qualities, hot, cold, dry and wet. But in the centuries after Galen the theory of the four humours surfaced again in various guises.

94 Hp. *Nat. Hom.* c. 4.

95 Hp. *Nat. Hom.* c. 9, *Epid.* 1.11, *Flat* c. 1. This principle of *contraria contrariis* or allopathy (treating a disease with drugs having an effect opposite to the symptoms) is the basis of Hippocratic healing, but in *Places in Man* (c. 42) there is also a reference to what is clearly homeopathy, treating a disease by minute doses of natural substances that in a healthy person would produce symptoms of that disease (*South African Concise Oxford Dictionary*). See in this regard Jouanna 1999, 342–3.

96 Passing remarks on individual humours are found in Celsus (*passim*) and a few paragraphs in the two pseudo-Hippocratic letters serving as introduction to Marcellus' *On drugs* (1968, 18–33), but nothing resembling this systematic discussion of the humours.

97 Schoch 1996, 123.

98 *Galen's commentary on Hippocrates' On the nature of man I, Intr. prooem.*11 CMG 5.9.1 p. 8.9 ff. and p. 8.19 ff. Reference in Jouanna 2006, 119 and n.16.

There is at present a lively debate on the date and authorship of the letter after some articles by the French scholar Jacques Jouanna, who dates it to the so-called second renaissance in Alexandria in the sixth century.[99] This immediately makes the authentication of the letter problematic. Reaction has come from various scholars, which cannot be discussed here due to lack of space; convincing arguments against Jouanna's view have, however, been forwarded by *inter alia*, Fabio Stok[100] and Francesco Fiorucci,[101] both of whom emphasize the complexity of the problem.

c. The *Gynecology*

The *Gynecology* is accepted as a work by Vindicianus. It is a very concise treatise on the anatomy of the human body, reproduction and the development of the embryo/fetus *in utero*, in the usual format of *a capite ad calcem*.[102] It was written with the professed aim of providing the knowledge normally gained by viewing the body during dissection,[103] which the Romans were no longer allowed to do.[104] The work is a good example of the eclectic approach of the Romans – my study of the *Gynecology* has indicated that Vindicianus excerpted passages from various Greek authors and combined them in his account of the anatomy of the human body and in the section on reproduction and embryology.[105] A number of other works on anatomy, said to be related to the *Gynecology*, have erroneously been ascribed to Vindicianus:

i. the so-called *Epitome Altera*,
ii. the fragment in the Codex Parisinus 7027 referred to as the *De natura humani* ('On the nature of mankind'), and
iii. the treatise referred to as the *De semine* ('On seed') in the Codex Bruxellensis 1348.[106]

99 Jouanna 2005, 138–167; 2006, 117–141.
100 Stok 2012, 138–143.
101 Fiorucci 2009, 67–90.
102 Text in Rose 1894, 426–463 and Schipper 1921, 13–22.
103 'And for other (sc. earlier) anatomists it was allowed to dissect a corpse and to attempt to come to know why they were exposed to danger or killed [...]. But we are not allowed to do this, since it is prohibited' (Manuscript G c. 2).
104 On dissection in the Greco-Roman world, see Von Staden (1989, 138–153).
105 Due to lack of space, it is unfortunately not possible to indicate all the sources used in the text of the *Gynecology*.
106 See Cilliers 2005, 154–155, for a concise overview regarding the relation of these manuscripts and their erroneous attribution to Vindicianus.

The *Gynecology* and the above-mentioned works were the standard texts on anatomy and physiology in the pre-Salernitan period (before the eleventh century), and among the most widely circulated and excerpted medical writings of Antiquity.[107] They were widely quoted in the early Middle Ages – the *Gynecology* was transmitted in at least thirteen manuscripts of widely different provenance.[108]

The title 'Gynaecia' ('Gynecology')

The Greek word *ta gynaikeia* means 'a female's genital organs', 'menstruation', 'female disorders' or 'therapies for female disorders'. In the Hippocratic Corpus it is the title of two long texts devoted to diseases of women – the Hippocratic writers were the first to give a relatively coherent view of female anatomy and physiology as well as the etiology of female diseases, and this resulted in the evolution of a new medical genre, the gynecological treatise.[109] In post-Hippocratic times this genre was called *ta gynaikeia* (in Latin *gynaecia*[110]) when gynecological recipes formed part of the treatise, and *gynaikeia nousoi* when it was a gynecological treatise. In later centuries, however, the title *ta gynaikeia* or *gynaecia* was preferred as the title for

107 Langslow 2000, 65. Lesky (1950, 64) adds: 'sie stellt eine Sammlung von gynäkologischen, embryologischen, anatomischen und physiologischen Lehren der Antike dar und hat nachhaltig auf mittelalterliche Schriften und Traktate medizinischen Inhalts eingewirkt' ('They represent a collection of gynecological, embryological, anatomical and physiological tenets of Antiquity and had a lasting influence on medieval writings and treatises with a medical content').
108 See for example the interpolations from the *Gynecology* in Isidore's *Etymologies* (11.1.20 and 28; 11.1.42 and 51; 11.1.108–9; 9.6.4). K.-D. Fischer (forthcoming 2019, 6–71) further refers to an *Epistola ypocratis de anatomia* (thirteenth century) in which various fragments of Vindicianus are quoted by Vincenz von Beauvais, and to references to Vindicianus in the 'Bamberger Chirurgie' (c. twelfth century, *Tract. De chirurg.*, c. 9 and 63). See also Ferckel (1914, 306), who states that Vindicianus' *Gynecology* was often ascribed to Hippocrates or Galen during the Middle Ages, and adds various references to Vindicianus in later writers, *inter alia,* his description of the development of the embryo, which appears unsourced in *Trotula, De mulierum passionibus* c. XII (end twelfth century). Various editions of a poem on healing attributed to Vindicianus (certainly spurious) were found in the library of the University of Leiden, *inter alia,* in the *Veterum quorundam bonorum scriptorum libri et singuli de materia et re medica, videl. Q. Sereni Sammonici de morborum curatione,* Lipsiae (1654), and in the *Poetae latini minores sive Gratii Falisci Cynegeticon*, ed. P. Burmannus, Leidae (1731). Even though this work was not written by Vindicianus, it shows that his name was famous enough to be connected with poems of which the author was unknown.
109 Hanson 1991, 96.
110 This is the meaning given by the *Thesaurus Linguae Latinae* (6.2.2382–2383 s.v.) of *gynaecia*: 'Those things which refer to women (sc. their diseases). It is the title of works translated in Greek or written by Mustio, Caelius Aurelianus, Vindicianus, Theodorus Priscianus.'

gynecological treatises in general. This genre spans more than 500 years from the Hippocratic treatises at the end of the fifth century BCE to Soranus' *Gynecology* in the late first century CE.

The subject of Vindicianus's *Gynecology* is basically human anatomy; in only six of the 24 chapters are reproductive anatomy, conception and the development of the embryo/fetus *in utero* discussed. The title is thus misleading and must have been given to some of the transmitted manuscripts during the Middle Ages – in fact, only two of the thirteen manuscripts have the title *Gynaecia*, and in both cases they are flanked by other therapeutically orientated gynecological treatises, which may have influenced the identification and naming of Vindicianus' manuscript.[111]

The format and presentation of the *Gynecology*

The *a capite ad calcem* ('from head to heel') presentation in the *Gynecology* was typical of medical literature in late Antiquity.[112] The description of the internal configuration of the body (cc. 1–17 in four of the MSS) is to a great extent presented in the same pattern (although not all the aspects mentioned below occur in the description of all the organs/parts):

1. the name of the organ or bodily part, sometimes with its etymological derivation;
2. the number of its constituent organs/parts or layers with their names;
3. the position of the organ or part in the body, and the organ/bodily part with which it is connected;
4. an identification of the organ by way of a brief description of its external appearance, with the number and position of openings (seldom);[113]
5. its function;
6. a sentence about the pathological condition of the organ (sometimes).[114]

It is interesting to note that this pattern of presentation bears a resemblance to Rufus of Ephesus' *De nominatione partium hominis* ('On the naming of

111 Green (1985, 189 n. 103) points out that there was a 'pronounced tendency [...] in early medieval manuscripts to group gynecological treatises together.'

112 Bujan 1982, 37. He points out that this practice already appeared in the Greek world.

113 Only the spleen (Vindicianus, *Gynecology* c. 12) and the female testes (c. 16) have adjectives describing their outward appearance: the spleen is 'oblong' and the testes 'shorter and more fragile'.

114 Perforation of the teeth due to a fluid constantly dripping on them from the head; choking; the uvula is referred to as a 'grape' (*uva*), which obviously describes a pathological condition of the normally finger-like flap that hangs at the back of the throat; and an exudation of the ears.

the parts of the human [body]').[115] It is quite possible that Vindicianus would have been familiar with the works of Rufus, who was one of the most prominent Greek physicians in the empire in the second century.[116] The description of the organs/parts is admittedly more detailed in the *Gynecology*, and more pathological conditions are described, but the general concise impression of the work does remind one of Rufus' presentation.

The intended readers

Vindicianus' *Gynecology* is unusual in that it is not dedicated to anyone and contains no explanatory introductory letter, in contrast with, for instance, Galen's *De dissectione uteri* ('On the anatomy of the uterus'), which was dedicated to an unnamed midwife, and Theodorus Priscianus' *Gynecology*, which was dedicated to a certain Victoria. Since it is not impossible that the *Gynecology* could be an abbreviated version of an originally longer text, the possibility exists that the original text may have contained a dedication, but, of course, only a small section of the whole work is on gynecological matters.

The question arises as to whether the *Gynecology* was written for midwives, physicians or a more general lay public. In discussing this matter, one must beware of assuming that the same sharp lines were drawn between these three groups as is the case today. Temkin points out that 'the domain of the ancient midwife extended beyond the field of obstetrics; it certainly included gynecology'.[117] On the other hand, there were physicians who were called gynecologists because they treated female illnesses.[118] And regarding the third group, the educated layman in Antiquity was 'much more likely to form his own judgment about medical matters [...] and to treat himself and his family.'[119]

The subject of Vindicianus' *Gynecology* is, then, not primarily gynecology. The body of the work consists of a brief overview of human anatomy. The emphasis is thus not on reproductive matters – as indicated above, only six of the 24 chapters are devoted to reproduction, conception and embryology. These six chapters contain a description of the anatomy of the reproductive organs (cc. 13, 16 and 17), a chapter on conception and the origin of seed (c.

115 In: Daremberg & Ruelle 1879.

116 See Haak 2013 for more information.

117 Temkin 1956, xxvii.

118 Soranus, *Gynaecia* 3.3.

119 Temkin 1956, xxxviii. Regarding this group see also Galen's view on the choice of the best doctor by the educated layman (Iskandar 1988), and Horstmanshoff's article on Galen and his patients (1995, 83–99).

18), followed in some of the manuscripts by a discourse on the importance of the number seven (c. 19).[120] Then there is a section on embryology, in which an outline is given of the development of the fetus (cc. 20–22). If one bears in mind Soranus' remark in his *Gynecology* that theoretical topics such as speculations on the origin of seed and reproduction are 'useless' (*Gynecology* 1.2), it seems clear that the section in Vindicianus' *Gynecology* on the origin of seed, the discourse on the importance of the number seven, and possibly even the discussion of the various stages in the development of the fetus would not have interested midwives whose main concern was obstetrics and gynecology. Vindicianus' treatise furthermore makes no mention of the treatment of the pregnant woman and the handling of parturition, abortion, difficult labor or female disorders, aspects that were of prime importance to midwives.

It thus seems that the original fourth-century text was rather intended for prospective and practicing physicians,[121] or as a *vademecum* for the laity[122] (the equivalent of our modern 'Pocket Edition'). Such readers would have derived much benefit from this short overview of anatomy containing an identification of the bodily organs and their respective positions and functions, and also from the number of brief references to pathological anatomy where diseased organs are described. The section on reproduction, conception and embryology would have provided handy background knowledge to impress patients and colleagues – theoretical information that would not have been of direct practical use for midwives. And in later centuries the snippets on pathological anatomy may have been very useful

120 The number seven played as important a role in ancient times as in all cultures of the world today; its origin can according to a treatise from the fifth century BCE be traced back to ancient Iranian and Persian speculation (Lesky 1950, 10). It occurs 700 times in the Bible, and 54 times in the Book of Revelation. In Greco-Roman times it was a significant figure – one need only think of the seven kings of Rome, the seven hills of Rome, the seven Greek sages, the seven wonders of the world, and the like. The Roman polymath Varro left a biographical work *Hebdomadas* (lit. 'a group of seven') in fifteen books, illustrated by 700 portraits. In c. 19 of one of the manuscripts of Vindicianus' *Gynecology* (B 1348) there is a long description of the importance of the number seven in the various stages of the development of the infant: it starts to get milk-teeth at the age of seven months, sheds them at the age of seven years, girls reach puberty at two times seven years and develop breasts and so on.

121 Thus too Fischer 1998a, 24.

122 See Green (1985, 81): 'Just as lawyers needed legal compendia and synopses, so physicians needed a thorough, yet not too substantial handbook they could take with them on their travels.' See Paul of Aegina's *Pragmateia* and Oribasius's *Synopsis*, which were also handbooks for the traveller. The physician Luke who accompanied St. Paul is of course a classic example of a doctor as companion of a traveller.

to the monks who transcribed the manuscripts, since caring for the sick was one of the important tasks in the monasteries.[123]

Conclusion

Vivian Nutton stated in one of his contributions that, in contrast with the great names of the second century (for instance, Galen, Rufus, Soranus) 'the fourth and later centuries present us with a dull and narrow range of authors – the summarizers, the encyclopaedists – who have been studied not for themselves but for the earlier sources that they happen to encapsulate'.[124] However, as has already been stated, had it not been for these late-fourth- and early-fifth-century medical writers, a great part of the medical heritage of Greece would have been lost. And at the helm of the endeavour to translate Greek works was Vindicianus, a physician, who, because of his prestige, rose to the highest level in the medical world, and thereafter was appointed proconsul in one of the most important provinces in the Roman Empire. Thanks to the initiative of this remarkable man, the process of translating Greek works was begun, and, due to his reputation – which, according to one of his students, was even greater after his death – was carried on by his students. It is clear that he was also an inspiring and sympathetic mentor, as St. Augustine experienced. If the late-fourth-century authors seem 'dull' to some scholars, then surely the contribution of Helvius Vindicianus has not been taken into account.

123 See the important Rule in the Benedictine Cloisters to look after the ill, as pointed out by Green (1985, 200).
124 Nutton 1984a, 2.

6. Theodorus Priscianus on drugs and therapies

The medical texts that were produced in the fourth and fifth centuries CE in North Africa were not original research, but translations/adaptations of the Greek texts of the masters of old. The writers would have been faced by two questions: which of the treasures of the past should be translated, and in how much detail? Fortunately the Romans, being traditionalists to the marrow, had a pattern to follow: Latin medical authors in previous centuries – Cato, Pliny and Celsus – had set a trend that could be be followed by the writers of the fourth and fifth centuries,namely a disregard for theoretical reflection, and a preference for practicality and brevity. This approach determined the choice of the author: rather than the theoretical and polemical approach of Galen (129–c. 210), whose discursive philosophical works dominated the approach taken in the East, the Romans preferred the mild and practical approach of the renowned second century CE physician Soranus of Ephesus. However, in contrast to Galen who left an enormous body of medical and philosophical works,[1] the only work of Soranus of which the complete Greek text has survived is his *Gynecology*,[2] a guidebook for midwives with remedies/recipes for the most important female diseases.

The author

We know very little about Theodorus Priscianus, apart from his own statement in *Physica* c. 3 that he was a student of the famous Carthaginian physician Vindicianus[3] (late fourth century CE), the subject of the preceding chapter. This implies that Theodorus was probably also a native of North Africa[4] and lived in the late fourth and early fifth centuries. We can also

1 Despite some major losses (a fire in Rome) his works take up twenty two volumes of the Kühn edition, apart from the works that were translated and survived only in Arabic, Hebrew, Syriac and Latin (Gourevitch 1998, 125).

2 Text and translation in Temkin 1956.

3 *Physica* c.1. In his *Gynecology* (c. 21) Theodorus also refers to *magister meus* when quoting a recipe, but does not specifically name Vindicianus.

4 For Vindicianus' African connection see Chapter 5 on Vindicianus. Sabbah (1998, 138) further refers to Theodorus' use of some African words, which shows that he had written for the Romans of Africa, who would have been familiar with them.

deduce that he was a professional doctor.[5] Scarborough believes, in addition, that he was probably 'a member of the social and economic levels associated with the royal house in the western empire'.[6] The work for which Theodorus is known is the *Euporiston*, which consists of four books of medical recipes:[7] the *Faenomenon*, in which he discusses the treatment of external diseases, the *Logicus*, in which treatments for invisible internal diseases (13 acute and 29 chronic) are discussed, and the *Gynecology*, which contains treatments for women's diseases. Of the fourth book, the *Physica*, a collection of magical remedies, we only have a fragment containing a chapter on headaches and part of a chapter on epilepsy. Due to its practical applicability, the *Euporiston*[8] was very popular in the later Middle Ages; this is proven by the fact that it was excerpted on numerous occasions.[9] The *Gynecology's* popularity is evidenced by the fact that it often circulated independently of the *Euporiston*.[10]

The professed aim and intended readers of the *Gynecology*

The *Gynecology* is dedicated to a midwife, a certain Victoria.[11] In the preface, Theodorus states that he wants to 'support her with his knowledge', and he requests her to 'faithfully, diligently and carefully [...] carry into effect the remedies for female ailments' as set out in his treatise.[12] This knowledge

5 In *Faenomenon* c. 1 Theodorus refers to his 'colleague' Olympios who was a teacher in Byzantium, and in c. 4 he humbly refers to himself as *quantulaecunque scientiae medicus* ('a doctor of some little knowledge').

6 Scarborough 2008, 787. Diepgen (1937, 109) believes that Theodorus was the personal physician of the emperor Gratian (r. 359–363).

7 The edition used is that of Rose 1894, 224–248.

8 Or '*Euporista*', Latin '*Parabilia*', meaning easily obtainable drugs that need not be produced by specialists. 'They were available above all to those who were not without a certain degree of education but who were not in a position to consult a doctor, whether because they were travelling or because they lived on their estates far from any city or town' (Formisano 2004, 127).

9 Langslow 2000, 55.

10 Hanson & Green 1996, 1057. Due to lack of space only the *Gynecology* will be discussed.

11 Meyer-Steinegg (1909, 72) is probably correct in stating that since Victoria is called by Theodorus 'the dear assistant in my art' in c. 1, she was probably more than an ordinary *obstetrix*, at least an 'educated midwife', if not a *medica*. This does however not affect the purpose or the intended readers of the book. The name may instead be Salbina (Langslow 2000, 54 n.164). The first two books are dedicated to an unknown 'dearest friend', and the *Physica* to Theodorus' son, Eusebius.

12 Theod. Prisc. *Gynaecia* c. 1. Her specialty seems to have been 'the prescription of drugs ensuring pregnancies' (Scarborough 2008, 788).

was then to be disseminated among midwives and other women to help them in treating ailing women.[13]

This differs from the intended readers of Soranus' *Gynecology*, one of Theodorus' main sources. The clientele of this renowned physician and gynecologist who practiced in Rome during the reigns of Trajan and Hadrian (early second century CE) were the elite Roman families who found Greek doctors more acceptable than Roman ones. The intended readers of Soranus' *Gynecology* (written in Greek) were therefore the higher echelons of society – doctors, educated midwives who had the status of doctors and educated laymen looking for a midwife.[14] However, by the late fourth and early fifth centuries when Theodorus' *Gynecology* appeared in North Africa, doctors and midwives could no longer read Greek, and educated midwives who were the equal of doctors were no longer to be found. It therefore had to be written in Latin, and had a different approach.

In the preface of the *Gynecology* Theodorus comes to the fore with an unusual view. He states that he had written 'a separate little book on women's diseases, not open to public scrutiny'. He points out that Victoria, being a woman, has an advantage that he does not have: that of being able to share women's secrets more easily. This view is unusual in that neither the Hippocratics nor Soranus had any qualms about discussing women's diseases. Green suggests that Theodorus, despite the fact that he was clearly quite knowledgeable about gynecology, had 'a sense that women's bodies were somehow beyond his ken', for he refers to menstruation as women's 'secrets', and he only discusses one aspect of menstrual disorders, although this was one of the most common problems to be discussed in other gynecological works.[15] He does not discuss obstetrical procedures either; his excuse is that Victoria will learn the details of the obstetrical practice better 'by doing than by reading'.[16] This must be a personal view, since Caelius Aurelianus and Muscio, who both used Soranus, were not squeamish about discussing women's bodies and ailments. Green points out that the idea of secrecy when

13 Cf. also Green (1985, 138), who states that the works of Theodorus Priscianus, Caelius Aurelianus and Muscio 'were not, it seems, written for learned doctors who might argue theoretical matters to win patients or merely for rhetorical show. On the contrary, all three treatises are expressly written for women – obstetricians, both experienced and inexperienced, who were the direct caretakers of women's illnesses.'

14 Baader 1991, 117.

15 Green 2000, 7. *Gynaecia* c. 21. Menstruation is referred to as 'purgation', and 'private parts' merely as 'parts' (*Gynaecia* c. 15).

16 Theod. Prisc. *Gynaecia* c. 32.

speaking about women's matters was a trend in specialized gynecological literature that only started in the later Middle Ages.[17]

The sources of the *Gynecology*

Theodorus, like his teacher Vindicianus, came from the still partly bilingual province of North Africa, and was therefore fluent in Greek.[18] In fact, he initially wrote the four books of the *Euporiston* in Greek to gain recognition in the larger medical community,[19] and then translated them into Latin himself to make them accessible to a broader readership. He himself states: 'I wrote them in Greek since those people have spread abroad the discipline of healing in their clear language. In the present volume, therefore, I will not aim for glory, and indeed in a scholarly work there is no need of eloquence, but of industry.'[20] It is possible that the translation was an abbreviated version, since he twice refers to the Greek original for more remedies.[21]

Theodorus was an eclectic as regards his sources: for internal diseases (the *Faenomenon*) he followed the approach of the Methodist sect,[22] but in the pathology of external diseases (the *Logicus*) he used the Hippocratic humoural theory.[23] He also mentions Hippocrates on various occasions.[24] The familiar way in which he refers to him as 'Hippocrates noster', gives the impression that he had some personal knowledge of his works.[25]

Galen was an important Greek source for Books I and II: there are resemblances between the *Faenomenon* and the Ps.-Galenic *Euporista*, and the latter's *materia medica* ('drug ingredients') were among those recommended

17 Green 2000, 5.

18 Langslow (2000, 126) believes that Greek was Theodorus' first language.

19 Theod. Prisc. *Faenomenon* c. 1; *Gynaecia* cc. 7 and 32; *Logicus* c. 29. Latin had not yet gained acknowledgement as a 'scientific' language; Pliny (*N. H.* 29.17) in the first century CE remarked: 'if medical treatises are written in a language other than Greek they have no prestige even among men ignorant of Greek.' Celsus, also first century CE, had broken the ice, as it were, with his *On medicine* in Latin, but had to develop a technical language to explain medicine to those who did not understand Greek. See Gourevitch 1998, 122.

20 Theod. Prisc. *Faenomenon* par. 1.

21 Theod. Prisc. *Faenomenon* c. 96 and *Logicus* c. 29.

22 See Chapter 5 on Vindicianus.

23 Migliorini 1991, 232.

24 Theod. Prisc. *Faenomenon* 1.48, *Logicus* 25 and 102 and 114 (re Hp. *Aphorisms*), *Faenomenon* 51 and 72 (re Hp. *Prognosis*) and *Gynecology* 28 (re Hp. *The Oath*).

25 Theod. Prisc. *Logicus* cc. 24 and 114.

in the *Logicus*.[26] For Book II (*Logicus*) Theodorus used Methodist sources (Caelius Aurelianus and Soranus) and the *Liber Byzantii*.[27]

Theodorus also specifically mentions Vindicianus, and calls him 'meus magister' (*Physica* c. 1). He would certainly have used his teacher's (now lost) collection of pharmaceutical recipes, *On proven remedies*. He would also have made use of Pliny's *Natural History* or the *Medicina Plinii*.[28] Migliorini[29] further refers to a few occasions when Thessalus of Tralles, the well-known first-century-CE physician at the court of the emperor Nero, could have been a source, and Langslow[30] adds that there are some parallels between the *Gynecology* and the *Liber Byzantii* (an anonymous handbook on acute and chronic diseases for travellers which still has to be evaluated).[31]

A careful study has revealed how heavily Theodorus relied on Dioscorides' *On drug ingredients*[32] in his recipes; without going into detail, it can be stated that the ingredients that he chose have all been documented by Dioscorides as relevant for the particular disease; to mention only one instance, Theodorus refers to the removal of impediments causing the retention of the menstrual flux, and the softening of indurations in the area of the uterus, also mentioned by Dioscorides.

As stated above, Soranus' *Gynecology* was one of the important sources of the *Gynecology*.[33] However, though Theodorus' direct use of Soranus was limited, he was faithful to many of the views of the Methodist sect that also underpinned Soranus' *Gynecology*:[34]

- Individual diseases are not identified but classified as either constricted or lax; they are treated according to the principle of *contraria contrariis*: if the body is constricted, it has to be relaxed; if suffering from a flux, the flux has to be controlled.[35]
- A distinction is made between acute and chronic diseases and each has its own specific treatment. If a disease has become chronic, the famous restorative and metasyncritic cyclical cure is applied.[36]

26 Meyer-Steinegg 1909, 31.
27 Fischer 1998b, 276–294.
28 Formisano 2004, 135–140.
29 Migliorini 1991, 238.
30 Langslow 2000, 54.
31 See Fischer 1998b, 276–294.
32 Text in Beck 2005.
33 See Rose 1894 *passim* for examples.
34 Temkin 1956, xxv–xxxvi; Gourevitch 1998, 112–115.
35 See Chapter 5 on Vindicianus for more information on this principle.
36 A medical procedure during which the patient's strength is first built up (the restorative phase), and then followed by the so-called metasyncretic phase, which is characterized by a

- In the employment of remedies, external applications such as poultices and plasters and baths are preferred to orally administered medicaments.
- Harsh and pungent remedies are avoided and only used in recalcitrant cases, but phlebotomy is often employed.
- There is very little interest in the etiology of diseases, since it is not regarded as useful; nor do physiology and anatomy play a role in Theodorus' works.
- The humoural theory and the testing of urine play an important role in Theodorus' pathology, but not observation of the pulse.

The recipe collection in Theodorus' *Gynecology*

Theodorus' *Gynecology* comprises numerous recipes for the ten female ailments he discusses. They are: engorgement of the breasts after parturition, swelling or contraction of the uterus, the mole, atresia, sterility, abortion, hemorrhage of the uterus, injuries to the uterus, the flux and gonorrhoea. Why he selected these ailments and omitted others that seem to have been more prevalent is impossible to ascertain. However, he does give a clue in the preface, when, as we have seen, it comes to the fore that he feels uncomfortable to discuss certain female problems.

Greek recipe collections can be traced back to the Hippocratic treatises.[37] Ilberg further refers to recipe collections by Diocles (fourth century BCE), Heraclides (first century BCE) and Antonius Mus (first century CE). Latin recipes occur in, *inter alia*, Cato (third/second century BCE), Celsus, Scribonius Largus and Pliny the Elder (all first century CE).[38] Theodorus Priscianus' *Gynecology*, however, was the first *Latin* recipe collection to be devoted solely to diseases of women. Other collections devoted to gynecological diseases (but written in Greek) are some of the Hippocratic gynecological treatises and of course Soranus' *Gynecology*. Stannard, who noted the frequency of this way of transmitting valuable information, even believed that recipe collections qualify as a genre.[39]

carefully directed diet (including acrid and pungent substances) and drastic local treatment (of a surgical or pharmacological nature) in order to eventually restore the equilibrium compatible with a state of health. The cycle is repeated if necessary (Temkin 1956, xxxv).

37 See the recent authoritative book on Hippocratic recipes by Totelin (2009).

38 Ilberg 1910, 457. Jones (1957, 460) believes that later authors such as Pliny the Younger, Gargilius Martialis, Serenus Sammonicus and Marcellus of Bordeaux were content with abstracts from Pliny the Elder.

39 Stannard 1982, 59.

Recipe collections were the standard way of transmitting medical knowledge. According to Rebecca Flemming, 'It is hard to overstate the importance of the recipe as the basic unit of medical knowledge, exchange and action, while that of the sophisticated surviving treatises of Galen and his colleagues are all too easy to overplay.'[40] Fischer emphasizes the importance of recipes for the laity when no doctor was available, 'sicher kein seltener Fall'.[41]

Stannard describes medieval recipes as consisting of the following:

i. the purpose of the recipe,
ii. the requisite ingredients and equipment,
iii. the rules of procedure,
iv. the application and administration,
v. the rationale,
vi. incidental data (not all recipes include the last two elements).[42]

In Theodorus' *Gynecology* the recipes contain very few of these items, as we shall see. The recipes immediately follow the very brief description of the symptoms of the disease. If we look at their constituent elements, we find that the purpose and the requisite ingredients are given. The procedure is also usually mentioned: 'If the uterus has for a long time been troubled with a swelling or contraction, I counteract it with all the above-mentioned remedies.'[43] This formulation is typical of the Hippocratic gynecological treatises, which also generally begin with a conditional clause: 'If a woman who has borne a child previously cannot bear a child: soda, resin, Ethiopian cumin and perfume; crush all together and apply.'[44]

The doctor at work: recipes, drugs and therapy

In order to illustrate Theodorus' approach and his use of medical recipes when prescribing medications and other treatments, his proposed therapy in the case of two of the female problems he identified will be looked at. Soranus will also be brought into the picture in order to evaluate Theodorus against a broader background.

40 Flemming 2007, 279.
41 Fischer 2017, par. 606.
42 Stannard 1982, 59.
43 Theod. Prisc. *Gynaecia* c. 9.
44 Hp. *Mul.* 1.75.

Abortion

Theodorus (*Gynecology* c. 23), following his source, Soranus (*Gynecology* 1.60), begins this section by stating his reservation about abortion. It was regarded as a crime in Antiquity, and in the Hippocratic Oath it was clearly stated that the physician may not give a woman an abortive pessary.[45] However, Theodorus qualifies this statement (following Soranus) by stating that induced abortion is indicated when the woman's life is in danger because of a physical defect of the uterus or age (if she is too young to bear or to carry the fetus to term). Then it was justifiable to 'buy' the pregnant woman's life at the cost of the baby's. Theodorus nevertheless still feels uncomfortable, and adds two images (the pruning of a tree and an overloaded ship) to prove that sometimes a part has to be sacrificed to benefit the whole (c. 23). It is also interesting to note that in cc. 25 and 26 where 'strong medicaments' are recommended, he quotes the recipes of 'other doctors' and uses the third person plural ('they') for the agents who prepare the medicament.[46]

Theodorus immediately continues with the recipes for abortifacients. Various pungent ingredients are to be mixed to make poultices and fomentations (c. 24); stronger medicaments (which, he says, do no harm) for bringing down the flux are then to be used, in the hope that it will also bring down the fetus (c. 25). Recipes for various draughts and pessaries and fomentations follow (cc. 24–25), some of which are quite drastic abortifacients that 'directly procure a miscarriage' (c. 25).[47] No advice is given on contraceptives.

45 'I will not give a deadly drug to anybody if asked for it, nor will I make a suggestion to this effect. Similarly I will not give to a woman an abortive remedy' (text in Edelstein 1967a, 6). Riddle (1991, 13) believes that the reason for this prohibition was probably because of the ulceration it was said to cause. Moral reasons only started playing a role in the Christian era and the Oath does not seem to have been widely known. In Republican and Imperial Rome the lawyers' motivation for opposing abortion was the father's loss of a future heir, not the right of the infant to live (Gourevitch 1990, 2105). See also Horstmanshoff & Van Everdingen (2003) on the Hippocratic Oath, and Edelstein (1967a, 4–63) for an extensive discussion of, *inter alia*, abortion in the Oath.

46 Green (1990, 53) mentions that in one of the manuscripts (twelfth century) a scribe has added the phrase '*non dando*' to the heading *De abortivo* ('On abortives [which ought not to be given]'), as a restatement of Hippocrates' directive.

47 See Riddle (1991, 3–32) for an overview of oral contraceptives and early-term abortifacients during Classical Antiquity and the Middle Ages. He refutes the view of Hopkins (1965, 124–151) that the majority of medicaments recommended were ineffectual. Scarborough (2010, 216) supports Riddle when he states that 'modern pharmacologists might be surprised at the biochemical and physiological properties (especially spermicidal) of such herbal preparations as oak gall, sumac, pomegranate, ginger and myrtle'. For a further evaluation of the effectiveness of ancient medications, see pp. 155–156 below.

Soranus (1.59–65) first differentiates between 'abortive' (*phthorion*), 'contraceptive' (*atokion*) and 'expulsive' (*ekbolion*) agents (1.60). Hippocrates, though prohibiting abortive pessaries, seems to have allowed the 'expulsive' approach (for instance, a woman leaping with her heels to her buttocks).[48] However, it is clear that there were opposing views on the issue of contraceptives and abortion even in Antiquity.[49] Soranus therefore introduces his recipes for abortifacients with the advice that 'it is much more advantageous not to conceive than to destroy the embryo' (1.61). For example, by not having intercourse during the periods favourable for conception, by *coitus interruptus,* and by the woman using pessaries that contract the uterus to prevent the seed from passing into the uterus. Various recipes for these pessaries are then given (1.62–63).

However, if conception has already taken place, Soranus again has some common sense advice: *inter alia,* violent exercise, shaking by riding in a horse-drawn carriage, carrying heavy things and purging the abdomen with relatively pungent clysters (1.64–65). If still unsuccessful, protracted baths and pessaries for relaxing the uterus are suggested, and then phlebotomy should be applied, for, as Hippocrates said: 'A pregnant woman, if bled, miscarries.'[50] If still not successful, the whole procedure should be repeated.

Hysterical suffocation

Hysterical suffocation, or the idea of 'the wandering womb', as it became known in popular parlance in Antiquity, was a common problem in the Greco-Roman world. Soranus (3.26) gives the following explanation: 'Hysterical suffocation (*hysterikê pnix*) has been named after both the affected organ [*hystera* the uterus] and one symptom, viz. suffocation [*pnix*].' He continues to give other symptoms – namely, 'obstructed respiration together with aphonia [inability to speak] and a seizure of the senses caused by some condition of the uterus'.

In the *Gynecology* (c. 6) Theodorus begins by giving the background against which the problems of the uterus he is going to discuss must be seen – namely, the Methodist view of the two main types of disease, those caused by constriction and those caused by flux. He does not,

48 Hp. *Nat. Puer.* c. 13.

49 See, for instance, Hanson (1992, 31–71). It is interesting to note that there is no mention of contraceptives in the work of Mustio either; Caelius Aurelianus, however, does mention contraceptives.

50 Hp. *Aph.* 5.31.

however, state how hysterical suffocation should be classified – it is possible that he thought it was obvious. Soranus, on the other hand, clearly states that the disease is 'of the constricted and violent class' (3.28). Theodorus mentions a few symptoms and distinguishes the condition from paralysis, which, to some extent, it resembles. Soranus, on the other hand, describes the symptoms in great detail, and adds that the disease is often preceded by problems such as recent miscarriages, long widowhood, the end of ordinary childbearing or inflation of the uterus (3.26). He also distinguishes it from other related diseases (3.27: epilepsy, catalepsy, lethargy, and so on).

Then, quite surprisingly, in c. 8, Theodorus comes to the fore with the old Hippocratic view of the treatment for the 'wandering womb': that it should be enticed by fragrant odours to lower parts of the body, or driven upwards with foul-smelling odours. This, despite the fact that Soranus (one of Theodorus' main sources) devotes a whole section to a refutation of this view, and explicitly states that 'the uterus does not issue forth like a wild animal from the lair, delighted by fragrant odours and fleeing bad odours' (III.29). Soranus also censures the ancients (Hippocrates, Diocles, Mantias, Xenophon and Asclepiades) for their proposed treatments (blowing air into the vagina, applying a sternutative, making noise by beating metal plates, the odiferous treatment, and so on), which not only cause the patient discomfort and pain, but also aggravate the situation.

The treatment recommended by Theodorus (c. 7) is of a very general nature: phlebotomy, purging of the stomach, the application of soothing poultices, plasters and pessaries, and thereafter the odour therapy (c. 8). When the symptoms have subsided, exercise, a change of climate and surroundings, pleasant food and baths are prescribed. Soranus too advises that 'the patient should be laid down in a room which is moderately warm and bright and, without hurting her, rouse her from the collapsed state.' One gets the impression that both physicians realized that hysterical suffocation was not only a physical problem, but also one of the mind.

The idea of the 'wandering womb' dates back to sixteenth-century-BCE Egypt. Lily Beck finds that the Egyptian Ebers papyrus discusses hysteria, and that the condition was referred to as, precisely, 'the wandering womb'.[51] Plato took over this idea and used the image of the uterus as a living creature wandering through the body, having no place of its own because the penis

51 Beck 2005, 28–29 n.49.

had no place of its own inside the body.[52] Hanson relates this view to the ailment called 'hysterical suffocation', which apparently particularly afflicted virgins, widows and women whose menstrual discharge is suppressed.[53] According to this view, the movement of the uterus to other places in the body in its search for moisture leads to overcrowding, which puts pressure on other sensitive organs. If it reaches the diaphragm, it obstructs breathing; hence the term 'hysterical suffocation'.

To understand the rationale of the odiferous treatment, one should keep in mind the Hippocratic view that there was a central tube (for alimentary and breathing purposes) from the mouth by way of the throat, stomach and intestines to the vagina.[54] This view, which was popular from the fourth century BCE onwards, pervaded the Hippocratic gynecological treatises.[55] Among later first-century-CE authors, Celsus tacitly distanced himself from it, Pliny was ambiguous, and there is no reference to the 'wandering womb' in Dioscorides or Scribonius Largus.[56] Galen rejected the idea of the displacement of the uterus,[57] yet he retained the odiferous therapy.[58] Caelius Aurelianus, a later contemporary of Theodorus, who also translated/adapted Soranus, remained faithful to the latter's negative view on the topic. Muscio, in the sixth century, again ascribed hysterical suffocation to a 'wandering womb', but repeated Soranus' censure of the odiferous therapies, which makes his adherence to the displacement of the uterus as incongruous as that of Galen.[59]

Finally, Beck updates the discussion of this interesting topic by stating that 'the modern English term for uterine suffocation is hysterics, though it is no longer used in psychiatric parlance. It has been replaced by "conversion symptom" on the grounds that in states of hysteria there is conversion from emotional to physical manifestations.'[60]

52 Pl. *Ti.* 91a and b. See Adair 1996, 153–163, and King 1998, 214–228, for a discussion of this theory.

53 Hanson 1991, 81–87.

54 King 1998, 72; Hanson 1991, 85–86.

55 For instance, *Mul.* 1.7; 2.123–126; *Nat. Mul.* 2.3 and 8. See also Lefkowitz 1981, 12–25, for a detailed discussion of this view.

56 Flemming 2000, 175–176.

57 Gal. *Ut. Diss.* 2.893 K.

58 Gal. *MMG* 11.1.15 K. and Green 1985, 47–48.

59 Green 1985, 135–136.

60 Beck 2005, 28–29.

The ingredients of the drugs in Theodorus' *Gynecology*

In the introduction to the first book of the *Euporiston*, Theodorus states that his drugs contain 'easily obtainable natural remedies' (*euporista*).[61] There will be no need to go to 'the Black Sea or the interior of Arabia in search of storax, beaver oil or the other treasures found in a far-away world'.[62] Nature has in common whatever herbs are necessary for healing. The *Euporiston* has a 'do-it-yourself' approach, a quintessentially Roman principle on which the Roman *paterfamilias* traditionally relied, as he prepared remedies for himself and his family members, slaves and livestock.[63]

The question is now whether the remedies in the *Gynecology* are really *euporista* (that is, easily obtainable). An investigation brings to light that some ingredients could be classified as rare and expensive, according to Totelin's study of exotica – conceding that ingredients that were rare and exotic in Hippocratic times could have lost their rarity and become locally available in the fourth and fifth centuries CE, for instance, castoreum, hyssop, cinnamon, amomum, storax, myrrh, cassia, galbanum and pomegranate.[64]

Some of the *materia medica* in the *Gynecology* have geographic epithets that, in Hippocratic times, indicated the high standard of the product, and were used by the doctors to impress audiences at a time when there was fierce competition among the great number of healers of all kinds.[65] However, the *Gynecology* was not written to impress readers, but to disseminate important Greek medical knowledge to Latin readers. The few ingredients with geographic epithets were most probably no longer linked to their respective places of origin, but could later merely have denoted a specific variety of the substance.[66]

The *Gynecology* does not include remedies based on superstition. The only 'purple patch' in this otherwise rational book of recipes is Theodorus' recommendation of the odiferous treatment for hysterical suffocation (c. 8), which Soranus had so thoroughly rejected (3.29). There are no ingredients of the typical 'Dreckapotheke' (medications containing, for example, animal

61 Various other medical authors (such as Galen) also wrote *euporista*, giving medical information in an understandable form with recipes of drugs consisting of easily obtainable ingredients.

62 Theod. Prisc. *Faenomenon* cc. 3-4. Ironically both these ingredients occur in Theodorus' recipes (storax in *Gynecology* c. 19 and castoreum in *Faenomenon* c. 8).

63 Formisano 2004, 136.

64 Totelin 2009, 145–196, *passim*.

65 Miller 1990, 14–17.

66 Illyrian sword–lily (c. 17), Indian nard (c. 18), Theban dates (c. 28), Chian mastic (c. 19), Pontic wax (c. 19), Syrian oak–apple (c. 28).

excretions) in the *Gynecology*, but Meyer avers that Theodorus does on occasion use such ingredients in the other books, but then mainly of plant and mineral origin.[67] The *Euporiston* is thus, according to Meyer, a 'typische Mischung rationell-empirischer und aber-glaubisch-volksmedizinischer Mittel' ('a typical rational-empirical and superstitious folk-medicine medicament').[68]

A conspicuous trait of the Hippocratic gynecological treatises, as pointed out by Totelin, is that the quantities of the ingredients are not given, nor the dosage to be administered to the patient, nor, in the case of an injection, the quantity to be injected.[69] Many other elements are also omitted – for instance, in the preparation of the medicament, the part of the plant (root, stem or leaves) to be used, and when and how it should be harvested. These details were therefore left to the doctor or the readers of the recipes, which implied that they had to have sufficient pharmacological knowledge and experience to make the right decision.

Six centuries later, Theodorus' recipes in the *Gynecology* also do not contain quantities of the ingredients, the dosage, or the frequency of the applications. On the whole, a general pharmacological knowledge on the part of the readers of the recipes is therefore presupposed.

Temkin believes that, regarding pharmacological practices, ancient physicians 'took what seemed good wherever they found it'.[70] Women, certainly midwives, but also prostitutes, very often provided physicians with recipes and advice on female ailments.[71] Their contribution in this regard can hardly be overstated. Remedies were traditionally transmitted from mothers to daughters from the earliest times; furthermore, women were the caretakers of their families throughout the ages; they learned through observation and experience what was beneficial and what was poisonous and when to harvest the plants, and in this way would have acquired a basic pharmacological knowledge. Riddle is of the opinion that medical knowledge about females belonged to 'a female culture'.[72] He refers to writers such as the sixth-century Greek physician Aëtius who, in his *Sixteen books*

67 Meyer 1909, 38.

68 Meyer 1909, 38–39.

69 Totelin 2009, 239–241.

70 Temkin 1956, xxxvi.

71 Flemming (2007, 263–4) points out that the main witness to female participation in the literary culture of medicine was Galen, especially in *On the composition of drugs according to places* (the part of the body to be treated), and *On the composition of drugs according to kind* (a generic classification of medicaments).

72 Riddle 1991, 27.

on medicine, frankly stated that he relied on what women told him about quantities, preparation and frequencies.

Other therapies and regimen

Apart from the medicaments prepared from the recipes, regimen also played an important role in the healing process. Not only diet, but exercise, rest, sexual activity, travelling abroad and the like, established in accordance with the patient's age, gender, habits, the season, the locale, and so on, complemented the drug therapy, because man was seen as a whole since Hippocratic times.[73]

The most important aspect of Theodorus' therapy, apart from the application of the *contraria contrariis* principle to neutralize constriction and relaxation as the cause of the main diseases, was his dietetic-hygienic approach.[74] Meyer, in his discussion of the whole of the *Euporiston*, mentions that in cases of serious illness, the patient is to be accommodated either in a sunny, warm room on a soft, warm bed, or in a cool, dark room on a cold, hard bed, in accordance with the *contraria contrariis* approach, and similarly, in other cases, the patient is to be exposed to the sun or protected from the sun.[75] In the case of fever, food is to be withheld at first, with the patient rinsing his mouth with ice-cold water, and thereafter he is to be given light, fluid nourishment. Among general therapies, massages, baths, orthopedic exercises of all kinds and the metasyncretic cycle[76] are prescribed, as well as, of course, phlebotomy. For female ailments Theodorus also recommended exercises, change of climate and surroundings and pleasant baths.[77] In the case of what we would call psychological problems, such as sleeplessness, nightmares and delirium, patients should be calmed down by anointing their heads with the oil of the poppy, mint or ivy plants; and those whose agitation causes them to move violently should be bound loosely and calmed with poppy oil.[78]

73 Stannard 1961, 516.

74 In the last chapter of the *Gynecology* (c. 32) Theodorus' final words are that 'the main diseases are caused by constriction and relaxation'.

75 Meyer 1909, 37.

76 See p. 145 n. 36 where this term is explained.

77 Theod. Prisc. *Gynaecia* c. 8, 11, 31. This is in line with those of Soranus, who also prescribes: 'bathing, varied food and wine, as well as rocking, promenading, active exercises and massage of the whole body' (*Gynaecia* 3.14).

78 Theod. Prisc. *Logicus* 2.11.

It cannot, however, be denied that Theodorus' approach is more impersonal and concise than that of Soranus. Perhaps the difference could be ascribed to the difference in their intended readers. Soranus was writing for his peers, the elite families in Rome, where his colleagues would have wanted a detailed explanation of the symptoms, and a motivation for the use of the specific therapy; husbands who attended his lectures would also have appreciated a sympathetic approach to the ailments of their wives. Theodorus' readers in North Africa some four centuries later, however, were doctors and midwives who could no longer understand Greek. Long motivations and explanations and sympathetic remarks were not called for.

On the efficacy of the drugs

Views regarding the efficacy of ancient drugs differ widely. The two extreme points of view are those of Heinrich von Staden and John Riddle: Von Staden comments that many therapeutic measures employed by the ancients were 'not only inefficacious but also harmful, and much seems to be outrageous and even amusing quackery'.[79] Riddle, on the other hand, believes that 'the correlation between the Hippocratic drugs and modern drugs available in Europe is [...] quite close'.[80] In his studies on contraception and abortion Riddle found that, according to modern biological research, three of the plants prescribed by the Hippocratics (the squirting cucumber, the pomegranate and pennyroyal) have contraceptive or abortifacient qualities.[81] Jones agrees and points out that the commonest form of folk prescription would have contained at least one actually beneficial ingredient, while some others would have been added to produce the right consistency for a poultice or pessary or the like, the rest being useless but pleasing and soothing. Some substances would have contained analgesic qualities that would at least have relieved the pain symptoms.[82]

79 Von Staden 1989, 397. Some years later, however, Von Staden mitigated his view and conceded that there is a 'possibility of therapeutic benefits, physical and other, of much ancient pharmacology' (1992, 52) – reference thanks to Totelin 2009, 220 n. 105.
80 Riddle 1987, 38.
81 See also p. 148 n. 47 above.
82 Jones 1957, 461–62; Jackson (1988, 80) is of the opinion that about 20 percent of the drugs prescribed in Imperial Rome might have had a positively beneficial effect, and that the remaining 80 percent could have had a beneficial placebo effect in patients. However, he adds that this is a mere estimate.

However, Riddle's conclusions have flaws, as King has pointed out.[83] Riddle experimented with animals that have different reproductive organs; in laboratory experiments concentrated essences are used whereas, in Antiquity, plants were taken orally in small amounts; the part of the plant tested is not necessarily the part recommended in ancient recipes. Totelin mentions other 'major problems': it is difficult to identify the ingredients in ancient drugs; the chemical make-up of the plant could have changed during the past two millennia; the part of the plant to be used is often not specified; quantities and dosages are not given, and so on. In short, determining the efficacy of a drug is a real problem.[84]

In contrast to modern doctors, who treat patients according to a specific disease, the ancients treated symptoms. The Methodists' generic approach of classifying diseases into two large groups (constricted and lax) made matters even more complicated and the chances of success in the treatment even smaller.

The remedies should, however, be seen in the cultural context of the time, some 2000 years ago. Some drugs could actually have been beneficial, but most would have had little or no effect other than psychosomatic, and here Theodorus' and Soranus' approach of treating the patient's body and mind would have played an important role. The role of the placebo effect should also be kept in mind: patients who believe that they can be healed, even today, have a greater chance of recovering, regardless of the treatment or lack of it. The ability of the body to heal itself despite the treatment should not be underestimated either – spontaneous cures are an important element in healing.

83 King 1998, 147–151.

84 Totelin 2009, 222–223.

7. More fifth-century Latinizers

Cassius Felix, Caelius Aurelianus and Muscio

Background

The late fourth and early fifth centuries CE were a remarkable period in the history of Roman North Africa. On the one hand there was the Vandal invasion of North Africa and the fall of Carthage in 439, with all that this disaster entailed on the social, economic and agricultural levels. On the other hand, in this very same period, we find an amazing productivity of medical texts, for which Vindicianus, proconsul and physician, his student Theodorus Priscianus, Caelius Aurelianus, the physician Cassius Felix and, somewhat later, Muscio were responsible.

If one were to look for an explanation for this interesting phenomenon, a few reasons come to mind. Rome was, in the first instance, no longer the official capital of the western Roman Empire (since 402 it was Ravenna), nor was it the intellectual and cultural centre that it had been in earlier times. The centre had gradually shifted south to Carthage, which had not been ravished by long drawn-out civil wars and invasions by barbarians during the previous two centuries. North Africa was peaceful and prosperous, at least until the Vandal invasion in 429. The social stability of the country meant that scholars had the opportunity to devote themselves to the study of the ancient Greek manuscripts, and the money to acquire the manuscripts. Travel was also still possible, retaining the possibility of contact with the medical school in Alexandria, which was still flourishing in the third and fourth centuries.[1] A more immediate reason was the fact that, thanks to the good schooling that children received in North Africa, there were still scholars who understood Greek in the late fourth and early fifth centuries, something that was becoming an exception in the rest of the western Roman Empire.[2]

The question arises whether the four medical writers mentioned above had anything in common, anything specifically 'African'? Was there, for instance, something 'African' in the drugs they recommended that caused them to be different from those in the Greek East? That does not seem

1 On the vicissitudes of Alexandria, see p. 108.

2 St. Augustine was still taught Greek in a small provincial town in North Africa (*Confessions* Bk. 1 c. 20).

to be the case. Sabbah points out that the plants from which the *materia medica* (drug ingredients) recommended by the North African authors derived are basically the same as those in the Mediterranean basin.[3] It was the weight of tradition and the respect for the Greek masters that was the link between these authors, causing them to reproduce their predecessors' recipes for the drugs (except in remedies that reveal an acquaintance with magic, where the authors innovated empirically and responded to the local demands). Their respect for the Hippocratic-Galenic tradition is clear from their implicit and explicit use of sources – works such as the Hippocratic *Aphorisms* and *Prognosis*, and the Galenic *On the composition of drugs according to kind* and *On the composition of drugs according to places*. It was thus, as Sabbah states, not 'un culte lointain [...] figées dans un passé révolu' ('a remote doctrine fashioned in a time long past') but still part of their daily medical practice.[4]

Sabbah's view that the intended readers of the works written by these authors were students has already been mentioned:[5] Vindicianus' *Letter to Pentadius* (a nephew who was starting his medical studies), Theodorus Priscianus' *Gynecology*, Muscio's *Gynecology* (midwives) and Cassius Felix' *On medicine* (young doctors). Another link might be found in these authors' adherence to a medical sect.[6] One could state that their main loyalty was to the great Greek masters of the past, to rational medicine, dominated by the theory of the four humours, and to views such as not to expose the patient to risk and to recognize the favourable time, *bono tempore*.[7] This view could, however, also be reconciled with an empiric view that was based on gentle therapy, adapted to the gender, age and strength of the patient – we see this in all four authors.[8] Only Caelius Aurelianus was a Methodist, following in the footsteps of Soranus, whose works he adapted/translated (see below).

3 Sabbah 1998, 146.

4 Sabbah 1998, 146.

5 Sabbah 1998, 145.

6 See Chapter 5, pp. 123–125 for a discussion of the various medical sects.

7 Sabbah 1998, 145. On the sect to which Vindicianus could have belonged, see Chapter 5, pp. 125–128.

8 See Vindicianus' respect for the *dignitas* of the patient when he prohibits the use of a clysma (*Epistula ad Valentinianum*), discussed in Chapter 5.

Cassius Felix (c. 400–450 CE)

Life

This was the intellectual background of Cassius Felix. From one of the manuscripts in which his *On medicine* was transmitted (the Parisinus 6114), we deduce that he was born in the ancient town of Cirta, the capital city of the Berber kingdom in Numidia (modern Algeria).[9] The city was destroyed in the beginning of the fourth century CE, but rebuilt shortly thereafter by the emperor Constantine the Great, who then gave his name – Constantine – to the new city (it is still the name of the city today). In the fifth century it was taken by the Vandals but a century later reconquered by Justinian. The Arabs finally destroyed it in 698; it only regained some of its importance many centuries later.

Cirta, situated c. 50 km southwest of Hippo Regius, was, from an economic, military and political point of view, an important Roman *colonia*. From the second century CE onwards there is evidence of Christian inhabitants, and in the third century it became the chief town of an ecclesiastical district. Cassius Felix was a Christian: in the preface of the *On medicine* he states that he wishes to write the book, 'the Almighty God being willing'.[10] Apart from that, a hagiographic text, the *De miraculis Sancti Stephani protomartyris*, mentions a widely admired *archiater*/city doctor from Carthage called Felix who, when summoned to a sickbed in a case of a facial paralysis, confided in the course of his consultation that he was guided in his work by the Almighty God.[11] This could very well have been the Cassius Felix under discussion. And, living so close to Hippo Regius, which was the see of the great St. Augustine, we can surmise that Cassius would at some stage in his life, while still in Cirta, have been in contact with his bishop.

The *On medicine* was published in 447, a few years into the Vandal occupation of the country.[12] Cirta is only c. 50 km from Hippo Regius, which

9 Further evidence of his African origin is given by Fraisse (2002, vii) – namely, that he mentions three recipes of his earlier contemporary, Vindicianus, that he uses several Punic or Semitic words, and refers to scars on the faces of the Mauri women, which gives the impression that he is familiar with the local population.

10 Cassius is the only one of the four authors who openly professed his Christian faith. On Vindicianus and Theodorus Priscianus, see Chapter 9.

11 *Patristica Latina* 41.833–854. Scarborough 2008, 208–9 mentions that this corresponds with a funerary inscription from Cirta (*CIL* VIII.7566), 'attesting an ancestral home, where he probably became a respected practitioner before going to Carthage'.

12 Codex Parisinus Lat.6114 (saec. XIII). Dedicated to the consuls of the year 447, Artaburus and Calepius.

was besieged by the Vandals in 430; its walls were razed and the city was partially destroyed; the Vandal leader, Geiseric, took up residence there for three years. Although we do not have evidence that Cirta was molested by the Vandals, the events so close by could not have failed to have an influence on the inhabitants of Cirta, and on Cassius, before he left the city for Carthage. Yet we read nothing about these circumstances in the *On medicine.*

The *On medicine*: content and characteristics[13]

In the preface of the *On medicine*, Cassius sets out his aim: 'to put together in writing, in an abridged form, in Latin, the theories concerning all the causes [of the diseases] taken over from the Greek authors of the Logic sect'.[14] He thus follows in the footsteps of Vindicianus and Theodorus Priscianus by translating into Latin the theories of the Greek masters of old, thus preserving the precious Greek medical heritage. He explicitly states that his treatise is 'in abridged form' (*in breviloquio*), thus making it available for practical use. However, two sentences later he warns his son, to whom it is dedicated, that the abridged form does not imply that anything must be added (or deleted, for that matter); in other words, the information contained in the book is complete as it is.

The book consists of 82 chapters in which diseases are treated in the traditional order *a capite ad calcem*. He starts with the head (scalp, face, ears, eyes, nose, teeth) and then moves downward (lungs, throat, stomach, spleen, liver, kidneys, bladder, intestines). Then he discusses cures for some common maladies and fevers, as well as for the bites of animals and scorpions, and ends with a few women's ailments.

The discussion follows a logical pattern: the Latin name of the disease is given, followed by the Greek equivalent and/or the etymology, then the symptoms, the causes, sometimes persons affected by it and the time favourable for the malady, and then the treatment. Various possible treatments are usually given (*aliud ... aliud*), often because Cassius' recipes are modifications or simplifications or more accessible versions of remedies taken over from, for instance, Hippocrates and Galen. The discussion centres on therapy with practically no theory, none of the speculation and criticism of earlier theories or physicians that so characterized the medical works of

13 Anne Fraisse's 2002 Budé critical edition, translation and commentary of Cassius Felix's *On medicine* is exhaustive and covers every possible aspect. I gratefully acknowledge the use of some of the information contained in her book.

14 Fraisse 2002, 3.

earlier centuries. The medications recommended are mostly herbal – for instance, fenugreek, dried figs, hyssop, myrrh, saffron, flowers of the wild pomegranate, cinnamon, coriander, parsley, pepper, a kind of sword lily, roses, aloes. Regular ingredients of recipes for women's ailments (cc. 77–82) were the juice of the balsam tree, bay leaves, birthwort and nard. For suffocation of the womb or hysteria[15] (c. 77.2): fumigation by way of fetid odors from above and pleasant odors from below to lure the womb to its proper place, vaginal pessaries made of various substances, a cupping glass on the painful area, poultices made of various substances – wine, olive oil, honey and oxymel (a mixture of vinegar and honey) – and phlebotomy done on specific places of the body.

Cassius' adherence to the Logic sect (Hippocrates *et al.*)[16] comes to the fore at times in, *inter alia,* his explanation of the cause of a disease when he states that it is caused by the melancholic humour (c. 9.1). Folk medicine also occasionally emerges in his recipes – for instance, the gall or blood of a bull, the fat of a goose or a little fox, donkey's or goat's milk, the blood of a pigeon, but very seldom do ingredients of the typical 'Dreckapotheke', such as the excrement of a mouse or a dog, appear.

Magical remedies that occur so frequently in other medical works are limited in the *On medicine*.[17] But among the few are two completely fantastic remedies: the bite of a serpent should be treated by putting a papyrus with the Greek word ASPIS (serpent) on the wound (c. 69), and against toothache a poultice consisting of fig and mustard should be applied not to the tooth but to the elbow opposite the tooth (c. 42). Other remedies against toothache are applying salt or coriander to the tooth before sunrise. No unusual or expensive remedies are recommended – he seems earnest in his attempt to recommend easily accessible remedies.

The intended readers

The *On medicine* differs from the writings of Vindicianus, Theodorus Priscianus and Marcellus of Bordeaux, which were written in the '*euporista*' tradition (simple, easily available medications for non-specialists to use to

15 See also p. 166 below. It is strange that Cassius still adheres to the idea of the 'wandering womb' that Soranus had already rejected. He clearly did not delve deeply into Methodist theories, else he would have read Soranus on this. See the remarks on the 'wandering womb' in Chapter 6 on Theodorus Priscianus.

16 See Chapter 5, pp. 123–125 for more information on the medical sects.

17 See, for instance, Theodorus' *Physica* and Marcellus' *On drugs*, in which no distinction is made between rational and magical recipes.

treat themselves). Cassius' work is interspersed with Greek terms; although they are mostly translations of the Latin names of the disease and do not require a knowledge of Greek from the reader, they do sometimes occur in the description of the symptoms and the explanations, which does not make for easy reading. The book is thus more for specialists than for the general public.[18] Fraisse is of the opinion that the intended readers may have been young doctors, basing her view on the absence of criticism against the medical corps, which had been castigated mercilessly since the earliest times and is a commonplace in Latin medical literature.[19]

Another argument supporting the view that the book is not written for the general public is the fact that magical remedies, so popular with the general public, are limited, as has been indicated above. Its discussion of surgery is also an indication that the book is not written for amateurs.

Surgery

The *On medicine* is unusual in that it is the first medical work after that of the first-century-CE medical writer Celsus to discuss surgery. But contrary to Book 7 of Celsus' encyclopedic work, also titled *On medicine*, Cassius is in his treatise to some extent more specific in giving clear indications for certain operations and even indicating the instruments to be used. Surgery is also absent from the *Compositiones* of Scribonius Largus and Marcellus of Bordeaux' work *On drugs*. In his letter to the emperor, Vindicianus judged the cutting of the eyelids and cauterisation too painful, while in Theodorus Priscianus' *Gynecology* the use of the knife is limited to phlebotomy. The operations described by Cassius are, admittedly, not complex or risky (such as amputation or trepanation or fractures), but are limited to the treatment of different kinds of abscesses (parotid glands and glandular swellings, c. 17.4; collections of pus, c. 18.4), and, of course, phlebotomy. A more delicate operation is the treatment of fistulas (c. 20), not by surgery but with a papyrus (c. 20.3); before giving instructions for the operation, Cassius describes how to prepare the papyrus for this unusual and delicate operation. Other instruments used for operations are also described in detail: a phlebotamum for phlebotomy, a syringe for operating on fistulas, a scalpel, spatulas, tweezers, and so on. He also describes how to make and use an injection needle (a

18 Thus too Fraisse 2002, xvi–xvii.

19 Fraisse 2002, xvi. The only criticism is against certain ignorant doctors in c. 29.12, but it is an isolated incident and does not condemn the medical corps as a whole. See Nutton 1988a, VII.30–58 for an extensive account of the criticism of doctors.<

Figure 7.1 A doctor's instruments; a cupping glass used for phlebotomy (top right), coins dating to 3rd century (2nd row), oculist's stamp on *collyrium* (compressed eye salve) (2nd row right), wound hook and scalpels below it (3rd row), pincers (to the right), pincer used in lithotomy (bottom right)

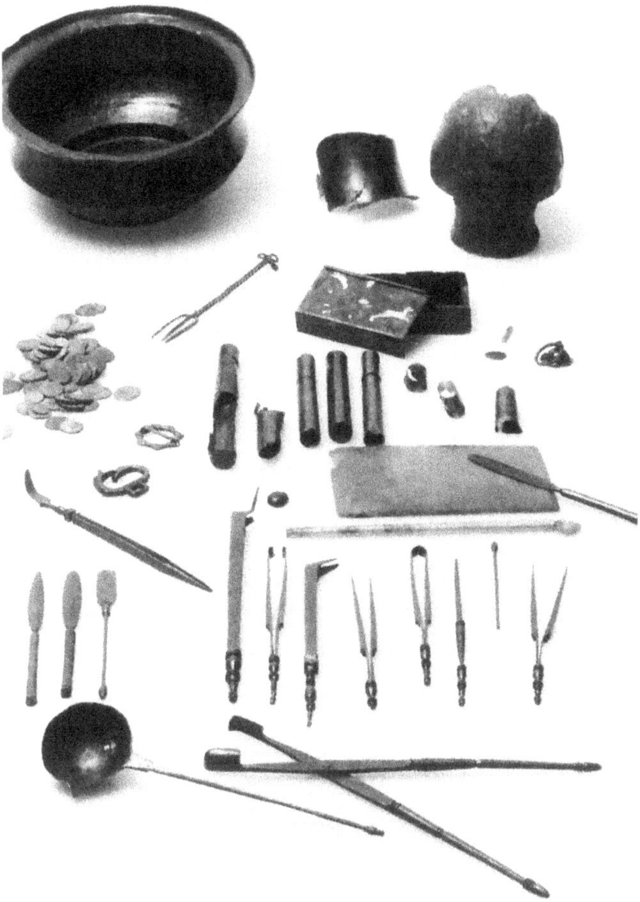

nozzle adapted to the bladder of a pig, c. 19.2) and a bellows for loosening the twisting of the intestines (c. 51.13). The development and crafting of these instruments required 'une certaine competence technologique'.[20]

Some two to three centuries later, surgery as practiced by Cassius had made a giant leap: Aëtius of Amida, who could possibly have been a physician

20 Fraisse 2002, xxiii.

in the court of the emperor Justinian (r. 527–565), and his wife, Theodora, describes some radical surgeries in his book, *Tetrabiblon*. In Book 16.86, a book that is mainly devoted to women's health and disease, he gives detailed accounts of, *inter alia*, mastectomies and what appears to be partial hysterectomies, the removal of cervical abscesses and other procedures.[21] A much-admired physician in the seventh century who was also known for his skill as surgeon was Paul of Aegina, who wrote a *Medical Compendium in Seven Books*. His views on gynecology, surgery and pediatrics were very influential, and the sixth book on surgery was used throughout the Middle Ages in Europe and the Arab world.[22]

Sources used by Cassius

a. Dogmatic/Logic

In the preface Cassius states that he is translating 'the theories of the Greek authors of the Logic School', the most important physicians of course being Hippocrates and Galen.

The *On medicine* is not, however, a mere translation of a Greek model into Latin, but is interspersed with his personal experiences as medical practitioner. Although Cassius often refers to Hippocrates (sometimes by way of other authors), he only makes use of two of his works: *Aphorisms* (with its cryptic formulation ideally suitable for use in a treatise in abridged form) and *Prognosis*. It does therefore seem as if he only knew Hippocrates second-hand – the two Hippocratic works have, for instance, been commented on by Galen.[23] The function of the allusions to Hippocrates was obviously to give prestige to the references – he is referred to as the *Dogmatum princeps* ('the leader of the Dogmatics') in cc. 1.3 and 65.1, and the honorary epithet *senior* ('venerable') is added to his name on five occasions. But beyond this veneration of the founding father of the medical profession, Roman medicine was slowly taking its own course on its way to the early Middle Ages. It is interesting to note that in two passages quoted from *Aphorisms*, Cassius adds an explanation of the medical expert Magnus (cc. 29.1 and 76.3); this is

21 Scarborough 2013, 745 n.16. Scarborough (p. 745) surmises that if Aëtius was indeed a court physician, 'one cannot escape the impression that Book XVI records his meticulous attention to the health and well-being of Theodora and her numerous attendants', taking into account the kind of surgeries and pharmaceuticals mentioned (Theodora came from the lowest class and was a prostitute before her marriage).

22 Pormann 2008, 629.

23 Temkin 1977a, 175; Fraisse 2002, xxix.

most probably Magnus of Nisibis, who belonged to the circle of Alexandrian physicians of the fourth century CE, which is evidence of the fact that there was contact between the physicians of North Africa and Alexandria.[24]

Cassius made much more use of Galen: he is cited seventeen times, but many extracts from Galen (especially those of a therapeutic nature) have been translated and integrated into the *On medicine* without acknowledgement. Four of Galen's books were used: *On the therapeutic method to Glaucon* (on fevers), *On the composition of drugs according to places* (grouping remedies *a capite ad calcem*), *On the composition of drugs according to type* (different types of remedies, their preparation and use), and *On the powers of simple drugs* (vegetable, mineral and animal). Cassius' use of the books varies – sometimes literal translations are made, and at other times a variant is added, perhaps because he had difficulty translating the Greek.[25]

Temkin describes Cassius Felix as 'one of those Roman physicians who may most nearly be considered representative of the Logicians'.[26] Fraisse takes this up by discussing Cassius' faithfulness to the principles of the Logic School.[27] The most basic tenet of the Hippocratics, the theory of the four humours, is regarded by Cassius as the origin of most of the diseases.[28] He also refers to the concepts of *crasis* (equilibrium), *acrasia* (absence of equilibrium) and *dyscrasia* (bad equilibrium). This disequilibrium must then be restored by various means: phlebotomy, scarification, purging, vomiting, fasting or following a regimen prohibiting certain foods that favour the malady.

Cassius also adhered to the theory of the critical days on which there is a decisive change in the course of a disease (c. 61.7), and followed the principle of allopathy (treating by contraries, *contraria contrariis*). Again in line with the Dogmatic principles, Cassius took into account the age, gender, season, place and time of the malady, and above all the principle of treating patients with gentleness.

24 Temkin 1977a, 175. Cassius also mentions Philagrius, a Greek medical writer of the third century. St. Augustine's account of the healing of Innocentius also shows that physicians in Carthage were frequently in contact with their counterparts in Alexandria (*City of God* 22.8.3).

25 Fraisse 2002, xvi.

26 Temkin 1977a, 175.

27 Fraisse 2002, xxxv–xxxvii.

28 Blood (*sanguis*), phlegm (*flegma*), yellow bile (*fel flavum/rubeum*), and black bile (*melancholicus humor/fel nigrum*).

b. Methodist

The practical approach of the Romans led Cassius to adopt theories from other medical schools as well, if they were found to be effective. Fraisse points out that there are numerous correspondences between Cassius' *On medicine* and the works of the two principal Methodist authors, Soranus (second century CE) and Caelius Aurelianus (? late fourth and early fifth centuries).[29] It is not certain whether Cassius used Soranus directly or through Caelius Aurelianus.[30] Fraisse (2002, xlv–xlviii) discusses some of the resemblances: Cassius' and Caelius' descriptions of the ileus, for instance, are nearly identical: the same symptoms are discussed in nearly the same terms (c. 51.2); on the other hand, Cassius' description of hysterical suffocation (c. 77) seems a literal translation of Soranus' *Gynecology* (3.4.26), in the same order and using the same terms.

It is, however, very strange that in the very next paragraph of Cassius' *On medicine,* when discussing the therapy for hysterical suffocation, he records the traditional scent treatment of the 'wandering womb' (c. 77.2), while Soranus has explicitly rejected this view.[31] The treatment mentioned by Cassius (c. 77.2) is then to lure the womb down again to avoid fetid odours presented from above, to pleasant odours presented below, and to settle it in its proper place (*in proprio loco*). The notion of female hysteria and its treatment haunted women for many hundreds of years in western Europe, but is of course no longer recognized by medical authorities as a medical disorder.[32]

Another Methodist theory adopted by Cassius was that of observing the symptoms of diseases to spot the common characteristic: it was found that diseases present themselves either as a relaxed state, a contracted state or a mixed state. In the treatment the rule of contraries was then followed: a relaxed state must be treated so that it becomes contracted and the other way round. Cassius often uses terms referring to contraction or loosening, as in cc. 51.1 and 72.7.

In contrast with the Dogmatics' theory of critical days in the course of a disease, the Methodists believed that there were four stages in the course

29 Fraisse 2002, xxxvii–xlii.

30 Sabbah (1998, 143) believes that Cassius, for his *breviloquium*, utilized the richer and more developed sources of Caelius, if we move the activity of Caelius back by one generation (see below, pp. 169–170).

31 'The uterus does not issue forth like a wild animal from the lair, delighted by fragrant odours and fleeing bad odours.' *Gynaecia* 3.4.28.

32 Now called 'dissociative disorder' or 'conversion'. See also Kumar & Clark 2002.

of a disease: the beginning (*initium*), development (*augmentum*), climax (*akme*) and decline (*declinatio*). These stages are referred to by Cassius in the *On medicine*. When he found Methodist theories useful, he used them, irrespective of their provenance: baths of hot, cold or tepid water, exposure of the patient to the sun, the air or darkness, physical exercise, and so on.

The language of the *On medicine*

One of the most striking characteristics of the *On medicine* is its massive use of Greek terms, contrary to the practical need of the abridged genre. Many of the Greek terms Cassius uses are words that had long been in circulation in medical works, such as the pathological terms alopecia (loss of hair), apoplexy (unconsciousness resulting from a stroke), dysentery (infection of the intestines resulting in severe diarrhea), hepatitis (a disease characterized by inflammation of the liver), or terms describing the medication or therapy, such as collyrium (an eye salve), cataplasma (a soft moist poultice to treat an aching part of the body), clyster (a fluid enema). On other occasions he simply transliterates Greek words, sometimes with a Greek flexion, sometimes with a Latin flexion. The discussion of a disease often starts with *id est* or *quod Graeci dicunt* ('as the Greeks say').[33]

Since Cassius' source texts are Greek, it is obvious that traces of the original will remain in his work. But there are also other reasons for the abundant use of Greek terms. Fraisse mentions a number, such as that the use of Greek gives the reader a means of controlling Cassius' translation, and of giving the reader the opportunity to refer to scholarly manuals and glossaries, of which a great many had been available since the third century CE.[34] The Greek medical terminology is, on the one hand, richer and more elaborate in comparison with medical Latin, which was still deficient and at that stage still in its infancy – Cassius sometimes had to make use of a long periphrasis that illustrates the relative poverty of Latin. On the other hand, Greek is more precise and concise than Latin, which is wordier and woollier.[35] The pedagogic motive for the use of Greek would also have played a role: Cassius' readers were probably young doctors, who would still have had some knowledge of Greek thanks to their good education in North Africa; from a didactic point of view he repeats the Latin name of the disease in Greek.

33 For a detailed discussion of the use of Greek, see Fraisse 2002, lvii–lxi.

34 Fraisse 2002, lix.

35 See also Langslow 2000, 121–124, and *passim*.

For a number of diseases, Cassius gives an etymological explanation of the name of the malady – for instance, pityriasis (c. 6.1) – usually when the Greek terms are confusing. When he wishes to explicate a difficult concept, he compares it to a concrete image – for instance, the fur of a fox to explain alopecia (c. 5.1). He is not, like Caelius Aurelianus, interested in philology or etymology as such, but wishes to adapt his sources to the Roman mentality by using concepts and images familiar to his countrymen.

On the whole, Cassius' style is simple and sober.[36] He knew how to avoid monotony by using variation, and he sometimes even used figures of style when he wanted to emphasize something important. Cassius' style has been investigated for possible signs of '*Africitas*', on the theory prevelant in the late 1800s that the Latin spoken and written in the African provinces in the later Empire should show some divergences from the Latin of the rest of the empire. The theory has, however, been rejected, and Cassius' Latin is now regarded as good, sober medical Latin.[37]

Caelius Aurelianus

'Caelius Aurelianus Methodicus Siccensis' is the heading of an early ninth-century manuscript from Leiden.[38] Two important bits of information are given here: namely, that Caelius Aurelianus was a Methodist – in fact the most important representative of this medical sect after Soranus – and that he was a native of Sicca in North Africa.[39]

Provenance and date

Sicca had been, in the third and second centuries BCE, an important town in the kingdom of Numidia in North Africa, probably of Phoenician origin. During Roman domination in later centuries, it was renamed Sicca Veneria

36 It is not, however, on the level of his first-century-CE predecessor Celsus, whose style was greatly admired in Antiquity – so much so that he was later referred to as a '*Cicero medicorum*' (Langslow 2000, 45–46).

37 Langslow 2000, 60.

38 Sabbah 1998, 141; Scarborough 2008, 201–202.

39 Rose (1870, 141) refers to Caelius as 'den historisch wichtigsten aller lateinischen Mediziner' ('From an historical point of view the most important of all the Latin doctors'). And Fischer (2019, par. 606) refers to the works of Caelius as 'das umfangreichste Textcorpus eines medizinischen Autors in lateinischer Sprache' ('The most comprehensive corpus of texts of one medical author in the Latin language').

Figure 7.2 Sicca Veneria, a metropolis in northwest Tunisia in Roman times and now an Arab town named Le Kef ('The Rock')

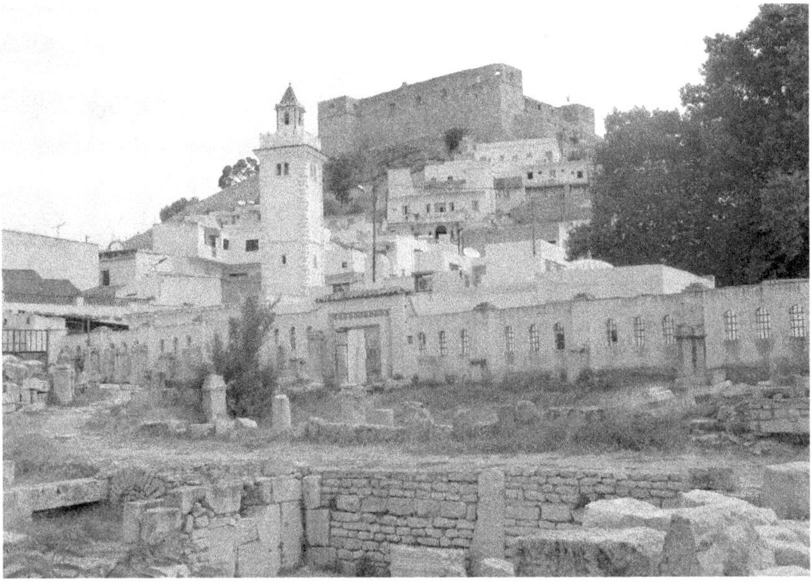

– the latter part of the name being derived from the goddess Venus, in whose temple the female inhabitants of this agricultural city supplemented their income.[40] Its modern name, Le Kef ('The Rock'), goes back to the sixteenth century and refers to the steep slope of rock on which the town is perched.[41]

The town, as many other towns in North Africa, also boasted a temple to Jupiter, Juno and Minerva, erected in the fifth century CE, as a sign of their loyalty to Rome, where these three gods were worshipped in a huge temple on the Capitolium. Sicca, on the crossroads between Carthage and Hippo Regius, was later incorporated into the province of Africa Proconsularis. This was the town where Caelius Aurelianus probably spent most of his life, and had his practice, if he was a practicing physician.[42]

Since there is no indication in Caelius' works, nor in references to his works by other authors, to when he lived, the problem of assigning him to a specific era has to be approached from a different angle. Although there are indications that he was a citizen of Sicca and probably had his practice

40 Val. Max. 2.6.15.

41 See *The Princeton Encyclopaedia of Classical Sites* in http://perseus.tufts.edu. Accessed 15/5/2017.

42 Uncertainty is also expressed by Van der Eijk 1999b, 415.

there, it was at one stage considered a possibility that he could have been established in Rome – an hypothesis deduced from a remark in Caelius' *On chronic diseases* (2.60) in which he refers to one of his works with the title *Letters to Praetextatus* (written in Greek).[43] Scarborough believes that the addressee was Rufus Praetextatus Postumianus, consul in 448, which would make Caelius a contemporary of Cassius Felix.[44] This, according to Scarborough, is a date 'consistent with Caelius' Latin, similar to the medical Latin of Cassius Felix'. Sabbah, on the other hand, believes that Praetextatus was the well-known aristocrat Vettius Agorius Praetextatus, City Prefect of Rome (367–8) and Praetorian Prefect of Illyria, Italy and Africa who died in 384, the year that he was elected as *consul designatus*.[45] This implies that the letter would have had to be written before 384, which would make Caelius a contemporary of Vindicianus. This suggestion is attractive because it would have connected Caelius (even by way of correspondence) with scholars such as Symmachus in a time when translations from Greek into Latin were in vogue – a lively intellectual milieu[46] and a pagan reaction against the emperor Theodosius' attempts to Christianize the Roman world that marked the last decades of the fourth century.[47] Caelius could have shared their pagan sympathies, as he shared their work as professional translator. Yet another argument in favour of this early date is that Symmachus and Vettius Agorius Praetextatus (mentioned above) are closely connected: in the year that the latter would have been consul (384), Symmachus was *Pontifex Maximus* – they thus 'held the two highest civilian offices in the West together'.[48] It seems logical that Caelius could have written to this Praetextatus, who also did a stint in North Africa in some capacity. However, none of the dates suggested above necessarily implies a long sojourn in Rome.

Medical works

We are fortunate to possess quite a number of Caelius' Latin translations/ adaptations of Soranus: two considerable portions of a medical catechism in question-and-answer form,[49] a fairly complete Latin version of Soranus'

43 Scarborough 2008, 201.

44 Scarborough 2008, 201.

45 Sabbah 1998, 141–142.

46 For the literary 'circle of Symmachus' see Cameron 2011, 360–383.

47 Sabbah 1998,141–142. Thus also Fischer 2018, 607.5 s.v. Caelius Aurelianus.

48 Cameron 2011, 298.

49 Caelius Aurelianus,*Medicinalium responsionum libri*, in Rose (no date) II.163–260. Fischer (2019, par. 607.5) notes that the section on surgery is amongst the portions that are lost.

two great works (lost) on diseases and their treatment (three books on the *Acute diseases* and five books on the *Chronic diseases*)[50] and substantial portions of a translation/adaptation of Soranus' *Gynecology*.[51]

The relationship between Caelius Aurelianus and Cassius Felix

There are many linguistic resemblances between the works of Caelius and Cassius Felix (see Scarborough above). These resemblances were – according to a theory based on a comparative stylistic analysis conducted in the late nineteenth century – ascribed to the fact that they were compatriots, since it was believed that African authors wrote a distinctive Latin. This theory has since been rejected, and it is now believed that the two authors used a common source, or, more likely, that one borrowed from the other.[52] If one accepts Sabbah's theory that Caelius was a contemporary of Vindicianus, then it is obvious that Cassius for his *breviloquium* borrowed from Caelius' richer and more developed work. This could also explain Cassius' advice (as a Christian) to his son in the preface of his *On medicine* not to look elsewhere for medical knowledge than in his own work – especially if Caelius was known to have shared the pagan sympathies of the circle of Symmachus and his friends.[53]

Caelius' works, to a greater extent than that of Cassius, reflect the late Latin vernacular language. His endeavour to translate Greek technical terms into Latin is conspicuous and shows his interest in the etymology of words, but as in the case of Cassius, and Oribasius and Alexander of Tralles later, it is also due to an attempt to be understood correctly.[54]

Soranus of Ephesus, the '*Methodicorum princeps*'

Caelius' works reveal that he was an adherent of the medical sect known as the Methodists, of which Soranus was the most important representative – as agreed by ancient and modern historians of medicine. In fact, he was not only the greatest of the Methodist physicians, but one of the greatest physicians of Antiquity, in a direct line beginning with Hippocrates, Herophilus and

50 Caelius Aurelianus, *On acute diseases* and *On chronic diseases*, transl. I.E. Drabkin (1950).

51 Caelius Aurelianus, *Gynecology*, ed. Drabkin & Drabkin (1951).

52 Sabbah 1998, 140 n. 48.

53 Sabbah 1998, 143.

54 In the Preface to *Acute diseases* Caelius remarks *ut, si qua forte a Graecis obscure dicta sunt, revelentur* ('So that, if perhaps any words said by the Greeks, are obscure, they will be made clear').

Erasistratus and culminating in Galen.[55] The respect with which Soranus was regarded in Antiquity is reflected in Caelius' reference to him as the *Methodicorum princeps*.[56] Although his fame far outlived him, only three works survive in Greek: the majority of the *Gynecology*, and fragments of *Bandages* and of *On signs of fractures*. Fortunately, we have a Latin version of the *Gynecology*, translated/adapted by Caelius and Mustio (see below), as well as Caelius' Latin version of Soranus' *Acute diseases* and his *Chronic diseases*.

Unlike the loquacious Galen, Soranus reveals nothing about himself in his works. But in the *Suda*, a tenth-century lexicon, we read that Soranus, a physician from Ephesus, spent time in Alexandria, where he perfected his medical knowledge (and would have come in contact with the writings of Herophilus and obstetrical practices) before going to Rome, where he practiced medicine in the time of the emperors Trajan and Hadrian, giving a *floruit* of 98–138 CE. His clientele were upper-class Roman families, the social elite, who in the second century preferred Greek physicians and 'sophisticated Hellenic medicine'.[57]

In writing the *Gynecology*, Soranus followed the example set by the fourth-century-BCE Greek physician Herophilus, who was the first to devote a book specifically to midwifery. In the book, *Maieutikon* ('On midwifery'), Herophilus did much to demystify female organs by showing that they operate in the same way as the organs in men's bodies – a view taken over by Soranus. His *Gynecology* consists of two parts, the first on the requirements of a midwife and the care of the newborn, and the second part about conditions particular to women – for instance, hysterical suffocation and hemorrhage, and sicknesses to be treated by medicaments and surgery. Throughout, Soranus battles against superstition, especially the lore surrounding birth. On the other hand, he is willing to accept popular practices and superstitious beliefs, such as allowing the parturient to keep her amulets in the birth chamber if it will make her more cheerful.[58] He rejects the odor therapy for hysterical suffocation as totally ineffective,[59]

55 Hanson & Green 1996, 969. Maire (2002, 216) states that Soranus was 'un des piliers de la medicine antique aux côtés d'Hippocrate et de Galien' ('One of the pillars of ancient medicine beside Hippocrates and Galen'). See also St. Augustine, who referred to Soranus as 'the most famous medical author' (*Contra Julianum* 5.14.51), and Tertullian, who regarded him as 'the most learned of the Methodist physicians' (*On the soul* c. 6).

56 Cael. Aur. *Tard.* 1.1.50.

57 Hanson & Green 1996, 970; Horstmanshoff 1999, 286–287.

58 Cael. Aur. *Gynaecia* 3.42.

59 Cael. Aur. *Gynaecia* 3.29.

and approves of contraceptives since it is safer to prevent conception than to induce abortion.[60]

Caelius' version of Soranus' *Gynecology*

Caelius' Latin version of Soranus' *Gynecology* was until quite recently known to us through incidental quotations in Oribasius, and in a small fragment of a manuscript of Apuleius' *De Herbis*.[61] However, in 1948 a thirteenth-century Latin manuscript containing gynecological works was offered for sale at an auction in Zürich. Fifteen leaves of this manuscript contained Caelius'/ Muscio's *Gynecology*, which then turned out to be a compilation made from two different translations and abridgements of Soranus' *Gynecology*, one by Caelius and the other by Muscio (see below). The main interest of this compilation lies in the fact that the original, Soranus' *Gynecology*, is still extant, which enables one to compare the two versions, and determine whether the Latin version is a mere translation or rather a reworking of the original.

M. F. and I. E. Drabkin have come to the conclusion that the manuscript containing the Latin version of Soranus' *Gynecology* is 'the result of a compilation or compilations made chiefly from two different translations and abridgements of Soranus' *Gynecology*, one by Caelius and the other by Muscio'.[62] According to them, the parts that are by Caelius are in the main 'quite literal renderings of Soranus', but sometimes it differs considerably from Soranus and seems entirely original with references not occurring in Soranus. The historical and doxographic material (see below) is omitted – it would not have interested midwives. Caelius' version is sometimes a paraphrase. If we have to single out Caelius' version, it is thus 'Soranian, if you will, not Soranus'.[63] In Muscio's sections the compiler sometimes excerpts a section, or quotes from the version he is using, or gives a free paraphrase. There is thus, as the Drabkins remark, a third element in the fragment: the work of the compiler himself.[64]

Caelius' *Gynecology* was transmitted in two books, the first on pregnancy, the birth of the child and some childrens' diseases, the second on diseases of the female genitalia. It looks as if the work is an abbreviated version of

60 Cael. Aur. *Gynaecia* 1.60–61.

61 The fourth-century medical writer and personal physician of the emperor Julian the Apostate (r. 361–363).

62 Drabkin & Drabkin 1951, viii and ix.

63 Hanson & Green 1996, 977.

64 Drabkin & Drabkin 1951, x.

Soranus' *Gynecology*, but Fischer points out that the abbreviation could also have been the work of a later compiler.[65]

It is interesting to note that whereas Soranus' *Gynecology* 'represented ancient gynecological and obstetrical practice at its height' and the profession of midwives was an accepted fact of life when it was written, Caelius, who lived about three centuries later, seems to have found it necessary to justify the profession of midwife.[66] In c. 1 of his *Gynecology* he points out that since the bodily functions of women and the illnesses resulting from them differ from those of men, and since women, due to their embarrassment at being examined by male doctors, often confess their illness too late, the state in former times saw to it that *medicae* (midwives/female doctors) were provided to treat gynecological problems.

The intended readers of Soranus' *Gynecology* were obviously midwives, but also included male doctors and *patres familiae*, heads of Roman households, who had to select midwives and wet nurses for their womenfolk.[67] The readers of Caelius' and especially Muscio's versions were more limited: midwives who no longer understood Greek. The age-old gender issue would have determined the approach – the patients would have been women who were reticent to discuss their problems with a male doctor and would more easily cxplain it to a midwife.[68]

Caelius' *On acute diseases* and *On chronic diseases*

Soranus' two great works, *On acute diseases* and *On chronic diseases*, were also Latinized by Caelius: *Acute diseases* in three books (14 acute diseases are discussed) and *Chronic diseases* in five books (44 diseases are discussed). These two books are a complete handbook for pathology, therapy and pharmacology, and provide information on symptomology, the techniques of diagnosis, on clinical examinations, on regimen (broadly speaking, one's way of life, habits, diet, and so on) and on practically all the diseases known at that stage.

65 Fischer 1999, 173ff.

66 Temkin 1956, xxv.

67 Hanson & Green 1996, 993.

68 See the introduction of Theodorus Priscianus' *Gynecology*, and his dedication of 'a separate little book on women's diseases' to the midwife, Victoria, who would be able to share women's 'secrets' more easily. See also Hippocrates, *Diseases of women*, 1.62 and 8.126.

The discussions of the diseases roughly follow the traditional *a capite ad calcem* order, but vary greatly in scope – some diseases are dismissed in a paragraph and others treated in detail.[69] The discussion of the disease usually includes:

i. The name of the disease and its etymology,
ii. The characteristics of the disease,
iii. The symptoms,
iv. How to recognize the disease and distinguish it from similar diseases
v. The part affected,
vi. The treatment employed by the Methodists,
vii. The treatment employed by others, followed by 'Replies', which invariably firmly refuted the treatment, sometimes very harshly (even those of predecessors among the Methodists).[70]

The latter section, the so-called 'doxographic' passages, is of particular importance, since they contain Caelius' account of the doctrines (*doxai*) and treatment of diseases by predecessors whose works are lost, like those of Diocles, Praxagoras, Themison, and so on.[71] This was a kind of medical history or historiography, important for contemporary medical practice – Caelius' contemporaries could learn from the mistakes of their predecessors. In these doxographic passages, Caelius/Soranus is following the example of ancient medical writers by disputing with the 'living presence' of their predecessors.[72]

At the end of his detailed chapter on medical doxography in Methodism, Van der Eijk makes the interesting suggestion that Caelius' vigorous polemic against his predecessors could have been inspired by an effort to reassert Methodist medicine in the fifth century, since Methodist views had been eclipsed by Galen and the Hippocratic-Galenic tradition for several centuries – they are, for instance, completely absent in the medical encyclopedias of Oribasius (fourth century), Alexander of Tralles (sixth century), Aëtius of Amida (sixth century) and Paul of Aegina (seventh century).[73]

69 Horstmanshoff (1999, 729) remarks that Caelius devoted a great part of the *Chronic diseases* to psychosomatic states, such as phrenitis, mania, melancholy, lethargy, and the like.

70 It is interesting to note that the cause of the disease is not one of the aspects included.

71 Van der Eijk (1999a, 432) notes that Caelius mentions no medical writers after Soranus; Galen, Aretaeus of Cappadocia and Archigenes, who all made valuable contributions, are thus not included in the doxographic passages.

72 Scarborough 2008, 202.

73 Van der Eijk 1999a, 452.

The relationship between Caelius and Soranus

Opinions are divided on the relationship between Caelius and Soranus. Some scholars believe that Caelius' works are translations, others that they are more independent and creative.[74] A distinction should, however, be made between Caelius' Latinization of Soranus' *Gynecology* on the one hand, and of his (no longer extant) rendition of Soranus' *Acute diseases* and *Chronic diseases* on the other hand. In the case of the *Gynecology*, Caelius' version varies between literal translation, paraphrase, different versions and original contributions, as has been indicated above. As to the *Acute diseases* and *Chronic diseases,* Van der Eijk, supported by most of the scholars who have worked on Caelius, argues that Caelius' version is 'substantially based on Soranus' works with the same titles', but that it is not a literal translation.[75] Caelius nowhere claims that he offers a translation of Soranus, neither that his whole work is based on the views of Soranus, nor that Soranus is the only authority from which he draws. Further evidence that Caelius' rendering of the *Acute diseases* and *Chronic diseases* is not a translation is given by Mudry, who states that it differs 'radicalement' not only from Soranus, but also from contemporaries such as Theodorus Priscianus and Marcellus of Bordeaux, as well as from the first-century medical writers Celsus and Scribonius Largus.[76] Whereas the latter two (and his own contemporaries) do on occasion include time-honoured popular remedies (though justifying their use with evidence that they are efficacious and do not harm[77]), knowing full well that the medicament is *extra medicinae professionem* (lit. 'outside the [limits of the] medical profession'), Caelius rejects popular knowledge as superstition, condemning it as irrational and without any value,[78] and states that it is ignorant people who attribute cures to incantations or amulets or luck.[79] Celsus and Scribonius, on the other hand, acknowledge the value of popular medicine, widespread in the Republic and early Empire,[80] and will

74 See in particular Pigeaud (1982, 105–117), who advocates a more independent role for Caelius, and criticizes Drabkin's English translation (1950) which, according to him, often attributes views to Soranus while they were actually views of Caelius.

75 Van der Eijk 1999a, 415–6 n.85.

76 Mudry 2006a, 179.

77 The Hippocratic admonishment in *Epid.* 1.2.5.

78 Cael. Aur. *Acut.* 3.137: 'But these notions, which are popularly thought to have been proven sound in actual practice, are obviously quite out of keeping with the medical art', being a comment on predecessors' advice for curing hydrophobia.

79 Cael. Aur. *Tard.* Praef. 1.

80 Scarborough (1969: 23–24) states that their approach is a mixture of Greek (i.e., rational) and national (i.e., popular) medicine.

recommend popular medicaments as a last resort in their attempt to help those who suffer.[81] How does one then explain the intransigent attitude of Caelius – even in the case of suffering? One answer could be that he merely reproduced his source, but since it is lost, such a solution is not verifiable, and from what we know about Soranus (for instance, his attitude to amulets in the birth chamber) it does not seem convincing. Mudry ascribes it to Caelius' fear that popular medicine will 'invade' rational medicine, as is clear from his section on epilepsy, in which he sees superstition in every predecessor's recommendation. To make his fear even worse, Marcellus of Bordeaux in his book *On drugs* cites 266 magical recipes without any indication that they differ from rational recipes. Caelius thus condemns any effort tending to the irrational as 'un coupable compromission'. Mudry concludes that in his haughty fidelity to the heritage of Greek medicine, Caelius goes against the medical tradition of Rome with its empirical medications, for which Celsus, Scribonius, Marcellus and Theodorus Priscianus gave a place, limited or large, even though their motivations may have differed.[82]

In the chapter on Theodorus Priscianus, the different attitudes towards patients of, respectively, Theodorus and Soranus were noticed – the rather more impersonal approach of Theodorus in contrast with the more sympathetic attitude of Soranus.[83] Sympathy or compassion is not an emotion which one would normally associate with the Romans, not even physicians, yet in an insightful article, Amber Porter points out that not only Soranus but also Caelius acknowledge patients' emotions and show 'compassion, understanding and flexibility of approach when dealing with patient issues'.[84] One example should suffice. When Caelius discusses *elephantiasis* (leprosy), a chronic disease and difficult to cure for ancient physicians, he criticizes the harsh current view that if the patient is a foreigner, he should be killed, and if a citizen, he should be sent into distant exile to protect the rest of the citizens from contracting the disease through contact with the patient.[85] Caelius' view is that such treatment amounts to abandonment and

81 See Scribonius (c. 17), who recommended the drinking of the blood of a slain gladiator for epileptics, admitting that it is *extra medicinae professionem*, but stating that it seemed beneficial to some. This advice also occurs in Celsus 3.23.7: 'Some have freed themselves from such a disease by drinking the hot blood from the cut throat of a gladiator: a miserable aid made an even more miserable disease tolerable'.

82 Mudry 2006a, 191.

83 See Chapter 6 on Theodorus Priscianus.

84 Porter 2016, 298–299. See however Vindicianus' sympathetic attitude in both cases, the patient suffering from constipation and the one with an eye disease (Chapter 5).

85 Cael. Aur. *Acut.* 4.13. See also Nutton's discussion of this case (1998, 233–242).

is 'foreign to the humanitarian principles of medicine'.[86] It thus seems that Caelius' attempt to maintain a high standard in prescribing medications to the point where he is accused of being anti-Roman did not mean that he lacked sympathy towards his patients.

Caelius' works on acute and chronic diseases were among the books that Cassiodorus, the sixth-century Roman statesman who later became a monk, included in his list of obligatory reading for his monks in his newly established monastery at Vivarium in southern Italy.[87] The detail and the correctness of the clinical information and the therapy in these two works were still greatly admired in the sixteenth to the eighteenth century, and are unrivalled in Latin medical literature.[88]

Muscio, unknown to us, but a great success in the Middle Ages

Nothing is known of Muscio, or Mustio,[89] other than that he was one of a number of medical writers who Latinized Soranus' *Gynecology*. It is believed, 'on the basis of several distinctive items in his vocabulary', that Muscio came from Africa and that he lived in the fifth or sixth century; one could add that Muscio must have had access to texts on gynecology that were available to him in Africa – for instance, those cited by Caelius. Muscio seems to have been ignorant of Caelius, since his Latinization duplicates that of Caelius' *Gynecology*.[90]

A Latin catechism (a work in question-and-answer format for students studying medicine) on women's diseases and midwifery with the title *Gynecology* or *De mulieribus passionibus* ('On women's diseases') survives[91] (as part of the compilation with Caelius discussed above), generally based on Soranus' *Gynecology*.[92] In the preface of this version Muscio states that

86 Other examples of compassion mentioned by Porter are, for instance, his advice on chronic headache that also affects the teeth (to keep warm mead or olive oil in the mouth, but if it nauseates the patient, not to give it, *Chron.* 1.10–11); phlebotomy (to draw blood from the arm opposite to the side where the pain is, *Chron.* 1.10–11), and the gentle handling of patients who suffer from mania (*Chron.* 1.56–57).

87 Cassiod. *Inst. Div. Litt.* 1.31.2 (reference in Fischer (2019, 607.5).

88 Fischer 2017, 607.5.

89 The alternate names are due to different versions in the manuscripts.

90 Rose (1882), reference in Hanson and Green (1996, 1046 n.292).

91 Text in V. Rose. 1882. *Gynaecia Muscionis.*

92 Hanson & Green (1996, 1042–1043) remark that it is ironical that Muscio's Latin rendition of Soranus was translated back into Greek in Byzantine times, then 'rediscovered' during the Renaissance, 'worthy to be translated into Latin'!

his aim is to Latinize the *Gynecology* for midwives who do not read Greek and who require an abridged and simplified version of the text, so that 'the weaker minds of the midwives may more easily understand it when read by another'. He explains his procedure by stating that he started using the *Triacontas* ('Thirties' – probably the full-length version of Soranus), but when he saw that it would be too long, he followed the *Cateperotiana* (gynecology in question-and-answer format). When, however, he realized that certain chapters were too short, he added information from the *Triacontas*. It is thus clear that Muscio's version is not a translation of Soranus. In fact, Maire suggests that it could be regarded as a new treatise/commentary, as Muscio himself states (*collectus commentarius,* line 15 of the Praefatio).[93]

Although Muscio generally stayed quite close to Soranus' text, as can be deduced from his sections in the surviving fragment, he deviated in his discussion of hysterical suffocation, where he too succumbed to the popular notion of odour therapy for the 'wandering womb'. Muscio's version furthermore differs from Soranus' in that it had different readers in mind. In contrast with Soranus, whose clientele were the elite of Rome in the first/second century, Muscio's intended readers in the fifth and sixth centuries were mainly midwives who were on a lower socioeconomic level than the readers of Soranus. While following in the master's footsteps by continuing to teach, Muscio adapted it to the public of his epoch.[94]

Muscio too, like Caelius, was 'anti-Roman' in rejecting popular medicine, but for a different reason. Maire points out that our author, in his attempt to raise the level of expertise of the midwives to that of veritable *medicae*, found it necessary to give a systematic rendition of gynecology, and to abandon 'toute pratique superstitieuse ou magique' ('Every superstitious or magic practice').[95] In order to realize this grand ambition and to establish gynecology and obstetrics in the cadre not of rustic and popular medicine, but of rational medicine, he had to extirpate, as it were, popular beliefs and magic from his system. It must, however, be added that in his justification of his rejection of a specific popular remedy, he was never as harsh and offensive as Caelius.

The influence of Muscio's *Gynecology* in later centuries was profound – not only were three adaptations made of this work, but thirteen complete or near complete manuscripts are still extant, and in the late medieval period

93 Maire 2001, 321. Maire points out that Rose's title *Gynaecia Muscionis ex Graecis Sorani in Latinum translata sermonem* ('The *Gynecology* of Muscio translated from the Greek versions of Soranus into the Latin language') (Leipzig 1882) is misleading.

94 Maire 2001, 322–323.

95 Maire 2002, 215–230.

they were translated into various new vernaculars. But due to the custom of compiling texts of the same author or the same topic, nothing Soranian was eventually recognizable.

Methodism as represented by Soranus proved to be more popular in the West than in the East, where Galen's works predominated. It was thus Soranus' works that became the basis of the Latinizations in North Africa. Not only the gynecological works of Caelius, Muscio and also Cassius Felix but also that of Theodorus Priscianus made use – to a greater or lesser extent – of Soranus' *Gynecology*. But while Soranus' works had a profound and long-lasting influence in the West, especially North Africa, Methodism in Europe and the East gradually moved to the background (as stated above). In none of the great Byzantine encyclopedias, with their distinct preference for Galenism, did Methodism figure. Hanson & Green surmise that that perhaps Methodism with its concepts and vocabulary had become too difficult and too foreign, since Greek was disappearing in the western empire.[96] But although the The Method dwindled into oblivion, Soranus' gynecological and obstetrical views lived on through Caelius, Muscio and later medical writers' versions, and formed an invaluable bridge between Classical and medieval medicine.

Gargilius Martialis (ca. 220–260 CE)

Chronologically, Gargilius Martialis, a native of the Roman province of Mauretania in North Africa, could have been mentioned much earlier, but has been saved for last because the remedies in his *Medicinae ex holeribus et pomis* ('Medicines from greens and fruits') only became popular in the early Middle Ages.[97] This work contains the therapeutic properties and medical applications of about 60 field and garden plants. Gargilius was probably not a doctor but a farm manager who had to treat illnesses and injuries.[98] In his work he recommended simple household remedies, or *euporista*, which would have been available in the running of the farm, and useful on farms and in monasteries in the Middle Ages. In this he followed in the footsteps of Cato, Varro and Columella.

96 Hanson & Green 1996, 1061.
97 Maire 2002, 215-230.
98 Riddle 1984, 408–429.

8. Augustine and the medical scene in Roman North Africa in the late fourth and early fifth centuries

Background

In 1919, archaeological excavations at Thamugadi (now Timgad) in North Africa brought to light a fragment of an inscription containing an invocation to *Christus Medicus* – 'Christ the Physician'. A second fragment completing the inscription was found nearby in 1923.[1] This unique epigraphic evidence dating to the end of the fourth and beginning of the fifth century CE confirms numerous references to this concept in Christian literature. Arbesmann indicates that it was popular in Roman North Africa since the time of Tertullian (second and third centuries CE), and occurs very frequently in St. Augustine's works, especially in his sermons as priest and later Bishop at Hippo Regius.[2] But before the reason for this African Church Father's use of the concept (which gives us an interesting glimpse of his personality) can be discussed, his life and his interest in the medical sciences have to be reviewed against the background of the era. The focus of this chapter is however not only Augustine himself; references to medicine in his voluminous writings allow us a wide-angle view of the whole medical scene in Roman North Africa in the late fourth and early fifth centuries CE.

Life

Augustine's childhood and his progress as a young man are well documented in what can, to some extent, be seen as his autobiography, the *Confessions*.[3] Aurelius Augustinus was born in 354 in the small town of Thagaste (now

1 Information on the inscriptions was published by P. Monceaux in two articles in *Comptes rendus l'Acad. des inscr.* 1920, 78 ff. and 1924, 78–81 (reference in Arbesmann 1954, 1–28). The inscription reads *Rogo te, Domine, subveni, C[h]riste, tu solus medicus sanctis et penitentibus* ('I beg you, Lord, come, Christ, you, the only healer, come to the aid of those who are holy and sinners who are repenting').

2 Arbesmann (1954, 1) mentions Augustine's 'extremely frequent use' of this concept.

3 The biography by Possidius, Bishop of Calama in Numidia, previous pupil and friend, also contains interesting details of Augustine's inner life.

Souk Ahras in Algeria) from middle-class parents.[4] His father, Patricius, about whom he has very little to say, was a pagan, but his mother, Monica, who had a great influence on him, was a Christian.[5] He had his first education in Thagaste, where he was, *inter alia*, taught Greek, but he himself states that he never properly mastered it.[6] At age eleven he went to Madauros (now Mdaourouch) for further schooling; he hated his time in school there, but enjoyed Latin, and Cicero's *Hortensius* sparked his interest in philosophy. Cicero, however, did not tell him about God, and finding the Bible disappointing because of the unskilful Latin translations that could not compare with Cicero's grand style, Augustine turned to the Manichees because of their appeal to reason and their erudition in the 'liberal arts' (see below).[7]

Augustine then went to Carthage to study rhetoric and philosophy, thanks to the financial aid of a fellow citizen, Romanianus. After completing his studies in Carthage, Augustine taught rhetoric in Thagaste for a year (an accepted way to escape municipal obligations) and during this time he formed a relationship with a young Christian woman from a neighbouring town; a son, whom he called Adeodatus, was born in 372. Thereafter he returned to Carthage, where he taught for some eight years, a time which he found extremely unpleasant due to the unruly behaviour of the students. It was during this period that he won a prize in a public literary contest and was crowned the winner by the proconsul Vindicianus.[8] Through the good offices of the City Prefect, Symmachus, he was soon appointed to a senior teaching post (in rhetoric and Latin) in Milan (384).[9] In the meantime he had joined the Manichees, a cult of which he was a member for some nine years.[10] Becoming disenchanted with the Manichees after

4 See Brown 2012, 151–154 for more information on his family's status.

5 An unusual name for a Roman woman, thus some scholars believe that she was of Berber origin (Power 1999, 353–354).

6 Aug. *Conf.* 1.13 and 1.14. However, De Labriolle (1968, 165) points out that Augustine at a later stage laboriously acquired knowledge of Greek, to the extent that in his old age he could read Greek works at sight without the help of Latin translations. As regards medical literature, De Labriolle (1968, 195) states that it is, for instance, certain that he read Soranus' *Gynecology* in Greek.

7 Aug. *Conf.* 3.5.

8 See Chapter 5 on Vindicianus.

9 Cameron (2011, 363) suggests that Symmachus, a pagan, deliberately selected this 'ardent young Manichee' (as he then was) in the hope that he 'would stir things up in the Catholic circles of the western capital'.

10 Manicheism was a developed form of Gnosticism; despite its being proscribed in the Roman Empire by Diocletian and later emperors as a subversive foreign cult, it spread rapidly in the West. Augustine was a hearer (the lowest rank) who by keeping simple rules could hope for rebirth as one of the Elect (Matthews 1996a, 917).

having met and questioned their leader, Faustus, Augustine broke with this sect, and under the influence of his pious mother and Ambrose, the intellectual and influential Bishop of Rome, he was 'nudged back into the arms of Christianity', and started attending the sermons of Ambrose.[11] It was an emotional time for Augustine, and in the turmoil he broke off the 13-year relationship with his concubine and agreed to his mother's proposal of a wedding with an 11-year-old girl from high-ranking parents. He soon took another concubine, however, and abandoned his arranged engagement. It was during this period that he uttered his well-known prayer: 'God, grant chastity and continence, but not yet'.[12]

Influenced by the community in Milan, Augustine started to study Platonism, and in particular the Platonic philosopher Plotinus, who became the lens that would help him in his interpretation of scripture. In the well-known passage in the *Confessions* Bk. 8.29, Augustine later recalled the moment in a garden in Milan when he was told by a voice to take up and read the Bible. This passage has by many scholars been seen as the moment of his conversion, but looking at the passage in Romans 13:14, it is clear that it is not about conversion, but that it contains an exhortation to renounce his profligate life.[13] He was, however, at that stage not yet ready to take up monastic life. It was after a retreat with his mother, son and some friends at Cassiciacum, a country estate of a friend near Milan, that Augustine's life took a drastic turn. He renounced his teaching position in Milan, and, now convinced of his Christian calling, decided to return to Africa.[14] During Passover 387 he and his son were baptized.[15]

On his way back (388), his mother Monica died at Ostia (probably of fever), and his son shortly afterwards, after he and his entourage had settled in his family home at Thagaste. These events deeply touched him.[16] Wishing to recreate the circumstances of Cassiciacum in Thagaste, he wanted to convert his family house into a monastic foundation (388–391), but soon

11 Wilson 2014, 11.

12 Aug. *Conf.* 8.17.

13 *Romans* 13:14: 'But put on the Lord Jesus Christ and make no provision for the flesh, to gratify its desires.' See Wilson 2014, 13–16, for more detail on this event.

14 Perhaps also because despite many dedications of works to influential people in Milan, no patron was found to subsidize him and his group further (Wilson 2014, 20).

15 Aug. *Conf.* 9.6. In accordance with the custom prevailing in the fourth century, his mother did not have him baptized at birth, 'foreseeing the temptations he would one day have to encounter' (De Labriolle 1924/1968, 395).

16 Boyce Gibson (1924, 258-271) is of the opinion that the loyalty and love Augustine showed to his son and the mother of his child was glossed over by the church for many centuries – this was not proper behaviour for a saint.

Figure 8.1 Saint Augustine

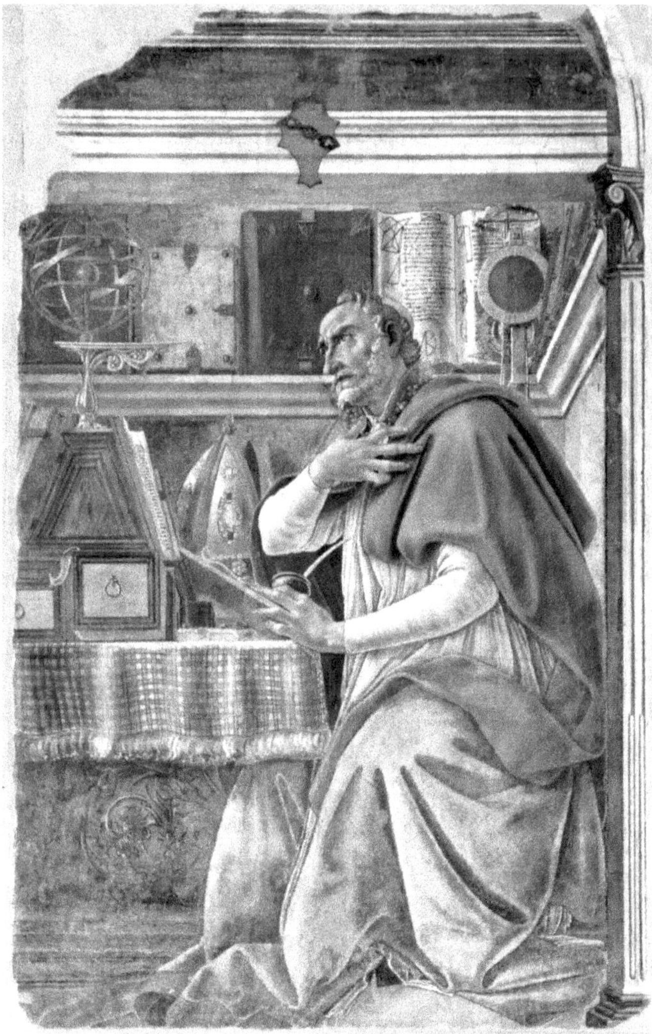

found that it was not possible to recreate his experience in Milan. Since he still lacked a patron and the leisure for studies and reflection, he eventually sold his patrimony and donated the proceeds to the poor.

In 391 Augustine visited Hippo Regius to found an ascetic convent.[17] He ended up being ordained as priest, and eventually in 396 as Bishop. He soon became a well-known preacher, and for nearly 35 years he guided the religious

17 On Hippo Regius, see Chapter 1.

thought of his age. He devoted the rest of his life to study, writing and teaching in the new young religious movement of Christianity. In 430 the Vandals overran Roman North Africa and besieged Hippo, where Augustine was in his final illness. He died on 28 August 430, 76 years old. Shortly afterwards the Vandals raised the siege, but then returned to burn the city. All of Hippo was destroyed except Augustine's cathedral and library. Tragically, he lived just long enough to see violence destroy his life's work in North Africa.[18]

Augustine was a prolific writer, and fortunately many of his works have survived. During the volatile fourth and fifth centuries, much of his energy was spent in polemic works combating movements that opposed Catholic Christianity, such as the Donatists, Manicheans, Arians and Pelagians. His important works include texts on Christian doctrine (*De doctrina Christiana*); the *De Trinitate*, in which he developed what has become known as the psychological analogy of the Trinity; the *De Civitate Dei* ('On the city of God'), consisting of 22 books, which he wrote to restore the confidence of his fellow Christians, who were devastated after the sack of Rome by the Visigoths in 410; the *De catechizandis rudibus* ('On the art of cathechising those who are ignorant of Christian doctrine'), many exegetical works such as commentaries on books of the Bible; and many sermons and letters. He is perhaps best known for his *Confessiones*, which is a kind of autobiography of his earlier life.

Augustine's knowledge of the medical sciences

The numerous allusions to the medical sciences in Augustine's writings raise the question of how and when he acquired this knowledge. In Roman culture, from earliest times, every intelligent layperson was expected to have at least some knowledge of medicine.[19] Medical knowledge was not limited to physicians; in fact, authors of practically every literary genre reveal remarkable medical insights. Philosophy in particular was closely related to medicine – Tertullian referred to it as the 'sister of philosophy'.[20]

18 Shaw 2011, 805.

19 See the discussion in Chapter 4 on the knowledge of doctors and in particular Galen's criticism of lay citizens who do not have enough knowledge to distinguish between a good and a bad physician.

20 Tert. *De anima* 2.6: *Sed et medicinam inspexi, sororem, ut aiunt, philosophiae* ('But when I consider medicine, it is, as they say, the sister of philosophy'). The idea of medicine being the healer of the body much as philosophy is the healer of the mind goes back to the Greeks (Democritus and Chrysippus) and is also found repeatedly in Cicero (especially the *Tusculan Disputations*), which is probably where Tertullian got this adage from (Waszink 1947).

Sister M. E. Keenan, who was one of the first to investigate the relation between Augustine and the medical profession,[21] believes that Augustine's medical knowledge derives from two sources: earlier Christian writers, particularly Origen and Tertullian, but also, and to a greater extent, philosophical works.[22] Cicero was a gold mine. The only medical writers whom Augustine would have consulted were the first-century-CE Latin authors Cornelius Celsus and Pliny the Elder, though Hippocrates was the only author mentioned by name (but this was borrowed from Cicero).[23]

Augustine shows remarkable knowledge of the medical sciences. It is impossible to discuss every aspect here, but some remarks may be useful. His insight into anatomy and physiology was at the level understood at the time: his knowledge of anatomy was restricted to body structures evident on external inspection – he was notably critical of anatomists who 'desecrated the body' by dissecting corpses.[24] The mechanisms of the bodily functions are beyond our comprehension, he said.[25] He was greatly interested in the precise nature of the soul, which he believed is separate from the body – an immortal component that continued to exist after death. On the question of which component ruled the body – the soul, mind, blood, brain or heart – he does not give a decisive answer.[26] He describes the process of respiration: our lungs are like a pair of bellows inhaling and exhaling air.[27] The air contains a nutriment that is necessary for the maintenance of human life, and it is only by breathing that it can be introduced into the body.[28] He was also interested in the growth and development of the human fetus; it is not certain what his view was on the time the soul entered the fetus.[29] He did take note of the Hippocratic concept of the four humours as the basis of bodily function and pathology: a superfluity of bile, he states, leads to outbursts of anger.[30] His concept of the limbs, brain, lungs, nerves and heart reflects the common wisdom of the day.[31] However, his statement that arteries contain air (not blood) indicates that he was unaware of Galen's

21 Keenan 1936, 168–190.

22 Keenan 1936, 189.

23 Augustine first heard of Hippocrates from the renowned physician Vindicianus (*Conf.* 4.3.5).

24 Aug. *Civ. Dei* 14.24.

25 Aug. *Ep.* 137.8.

26 Aug. *De anima et eius origine* 4.6–7; *Trin.* 10.9.10.

27 Aug. *De anima et eius origine* 3.4.

28 Aug. *De arbitrio* 9.

29 Keenan 1936, 187 n. 145.

30 Aug. *Ep.* 205.3; 9.4; *Civ. Dei* 11.34.

31 Aug. *De anima et eius origine* 4.6.7. See Keenan 1936, 185–188 for more information on Augustine's medical knowledge.

correction (second century CE) of this pre-Galenic misconception that the arteries contain air, not blood.[32]

Numerous diseases, mostly known from observation, are mentioned by Augustine. At the top of the list are fevers; one can imagine that malaria would have raged in the hot countryside and badly drained areas of North Africa.[33] He describes various cases, and states that in serious cases when it is accompanied by delirium, it can be fatal.[34] He himself suffered from it on more than one occasion, and his mother Monica at the age of 56 years died of fever, likely from malaria, in Ostia on their return to Africa.[35] Another possibly fatal disease was tuberculosis.[36] Leprosy, known as elephantiasis in Antiquity, which seems to have been endemic in Africa, is mentioned as incurable, due to the lack of hygiene.[37] Paralysis, hydropsy and fistulas were current. Other diseases mentioned are dropsy, pulmonary tuberculosis, cancer, which was considered fatal, rabies, which was considered incurable, the plague, gout, considered incurable and gall stones.[38] Augustine also mentions hemorrhoids, ulcers, headache and toothache. Eye diseases such as trachoma and ophthalmia were apparently widespread, as were intestinal diseases such as dysentery and cholera.[39] Epilepsy was usually attributed to demons, which were responsible for numerous maladies.[40] Infant mortality was high, often due to impure water and artificial feeding; frequent pregnancies and marriage at too early an age were the reason for the death of many young mothers. Augustine's disapproval of the use of contraceptives led to a

32 It is possible that Augustine had used only Cicero (*On the nature of the gods* 2.55.138) when making this remark and did not yet have sufficient knowledge of Greek to read Galen.

33 Retief & Cilliers 2004, 127–138, and 2006, 684–688.

34 Aug. *Serm.* 9.10; 19.6; *Ep.* 111.6; 113.2; 122.1; 158.10; 229.1.

35 Aug. *Ep.* 118.34; *Conf.* 5.9; 9.11. Keenan (1936, 180) believes that it was during Augustine's watches at her bedside that he could see the effects of fever, which he describes so frequently in his works.

36 Aug. *Serm.* 77.10.14.

37 Retief & Cilliers 2009, 1–11.

38 On dropsy: Retief & Cilliers 2009, 1–11; on pulmonary tuberculosis: Aug. *Serm.* 77.14; on cancer: Aug. *Civ. Dei* 22.8 – Dinocrates, a certain young man, died of cancer in his face. Keenan (1936, 181) states that the usual procedure was to abandon all remedies; on rabies: Aug. *City of God* 22.8; on plague: Aug. *Serm.* 169.11; on gout: Aug. *City of God* 22.8, *Serm.* 169.11; on gall stones: Aug. *City of God* 22.8.

39 Aug. *Conf.* 1.11.

40 Aug. *Civ. Dei* 22.8. Benseddik (1988, 677 n. 111), referring to *On the literal meaning of Genesis* (12.17.35), states that Augustine calls it an 'espèce d'alienation mentale ou de possession diabolique'('a kind of mental alienation or diabolic possession), and then gives a description of what seems to be epilepsy.

greater number of abortions, which became the method of birth control, despite its condemnation by Augustine and the penalties imposed by Christian emperors.[41] Temperance in marriage was advised, and sexual activity was permissible as long as it was not performed merely for sexual pleasure.[42]

We also find references to Augustine's own delicate health in his writings.[43] It seems that he had severe abdominal pains in his childhood that nearly caused his death but his mother did not permit that he be hurriedly baptized during one of these episodes, foreseeing that there would still be many temptations in the rest of his life (after baptism one is not supposed to sin again).[44] He also mentions a violent fever he once had in Rome.[45] In Milan he complained about pain in his chest and breathlessness that made speaking difficult; this may have been one of the reasons for abandoning his post as lecturer.[46] After his conversion he mentions the intense suffering he endured from toothache, but the most enduring complaint in his later life seems to have been hemorrhoids, which at times totally incapacitated him, preventing walking, sitting and standing.[47] We do not know what the reason for his death in 430 CE was – though he was 76 years old.

Medical and miraculous cures

Augustine also describes some cures. Keenan points out that baths were still 'part of the health regimen': Augustine prescribed that baths, which were normally permitted once a month to the nuns, could be taken more often should it be needed to alleviate a disease.[48] Warm mineral baths are also mentioned, and there are many references to recipes for poultices and plasters.[49] The traditional mode of managing illness in Roman times was by following a healthy lifestyle (called a *regimen*), which included a healthy diet. If this proved insufficient, pharmaceutical treatment followed, and

41 Aug. *De matrimonio* 1.15.
42 Aug. *De matrimonio* 17.15.
43 Aug. *Ep.* 10.1; 229 and 269.
44 Aug. *Conf.* 1.11.
45 Aug. *Conf.* 5.9.
46 Aug. *Conf.* 9.11.4.
47 Legewie 1931, 5–21.
48 Keenan 1936, 182.
49 Aug. *Ep.* 185.45; *De doctr. Christ.* 1.14.

ultimately surgery and cautery.[50] Augustine preferred medicaments provided by Nature – for instance, hyssop, which he describes as 'a humble little herb' which has medicinal virtues in that it purges the lungs, hellebore, which can be used as nutrition, a medicament and poison, and olive oil, which is salutary for the body.[51] However, he warned that drugs were often taken for superstitious and not for medical reasons – for instance, herbs and amulets hung around the neck, and mandragora taken for fecundity.[52] Astrology was another kind of superstition to which especially the rich were prone.[53] Augustine himself was tempted when teaching in Carthage, but thanks to the kind and fatherly advice of the proconsul, Vindicianus, who was himself at one stage tempted to become a professional astrologer as well as a doctor, he was dissuaded.[54]

Although the earlier Church Fathers believed that miraculous cures were confined to the Gospel era, and although Augustine rejected magic and superstition and accepted the principles of secular Hippocratic medicine, he did believe in miracles, of which a great number are described in Book 22.8 of his *City of God* – it looks as if Augustine wished to give maximum publicity in North Africa to the miraculous healings. Only a few miracles will be mentioned here: Innocentia, a pious lady in Carthage who was diagnosed with fatal breast cancer which needed surgical excision, was advised in a dream to be baptized at Easter and to draw a sign of the cross on her breast. She did this and the cancer miraculously disappeared. Many other miracle cures are also reported: a physician with gout and an actor from Corubis with paralysis: in both cases the illness disappeared after baptism. Hesperius, an ex-tribune, was cured after prolonged prayer and sacrifice, and a young virgin was cured after being salved with the tears of a priest. And then Possidius, Augustine's biographer, records that on his deathbed Augustine was requested to lay his hands on a sick man who had a dream that this would cure him. Augustine acceded and the man was healed.[55]

50 In this Augustine followed Scribonius Largus *Praef.* 6.

51 On hyssop: Aug. *Serm.* 126.8; *Enarrationes in Psalmos* 50.12; on hellebore and olive oil: Aug. *De Genesi contra Manichaeos* 8.12.

52 Aug. *Contra Faustum* 22.56; *De doctr. Christ.* 29.2.45.

53 Predicting the future by scanning the sky 'in an attempt to detect (in the shifts in the relations between the individual planets, traced against the background of the Zodiac) the fortunes and misfortunes of human beings'. Brown (2012, 203) states that astrology 'was the default religion of the upper classes of the later empire'.

54 Aug. *Conf.* 4.3.5. See also Chapter 5.

55 Weiskotten 2008, 43.

Contemporary physicians

In Augustine's letters and sermons we also meet quite a number of physicians. By the fourth century CE, physicians in the West had come to be regarded as influential persons and were often leaders in the community.[56] Vindicianus was not only proconsul of the province of Africa Proconsularis, but also Count of the Council of Physicians in Rome. His student, Theodorus Priscianus, also a physician, who had a great admiration for his master, stated that his fame after his death was even greater than during his lifetime.[57] Another prominent physician was Hilarinus, *archiater* (city physician) and *principalis* (head of the municipal senate in Carthage), whom Augustine in a letter recommends to Aurelius, bishop of Carthage.[58] In a letter to his friend and fellow bishop, Augustine describes the unusual conversion of Dioscurus, the head physician at Hippo Regius. He was initially a non-Christian; when his daughter was dying, he made promises to the church that he did not keep; eventually, after divine punishment with blindness and paralysis, he converted.[59] Gennadius, formerly a practitioner in Rome and later in Carthage, was a good friend of Augustine. In a letter to Alypius, Augustine describes him as a religious person, generous and compassionate in his care for the poor.[60] Another close friend of Augustine was the physician Lucillus, bishop of Sinita – he is referred to as *familiarissimus suus medicus* by Augustine. Confirmation of the view that there was contact between the physicians in Carthage and those in Alexandria is found in an incident in the house of *Innocentius*, a notable person in Carthage. After having been treated by numerous physicians in Carthage without success, a famous Alexandrian physician was called. The latter, after examining the procedure of the local physicians, commended their skill, and persuaded the patient to let them continue with the case. They thus performed the operation in the presence of the *chirurgus mirabilis*, as Augustine refers to him, and it was successful.[61] Also involved in this case was Ammonius, who is mentioned in another story about an official in the Pope's office who was cured of

56 See Nutton (1984, 12): 'Compared with the first three centuries of the Roman Empire, the doctor in late antiquity has a much greater public profile beyond the confines of his city and civic life. He becomes a bishop, a church leader, even a saint; an ambassador, a provincial governor, even Master of Offices.' On Vindicianus see Augustine *Conf.* 4.3; *Ep.* 138.

57 Theodorus Priscianus, *Physica* Preface.

58 Aug. *Ep.* 41.2.

59 Aug. *Ep.* 227.

60 Aug. *Ep.* 159.3.

61 Aug. *Civ. Dei* 22.8.

hemorrhoids.[62] Maximus was yet another physician who enjoyed high social standing; he had recently converted from Arianism to Christianity.[63] We furthermore read of the presence of one or more physicians in the monastery at Hippo.[64] And in a sermon Augustine tells the moving story of the founding of a *xenodochium* (hospital) in Hippo, built on the instigation of Leporius, one of his priests.[65]

It is interesting that nowhere does Augustine refer to unprincipled physicians.[66] Professional medical standards seem to be high. He does, however, speak ill of midwives, regarding them as 'frequently ignorant, unprincipled, and lacking in skill'.[67] Regarding therapy, there are frequent references to cutting and cauterizing.[68] Surgical operations – for cancer, fistulas and blindness, for instance – seem to have been done in the home, and required a high degree of skill on the part of the surgeon.[69] Keenan reports that physicians were also experts in bone setting, as well as in the treatment of wounds; the principle in healing was the application of contraries, *contraria contrariis*.[70] The bandaging of wounds was developed into a fine art, and there were many recipes for poultices. Regarding the daily routine of a physician, Augustine mentions the following: visits to the patient, consultations, the diagnosis and prognosis of disease, the prescription of remedies, and the alleviation of pain.[71]

When Augustine established a monastery for lay people in Hippo in 397, he used the *Ordo Monasterii*, or institutional guide, compiled by Alypius, as a directive, but wrote the *Rule* himself; in this, in contrast to other similar documents, he paid attention to bodily health. Some of the regulations include the following: emphasis on personal hygiene; in case of illness a

62 Aug. *Civ. Dei* 22.8.

63 Aug. *Ep.* 170.10.

64 Benseddik 1988, 673–674.

65 Aug. *Serm.* 356. In par. 10 of this long sermon, Augustine explains at length how the *xenodochium* (a wider concept than a hospital, it also included space for travellers, the homeless, and the like) came about. It was built at the instigation of the priest Leporius, who started building it using the money given to the Church; eventually, when the money proved to be insufficient, and the congregation saw the building rise, they started to donate money, and he was able finish it.

66 Keenan 1936, 173.

67 Aug. *Civ. Dei* 3.18.

68 Cutting: Aug. *Ep.* 73.4; 93.8; 104.7; 211.11; *Serm.* 80.3; 87.3; 278.4. Cauterizing: *Ep.* 104.7; *Serm.* 80.3; 87.3; *Enarrationes in Psalmos* 6.3.

69 Keenan 1936, 174.

70 Keenan 1936, 175-6; *Enarrationes in Psalmos* 146.6 and 125.14.

71 Visits to the patient: Aug. *Ep.* 158.10. Consultations: Aug. *Civ. Dei* 10.32. Diagnosis: Aug. *Ep.* 138.31, 48.10; *Serm.* 77.10.14; 80.3. Prognosis: Aug. *Civ. Dei* 10.32. Prescriptions: Aug. *Serm.* 156.2; *Civ. Dei* 22.8; *Ep.* 211.13. Alleviation of pain: Aug. *Ep.* 138.3; *De doct. Christ.* 1.13.

physician should be called and his advice should be heeded. Fasting was advised as long as it did not cause harm. Patients should not be denied the right to visit public baths, and if advised by a doctor, they should comply even if they do not feel like it. A proper diet for each individual was necessary and the caretaker should have direct access to the kitchen to acquire food for the sick.[72]

The *Christus Medicus* concept and Augustine's use thereof

The frequent use of the *Christus Medicus* concept (despite the pagan roots of this expression) by Christian authors in the third and fourth centuries CE must be seen against the background of the intense struggle of Christians against the Greek god of medicine, Asclepius.[73] Worried about the great number of pilgrims who flocked to the famous shrines of the pagan healer and saviour, and greatly disturbed by the many similarities between Asclepius and Jesus pointed out to them, Christian apologists attacked Asclepius fiercely.[74] Tertullian called Asclepius 'a bastard' and 'a beast so dangerous to the world'.[75] Lactantius referred to him as 'the archdemon'.[76] Eusebius called the Greek god a 'downright destroyer of souls, drawing them away from the true Saviour'.[77] In contrast, Jesus was called the Great Physician, *Christus Medicus*, the *Verus Medicus*, the *Solus Medicus* ('Christ the Physician, the True Physician, the Only Physician'). It was Tertullian who introduced the concept of Christ as a healer into Christian Latin literature – a healer who, as a human physician, often has to be cruel by cutting and cauterising in order to heal.[78] St. Cyprian, bishop of Carthage, also described Christ's mission on earth as that of a Divine Physician who healed the wounds inflicted on mankind by Adam's fall.[79] Ambrose emphasized the close bond between the physician and the patient, and Jerome (as had Origines before him) called Jesus the *Verus Medicus*.[80]

72 Van Geest 2002, 32.

73 See also the discussion in Schulze 2005, 156–162 of 'Der "Arzt" als Metapher'. The Christian struggle against Asclepius is discussed in Chapter 9.

74 Just. *Apologia* 22.6, Testimony 94 in Edelstein & Edelstein 1998, 48–49. See also Chapter 9.

75 Tert. *Ad nationes* 2.14 (reference in Arbesman 1954, 3 n.18).

76 Lact. *Inst.* 2.16.12 (reference in Arbesman 1954, 4 n. 22).

77 Eusebius, *Vita Constantini* 3.56 (reference in Arbesman 1954, 4 n.23).

78 Arbesmann 1954, 6, and note 38. Tertullian quoted *Isaias* 50.10, 53.4, where Christ's work on earth is seen as that of a preacher and a healer.

79 Cypr. *De opera et eleemosynis* 1('On work and mercy', reference in Arbesmann 1954, 7 n. 44).

80 Van Geest 2002, 31 n. 10.

It is, however, interesting that in the course of the fourth century the situation changed; Arbesmann remarks that Asclepius was no longer the target of the Christian writers, 'but the Oriental cults of Isis, Mithras, and Serapis, which now fascinate the masses by the magic spells of their gorgeous and mysterious ritual and especially their promise of deliverance and immortality'.[81] We no longer find the vituperative language used by Tertullian and the other Christian fathers in their attacks on Asclepius; he is now criticized along with the other pagan gods. Augustine, for instance, mentions Asclepius in various passages in the *City of God*, but does not treat him differently from the other pagan gods.[82]

The fear of the pagan god seems to have subsided, and with that the frequently used concept of Christ the Physician. In Augustine's works, however, it still occurs frequently. Arbesmann believes that it may be due to its popularity among the African people at large – the notion is mainly confined to his sermons, where he would have addressed a large gathering of people.[83]

The impact of his sermons

Hippo Regius was a large urban port and had a mixed congregation that would have made preaching difficult: there would have been dock workers, but also traders, artisans, shopkeepers, landowners, even town councillors – people whom Peter Brown refers to as the *plebs media*, the 'middle class'.[84] Not many of them would have been distinguished by their education, however. Then there was the language barrier, which would have impeded a great number of the congregants from understanding the sermons because of their poor grasp of Latin. Latin and some Greek were spoken in the cities, but among the rural population outside cities, the language was mainly Punic.[85]

Brent Shaw draws our attention to the circumstances Augustine had to face in his congregation some 1500 years ago in Hippo Regius.[86] In view of his audience, Augustine soon had to adapt his elite rhetorical training to a more direct way of communicating with his congregation, which implied

81 Arbesmann 1954, 4.
82 Aug. *Civ. Dei* 3.12; 8.5; 10.6; 17; 4.21; 22; 26; 27 (references in Van Geest 2002, 31).
83 Arbesmann 1954, 6–23.
84 Brown 2012, 342–347.
85 Shaw 2011, 427–431. See also Chapter 1.
86 Shaw 2011, 4– 423.

using colloquial Latin and expressing his thoughts on a level where he would share their experiences.[87] He also had to get used to the fact that he was not the only one speaking – the congregation talked back, whispered, chanted, registering their feelings in a very audible way. And then he had to take note of the fact that the audience was standing 'in the heat of a confined space', and would soon get exhausted, so that he sometimes had to cut his sermon short.[88] Shaw states that especially the women were not willing to put up with lengthy and 'irrelevant' sermons.[89] And lack of attention was not the only problem, there was also misunderstanding, and the ignorance of the local population.

In adapting his sermons to the level of his congregation, Augustine's interest in and knowledge of medicine served him well. He saw the relation between man and God in terms of a patient and a physician: man in his imperfection is likened to a disease and God's mercy is compared to healing. Thus, rather than explain, for instance, the abstract redemption theory in philosophical terms, he relates sin to a disease that is healed by a physician. And to explain why man sometimes has to suffer, Augustine uses the image of a doctor who sometimes has to cauterize and cut deeply in order to eradicate the cause of the disease. This is where the *Christus Medicus* concept comes into play. Man cannot by himself eliminate the evil; only the Divine Physician can.[90]

Augustine also used medical images to bring his congregation to the realization of their sinfulness – their greatest sin being the deadly tumor of pride. He himself knew it all too well – for years he was impressed by the intellectual pride that characterized the ethical ideals of the Stoics and Platonists, until he started studying St. Paul, and learned that only a humble soul could follow Christ.[91] The basis of man's imperfection is his pride, which is portrayed as a disease that only the mercy of Christ the Healer can heal.[92] Once man realizes his imperfection, he will be more receptive of God's mercy, which will heal him. Augustine does not shy away from using

87 Rebillard (2012, 63) remarks that numerous features prove that Augustine's sermons were to a great extent 'delivered extemporaneously'. They were 'recorded by stenographers who took notes in shorthand during the delivery and then transcribed them in longhand'.

88 Shaw 2011, 414.

89 Shaw 2011, 414.

90 Aug. *De doctr. Christ.* 1.14.13.

91 Aug. *Conf.* 7.18.24. Arbesmann (1954, 9) points out that Augustine's conversion was 'not only the outcome of a struggle for truth and against the weakness of the flesh, but it needed all his moral strength to overcome that intellectual pride which was the mark of ancient philosophy'.

92 Aug. *Serm.* 80.2.

the well-worn image of *Christus Medicus* even though he knows that many members of his congregation will have heard it before. In *Sermon* 250.3 he says, 'Many have forgotten, and some have not heard it: but those who have not forgotten and have heard it, must bear it patiently, so that others may be reminded and instructed'.[93]

These are but a few examples of the way Augustine applied the principles of professional health care to his teaching of Christianity. After Augustine, the use of this motif diminished. The ingenious way he employed not only the *Christus Medicus* concept but also many other medical images to explain difficult theological doctrines to his parishioners in Hippo Regius is nonetheless remarkable.

Conclusion

Augustine had a far-reaching influence on Western theological thought and on the interpretation of the sacraments, sin, and predestination that 'determined the attitudes of Reformers and Catholics in the Reformation', views that were only successfully challenged under the crisis of war in the first decades of the twentieth century.[94] When considering this, one tends to forget his role as preacher and pastor, and the profound influence he must have had on his congregation with his interest in and knowledge of medicine in his more than 4500 sermons over 35 years as bishop.[95] It is said that on his deathbed this 'greatest African' tragically saw the world he was trying so hard to reform going up in flames, but he also saw on the wall of his cell the penitential psalms he had inscribed in huge letters. He was ready to enter the City of God.[96]

It is interesting to note that the rise and fall of Roman North Africa was marked by two outstanding North African figures in crisis situations: Hannibal, the brilliant young Carthaginian general, who at the end of the third century BCE nearly brought the young, upcoming Roman Republic to its knees, and some six centuries later Augustine, who did indeed see the Roman Empire collapse.

93 Many aspects of the *Christus medicus* theme are commonplace ideas, as pointed out by Arbesmann (1954, 25) and Van Geest (2002, *passim*): it was used by, *inter alia*, Eusebius, Ambrose, John Chrysostomus, Origen and Jerome.

94 Merrills 2004, 259.

95 Shaw 2011, 417.

96 Raven 1969, 144.

9. Reciprocal influences

Greco-Roman and Christian views of healing

Christianity was one of a great many religions in Roman North Africa during the early Empire. Initially the religion of Rome, with its pantheon of gods (especially Jupiter, Juno, Venus and Mars), dominated. Later there was also the emperor's cult, which had to be held in reverence by all. In the coastal cities of North Africa, Punic religious traditions continued to exist, often in Roman garb – Saturn (the local Baal with a Roman name), for instance, was prominent in the religions of North Africa. The native Berber and Libyan cults also still existed, mostly with a Roman overlay. There were also gods of other parts of the empire: the African author Apuleius, for instance, was an adherent of the cult of the Egyptian goddess Isis. Then there were also Jewish communities with their monotheistic religion of Yahweh. Healing was a characteristic of some of these religions; among them the cult of the healing god Asclepius was the most important and widespread.

Each of these religions was part of a culture that had its own management of health care, a wide variety of medical care was thus available to the sick in Roman North Africa. Ferngren refers to the existence of medical, religious, folk and magical traditions.[1] In these traditions, Lloyd points out, the actual healers could be root cutters, drug sellers, midwives, religious healers, or the more rational kind of physicians represented in the Hippocratic texts.[2]

This was the pluralistic religious scene in Roman North Africa during Imperial times. The Christian view of life may have brought about a great change in health care, but much of what is believed to be inherent in Christianity was actually inherited from pagan practices and beliefs and adapted to the new religion.

1 Ferngren 2009, 37.

2 Lloyd 1979, 38.

Greco-Roman medical views

When discussing the medical views of the Greeks or the Romans, the Jews or the Christians, it is important to keep in mind that none of these groups should be regarded as monolithic – they were as diverse in their views within each group as they were in their opposition to the other groups.[3] It should also be pointed out that there was no organized Jewish health care system, nor a coordinated Christian health care system. The Greek system, which eventually became Greco-Roman, had by the time of the early Empire spread over the whole Mediterranean world.

From Hippocrates to Celsus

After centuries during which diseases were ascribed to the wrath of the gods, Greek medicine entered a more scientific phase in the fifth and fourth centuries BCE, when doctors of the Hippocratic school began to explain disease in terms of natural causation. It was believed that the body contained four fluids or humours (blood, phlegm, black bile and yellow bile), and that disease was caused by an imbalance of these humours. With this theoretically based physiological approach, supernatural powers, magic and superstition were pushed to the background, although belief in them was not and will never be totally eradicated. During the third century BCE great progress was made at the medical school in Alexandria when dissection was for a brief period permitted by the first two Ptolemies; two famous physicians working in Alexandria during this period were Herophilus of Chalcedon, best known for his discoveries in anatomy, and Erasistratus of Ceos, known for his work in physiology.[4] After the conquest of Greece in 146 BCE, Greek culture, including medicine, soon spread to Rome. At that stage the medical setup in Italy and Rome was still rather primitive, consisting of folk medicine and magic, which, in fact, still remained popular for many centuries.[5]

Therapeutic strategies involved restoring the presumed imbalance of the four bodily humours proposed by Hippocrates. In Roman times the medical writer Cornelius Celsus distinguished three branches of medicine: regimen (including dietetics), pharmacology and surgery. This was in fact

3 Van der Eijk 2014, 340.

4 Nutton 2004/2013, 131–135.

5 Various authors recorded these folk recipes; for instance, Pliny the Elder and Cornelius Celsus (first century CE), as well as the Gallic nobleman Marcellus of Bordeaux (fourth and fifth centuries CE).

Figure 9.1 Doctor treating a patient; on the bed a patient in the temple of Asclepius (note the snake on the patient's shoulder)

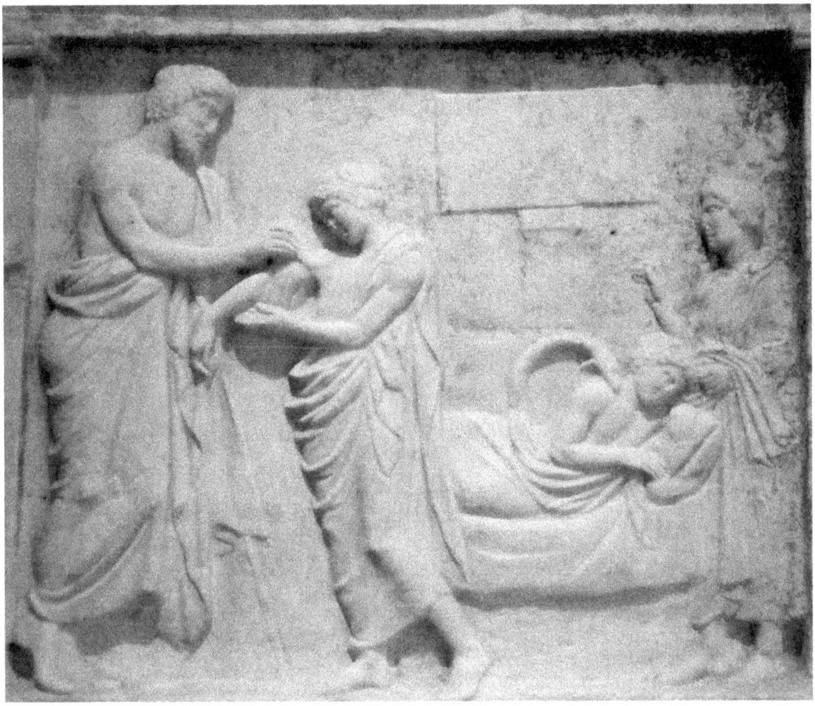

the steps the sick would follow: if one's lifestyle was not healthy, drugs (of which there were a great many, but most of them ineffectual) would be taken, and if that did not help, a physician would be consulted (of which there were many, but not all of the same quality) and finally surgery.[6] Many physicians had their consulting rooms in the cities, but the wealthy were visited at home.[7] Acute diseases would be treated by the physicians, but patients with chronic diseases and those who were regarded as hopeless cases had one last option: to visit a sanctuary of the healing god Asclepius.[8]

6 See in this regard Galen's advice on how to distinguish between the best and the worst physicians, *On examinations by which the best physicians are recognized* (c. 4). See also Marcellus' work *On drugs*, a self-help guide to enable lay people to heal themselves without having to consult a physician.

7 Horstmanshoff 1995, 83–99.

8 In the cases of certain chronic or terminal diseases, doctors were advised not to treat them, even though it clashed with popular conceptions of ethical conduct; in this debate one of the Hippocratic writers state that doctors should know their limitations (Hp. *Morb.* 1.6 and *De Arte* 3.5–8). In *De arte* (c. 3) doctors are advised 'to refuse to treat those who are overmastered by

Asclepius

The cult of Asclepius was the most important and widespread of the pagan cults in the Roman Empire. Attested since the fifth century BCE in Epidaurus, the cult spread rapidly across Greece and soon had sanctuaries in all the major cities.[9] It became established in Rome in 291 BCE in response to an epidemic, and reached its zenith in the second century CE, with more than 400 temples or shrines all over the Mediterranean world.[10] Pilgrims seeking miraculous healing came from afar. The healing procedure basically consisted of incubation: sleeping in the sacred precinct of the temple, where it was believed that the god would appear to the incubant in a dream and effect a cure or give advice regarding a remedy.[11] No admission fee was charged, but a small donation of some or other kind as a token of gratitude for healing was customary. The cult was 'advertised' by the votives of the patients consisting of brief descriptions of the disease and the healing on stone slabs (*iamata*) in the entrance, often accompanied by an image of the healed body part, formulaic but sufficiently convincing to draw those who could not obtain healing through secular medicine and physicians. Asclepius was very popular in the Roman world, and the sanctuaries were visited not only by the poor but also by emperors (Hadrian, possibly Marcus Aurelius, and Caracalla), the only prerequisite being purity of mind.[12]

In North Africa there was an Aesculapium in Carthage[13] and also one in Lambaesis, the military headquarters of the province of Africa Proconsularis, where 1400 inscriptions of grateful patients were unearthed.[14]

their diseases, realising that in such cases medicine is powerless'. It was an ethical dilemma for doctors, whatever they decided, since their reputation was at stake, and one's reputation was one's 'papers'. But in the Hippocratic treatises taking on a critically ill patient was described as inappropriate, reckless and irresponsible. See also the discussion in the article of Rosen in this regard, retrieved from http://repository.upenn.edu/classics_papers/10 on 17/11/2017.

9 See Edelstein & Edelstein 1998, II. 65–138, for a detailed discussion of the cult of Asclepius.

10 Ferngren & Amundsen 1996, 2959.

11 Cilliers & Retief 2013, 75–78.

12 Asclepius was called *philanthropotatos* by the author Aelian (*NA* 2.33). Porphyry, *De abstinentia* 2.19 stated: 'It is seemly then that those who want to sacrifice go purified in their moral character.'

13 Liv. 41.22.2, and Str. 17.3.14. References in Edelstein & Edelstein 1998, I, Testimonia 832 and 834.

14 MacKendrick 1980, 224–226. One inscription pithily states: *bonus intra, melior exi* ('go in good, come out better'). See also Chapter 2 on health facilities.

Figure 9.2 Votives of healed body parts on marble slabs in Asklepieion

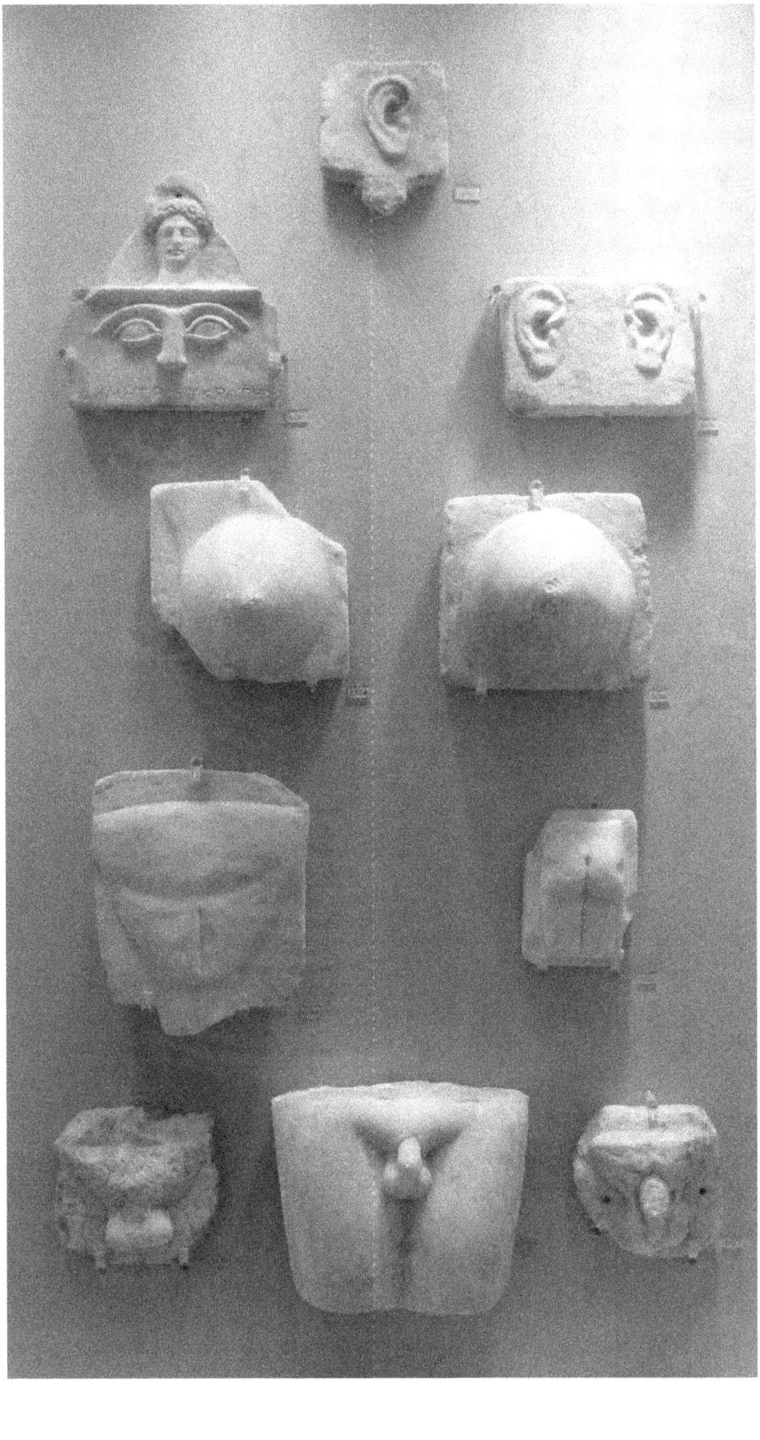

Figure 9.3 Asclepius

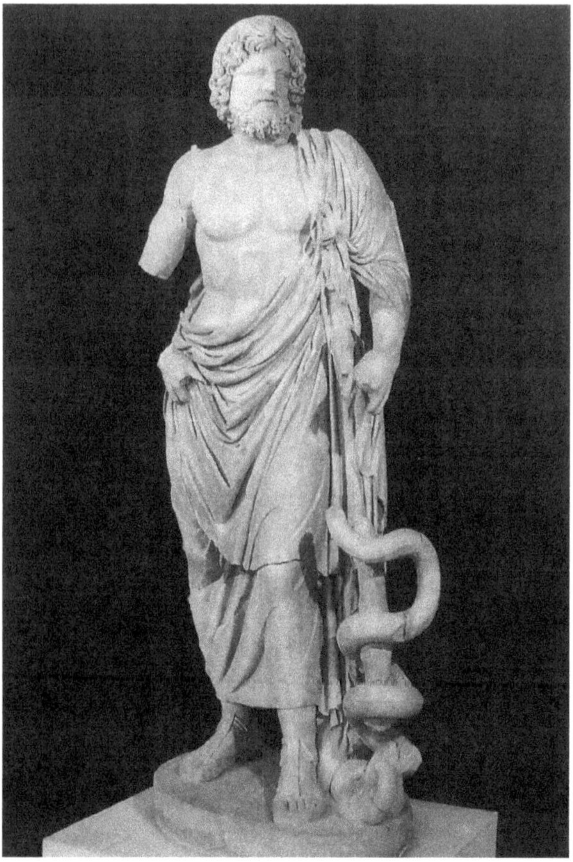

Asclepius and Jesus

Even in Antiquity it was noted that there were many resemblances between Asclepius and Jesus; in fact, their lives and activities were so alike that it greatly disturbed the Church Fathers, who realized that of all the Greek and Roman gods, Asclepius was their strongest enemy.[15]

– It was when Jesus started healing diseases and resurrecting the dead that the resemblance became apparent. The Christian author Justin stated that it seems that one is 'mentioning deeds similar to and even identical with those which were said to have been performed by Asclepius'.[16]

15 Asclepius was vilified by some of the Church Fathers (see p. 192)
16 Just. *Apologia* 22.6, Test. 94 in Edelstein & Edelstein (1998).

- There were other resemblances, too. Some of those mentioned by the Edelsteins are: Jesus, like Asclepius, was the son of a god and a mortal (virgin) woman;
- like Asclepius, Jesus rose to heaven after a tragic death and became immortal;
- both were human and divine at the same time;
- both came to earth as a helper of men; both lived a blameless life.[17]

The similarity between Asclepius and Jesus seemed to be rooted in the very essence of their lives.

Despite these resemblances, however, there was a difference between the cult of Asclepius and the religion of the Christians.

- Over the entrance of the temple of Asclepius at Epidaurus there was the inscription: 'Pure must be he who enters the fragrant temple; purity means to think nothing but holy thoughts'.[18] It must be noted that this inscription refers to purity in thought, not in the body, since the sick were admitted to the temple. This inscription resembles the purity of mind represented in Matthew 18:3 where Jesus says that 'unless you turn and become like children, you will never enter the kingdom of heaven'. But this is where the resemblance ends. While Asclepius healed the body, Jesus healed both body and soul.
- The uniqueness of Christianity lies in Jesus' mission being not to preach for those who are pure of heart, but to heal the impure, those sick in body and mind, those banned from Asclepius' temples. Jesus associated with sinners and the hated Roman publicans.
- Another marked difference is that He showed compassion to the fallen; the inscriptions of healed patients on the stone slabs at Epidaurus are impressive, but there is no record of the many thousands who were not healed, and lived in anguish for the rest of their lives. Nor do we read about compassion from the god or his priests. It was these who were picked up by Jesus in his compassion. Miraculous healing is one thing, but long-term care during suffering and sickness is another.

However, of all the pagan religions in the Greco-Roman world, Asclepius' cult came closest to being a precursor of Christianity, and his cult endured the longest. During the third century CE it started losing ground – the sanctuary at Pergamum was destroyed in c. 255 by an earthquake and was

17 Edelstein & Edelstein 1998, II.135–136.

18 Porph. *Abst.* 2.19. Text 318 in Edelstein & Edelstein (1998).

not rebuilt. The legalization of Christianity in 313 dealt the cult another blow (the last inscription at Epidaurus is dated to 355), after having persisted for close on ten centuries.[19]

Judaism

Christianity's health-care concepts were molded on traditional Jewish views of health, as set out in the Biblical book of Leviticus. At the core of the Jews' monotheistic religion lay the belief that Yahweh is holy, and therefore His chosen people must also be holy, and thus practice a holy lifestyle.[20] Linked to this was the belief that man is an image of God, and thus has intrinsic value by virtue of his divine endowment.[21] This found expression in more than 600 commandments and bans, laid down by a Priestly Code, of which 213 are described in the book Leviticus. Among these commandments are those determining health care.

Yahweh alone was in control of illness, although in most forms of Judaism it was believed that demons were the cause of disease.[22] Many Jews did also call upon other deities or consult Greek doctors, though it was forbidden by the Bible.[23]

As is the case in the Asclepian cult, purity was a prerequisite, but in the Judaic religion it was purity in body, not in mind.[24] Illness and deformity and any other deviation from normality thus made man impure. This had as consequence that a large group of people, those who most needed health care, like lepers, the blind, and the lame, were banned not only from the temple but also from the community – not because they were contagious, but because they did not reflect the image of God.[25] The Priestly Code also

19 Edelstein & Edelstein 1998, II. 355–356.

20 *Lev.* 11:44: 'For I am the Lord your God. Consecrate yourselves therefore and be holy, for I am holy.' Discussed in Wasserman 1997, 51–65.

21 Ferngren 2009, 98.

22 Avalos 1999, 63. Early Christianity also assumed that demons could cause disease, as is attested in numerous cases of demon possession in the New Testament.

23 See the rebuke of Asa for consulting 'healers' (2 *Chron.* 16:12). Reference in Avalos 1999, 78.

24 See *Lev.* 21:17–22: 'None of your offspring throughout their generations who has a blemish may approach to offer the bread of his God […] none who has a blemish shall draw near, a man blind or lame, or one who has a mutilated face or a limb too long, or a man who has an injured foot or and injured hand, or a hunchback, or a dwarf, or a man with a defect in his sight or an itching disease or scabs or crushed testicles.'

25 It is now generally agreed that *tsara'at*, the Hebrew word later mistranslated as 'leprosy', originally referred to a variety of non-specific skin afflictions and not to leprosy as we know

'evaluated persons by their monetary worth and their productivity':[26] the chronically ill and deformed were not productive and could not contribute to the social and economic welfare of the state,[27] thus they were classified as impure and as a burden.[28] This banning order created a socioeconomic problem: not only could the impure not work and earn money to provide for themselves, but they were also excluded from the health care the community could offer and even from their own families. It does indeed look as if the Levitical health care system was 'not geared toward the needs of individual patients' but seemed designed to get rid of the sick and the poor.[29]

Therapeutic strategies would include a prayer to Yahweh in which confessing one's sins was the most important item.[30] A second option was self-help, using natural remedies such as herbs or pharmaceuticals. If this did not help, a (legitimate) healer would be consulted, which would usually have been a prophet, though there were professional Jewish physicians, as is shown by archaeological finds on Mt. Masada, *inter alia,* a cupping vessel for phlebotomy.[31] Despite their strict monotheistic religion, many Hebrews visited sorcerers and made use of minor gods, figurines and amulets as curing aids. By the second century BCE, however, Jewish medical practitioners who had adopted Greek empiric medicine, as far as it was not antithetical to Jewish religion, were common.[32]

it today (Hansen's disease). See Retief & Cilliers (2009, 1–11) on leprosy in Antiquity. Blindness was common in Israel, the Middle East and Asia in Antiquity (Wasserman 1997, 104). Trachoma, a virus disease, was an important cause of blindness, and often the result of a low standard of living and poor hygiene. We read of at least ten cases of blindness in the New Testament (Wasserman 1997, 104).

26 Avalos 1999, 35–36.

27 Fertility was also a matter of concern for the Priestly writers: a menstruating woman would also have been regarded as impure, not because of the loss of blood, but because she was not (re)productive.

28 Illness also conferred a stigma: in the book Job we read that only his wife and three close friends visited him, and the latter three showed no pity, but believed that his illness was a sign of sin and urged him to repent.

29 Avalos 1999, 45. Those affected by these bans suffered great hardhips; Jesus, himself a Jew, contravened many of them by healing lepers, the lame and the blind, setting a precedent for his Christian followers. See also below on Christian health care.

30 Avalos (1999, 38) states that 'patients spent time reminiscing about their lives and attempting to identify possible sins'.

31 Avalos 1999, 78.

32 Ferngren & Amundsen 1996:, 2958.

Christianity

Christian health care

Christianity, like Judaism, emphasized the role of an omnipotent God who controls all illnesses. During his ministry on earth, Jesus cured many persons from a variety of illnesses and also raised people from the dead. These were accepted as miraculous cures, and after his death his followers continued to cure people in the name of God. The New Testament also mentions anointment, laying on of hands and fasting as therapy.[33] It must, however, again be pointed out that there was no specific 'Christian medicine' – health therapies were those established by the Greco-Roman way of thinking over centuries. Ferngren illustrates this point by referring to the Christian physician Luke, who, when travelling throughout the Roman Empire with St. Paul on his missionary journeys, would have felt no 'cultural boundaries' – his views reflected those of his medical colleagues who had grown up in a Greco-Roman world.[34]

The question may arise as to why the Christians had this unusual interest in medicine – as also revealed in Chapter 8 on Augustine. In his discussion of this matter, Schulze suggests some reasons: the Gospels are interspersed with the injunction to love one's neighbour, with emphasis on the idea of caring for the sick (for instance, Matthew 25:36); then there is the age-old connection between medicine and philosophy.[35] Schulze further mentions that man's body is created by God and must be cared for (sc. by a physician), and finally there is the setting of early Christianity in a world permeated by the Asclepian healing cult.

The influence of Greco-Roman views of healing on Christian views

We first hear of Christianity in Roman North Africa in the late second century CE when mention is made of the martyrdom of seven Christians from the little village of Scilli, near Carthage.[36] By then, Greco-Roman culture and its medical views had reached North Africa and were part of everyday life in the Roman Empire. Since medical views did not depend

33 Anointment is mentioned in *James* 5:15; laying on of hands in *Mark* 16:18; and fasting in *Mark* 9:29.

34 Ferngren 2009, 10.

35 Schulze 2005, 163–164.

36 Isichei 1995, 34.

on the current polytheistic world view, they were compatible with the tenets of many Jews and Christians, and accepted by the majority of the population. In fact, Ferngren states that 'there exists in the New Testament no condemnation of physicians, either specific or implied', thus one can accept that the views the physicians represented were also regarded as compatible.[37] Christians continued to use traditional means of healing – for instance, St. Paul's advice to Timothy to take a little wine for his stomach.[38] Christians' view of medicine thus reflected those of the Mediterranean world – Greco-Roman, Jewish and Christian.

The comments of the Church Fathers on Greco-Roman medicine are nuanced, but most of them praised the utility and efficacy of the medical art.[39] There were, however, Fathers like Ambrose who reprimanded Christians who prayed for healing only when physicians had failed to cure them. However, all of the Fathers, without exception, reminded Christians that when they used medicine, ultimately it is God who heals.[40]

Perhaps the greatest indication of the influence of Greco-Roman views are the examples of Christian borrowings from pagan healing views. Vivian Nutton points out that a great number of pagan medical analogues were taken over by the Christians and became an important part of Christian theological exegesis.[41] The aforementioned metaphor *Christus Medicus* as a title for Jesus, for instance, became commonplace in Christian literature since the second century.[42] Medical terminology also became frequent in exegesis: Clement of Alexandria and Tertullian were especially fond of using medical analogues and applying them to the soul.[43] Pagan iconography became transformed: Asclepius became Jesus, as can be seen in the famous image of Christ bearing a lamb, which was a favourite Asclepian image. Pagan sites were taken over: a Christian basilica was built in Epidaurus, and the pagan Asclepian slave hospital on the Tiber Island in Rome became the hospital of St. Bartholomew.[44]

37 Ferngren 2009, 48.

38 1 *Tim.* 4:23.

39 Some of the Church Fathers, like Eusebius, Gregory of Nyssa and Ambrose, were to varying degrees 'receptive of Greco-Roman medical and physiological ideas' (Van der Eijk 2014, 339).

40 Ferngren 2009, 140–141.

41 Nutton 1984, 7. See also Schulze (2005, 155) who notes 'wie die Patres auf verschiedenste Weise medizinishes Gedankengut in ihre opera inkorporiert haben' ('As the [Church] Fathers incorporated medical ideas into their works in many different ways').

42 See Chapter 8 on Augustine and also Schulze (2005, 156), who devotes a whole section to 'Der "Arzt" als Metapher'.

43 Ferngren and Amundsen 1996, 2964.

44 Schulze (2005, 165) indicates that there is archaeological and literary evidence of more than 400 Asklepieia which later became Christian churches.

Figure 9.4 Christ bearing a lamb

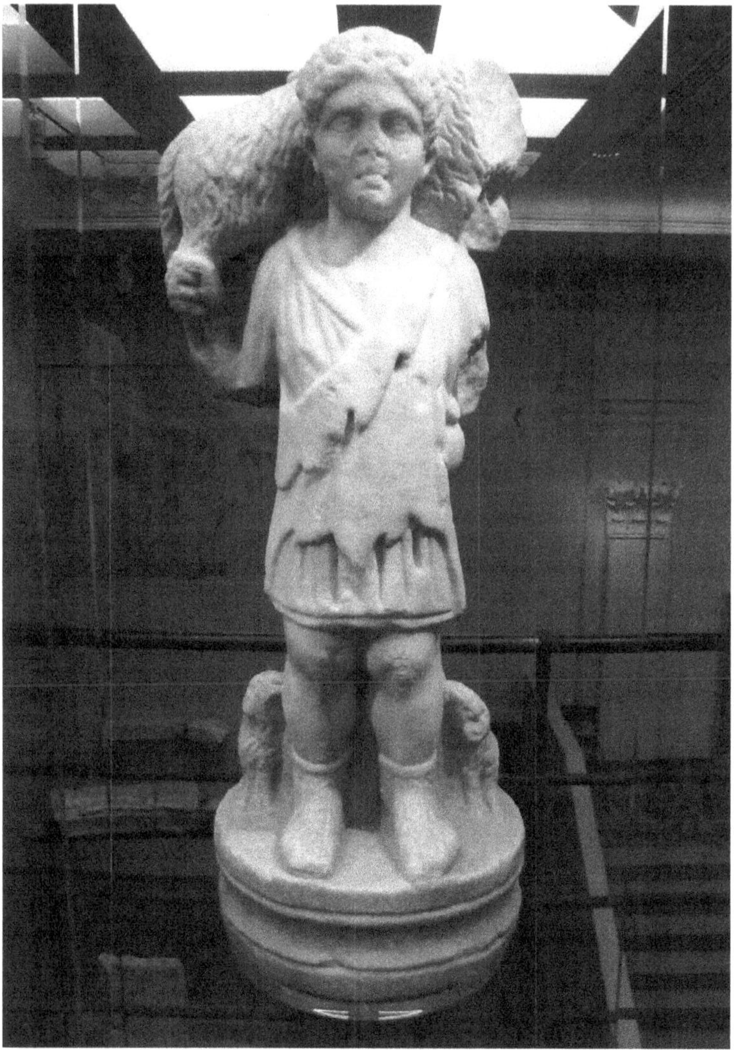

The influence of Christianity on Greco-Roman views of healing: *philanthropia* vs agapê

To understand the shift in the mental attitude of those who converted to Christianity and the far-reaching influence of this new religion, a short excursus on the Greco-Roman view of mankind is necessary. A conspicuous feature that Greco-Roman health care shares with other pagan cults is a lack of compassion and care. There is evidence of this attitude in one of

Figure 9.5 Asclepius bearing a calf

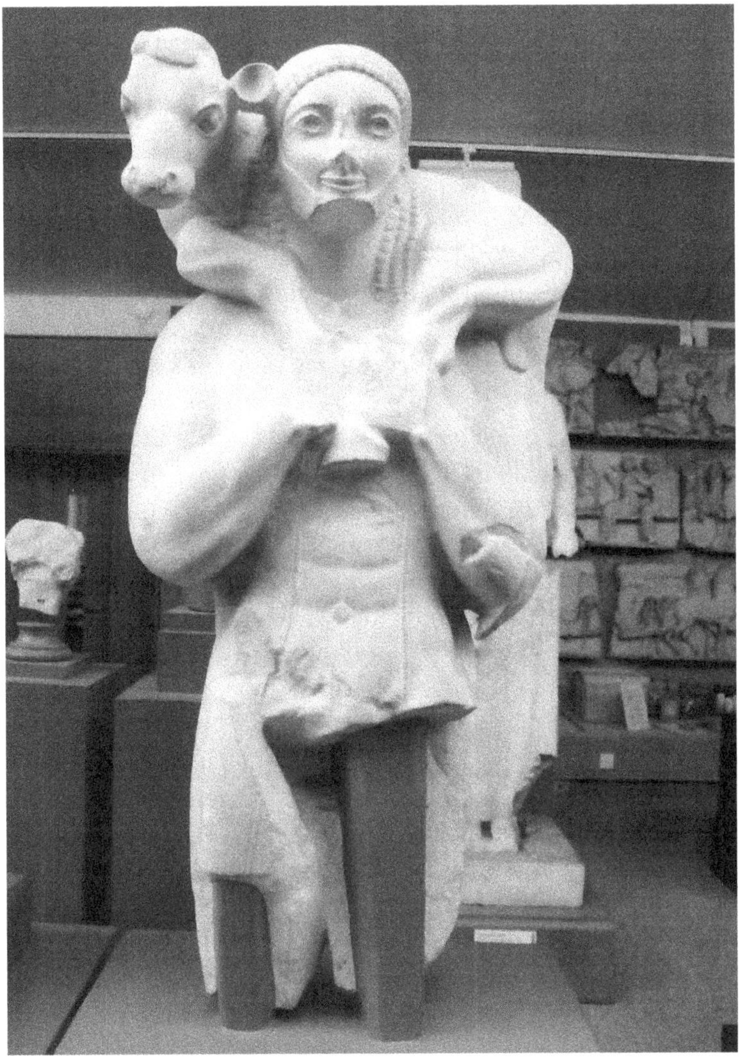

the fifth-century-BCE Hippocratic treatises, where the author recounts the case of a girl in Abdera in Greece who lay sick in the Sacred Way for 27 days, and Anaxion who lay sick of acute fever by the Thracian Gate in Abdera for 34 days – one assumes that these patients were probably set out to die, or were destitute and had no relatives caring for them, and that they died after respectively 27 and 34 days.[45] We also see this lack of compassion

45 Hp. *Epid.* 3 case 8.

in fifth-century-BCE Greece when the historian Thucydides describes the plague that ravaged Athens in 429 – the dead lie heaped up in the streets, and people flee from those closest to them.[46] We see it again in the description of the effect of the plague of St. Cyprian in 250 CE when neither municipal officials nor individuals took care of the sick.[47] Ferngren describes this as 'the traditional attitude of those brought up within a classical culture in which neither philosophy nor religion encouraged a compassionate response to human suffering'.[48] In Rome one finds the same situation. There was no shelter for the homeless – they lived on the streets, in porches, in temples or, during winter, in the public baths for some heat. In an epigram, the poet Martial (first century CE) gives a description of a dying person who is listening to the dogs howling in anticipation of eating his corpse, while he desperately tries to ward off birds of prey by flapping his rags.[49]

There is a Greek word, '*philanthropia*', taken over in the Latin vocabulary, which means 'love of mankind' in general (*humanitas* in Latin), a humane virtue educated men were supposed to possess. It did not imply private charity or a personal concern for those in need. Pity was not a 'desirable emotional response' to need and suffering as a motive for charity, says Ferngren.[50] The Stoic doctrine of indifference to human suffering has much to do with this attitude. There was a hardness in Stoic philosophy that left little room for the gentler virtues.[51] Almsgiving, an obligation in Jewish religion, took the form of a public donation in the Roman world – civic beneficence or *euergesia*; the rich would show their civic patriotism by sharing their wealth not with the poor, but with their fellow citizens, for which an enhancement of their reputation was expected. This is evident in many of the buildings erected by the aristocracy in cities in North Africa.

In contrast, Jesus' parable of the Good Samaritan sets a paradigm for his followers. Already in the first century the indifferent Greco-Roman concept of *philanthropia* acquired a new name, *agapê*, with a new content, meaning unlimited love of one's neighbour, given freely and without regard to the object. Ferngren points out that this version of love of one's neighbour linked up with the Christian understanding of the concept of *imago Dei* (man as the image of God), which they had taken over from Judaism.[52] This

46 Th. 2.7.
47 Cypr. *De mortalitate* cc. 15–20.
48 Ferngren 2009, 150.
49 Mart. 10.5.11 ff.
50 Ferngren 2009, 87.
51 Ferngren 2009, 97.
52 Ferngren 2009, 98–103.

had far-reaching consequences; in fact, it represents 'a radical departure from the social ethics of classical paganism'. It gave, in the first instance, an impetus to Christian charity, in contrast with the Greco-Roman world, where there was no religious impulse to private charity.[53] Furthermore, almsgiving, a duty in Judaic religion, became an outgrowth of Christian *agapê* and extended beyond one's own community. A further consequence of the Christian interpretation of the *imago Dei* concept was that every human's life has intrinsic value, in contrast with the Judaic and Greco-Roman view that the sick and disabled have no worth. This had the implication that there was now a redefinition of the sick and the poor. Everyone shared in the divine image, even the diseased body of the leper.

The influence of Christianity on the practice of medicine

Seen against this background, only one physician (not a Christian), Scribonius Largus (first century CE), stated that, apart from competence, compassion should be required of a doctor.[54] The famous physician Galen (not a Christian) believed that by being competent, a good doctor would be able to relieve suffering and show *philanthropia*, but his ideal doctor was not in the first instance compassionate. Ferngren draws attention to an interesting case where the Greco-Roman and Christian views on the ideal doctor come together in two documents by the same person, Cassiodorus (c. 487–583). In the first document, written when he was still serving in the administration of the Ostrogothic king, Theoderic, Hippocratic values and the usefulness of the art of medicine dominate. In the second, written after his retirement and after he had founded a monastery in Vivarium in southern Italy, Cassiodorus admonishes his monks to put their hope in the Lord rather than in the art of medicine, and urges them to be motivated by compassion.[55]

What then was the influence of Christianity on the practice of medicine by the ordinary physician? Since there was not, as has been stated above, a specific Christian kind of health care, it is obvious that doctors, even Christian doctors, would still follow the Hippocratic precepts or the therapeutic strategies as determined by the sect of which they were adherents.[56] Ferngren

53 Christian preachers had a hard time to change the attitude of their parishioners from giving only for their own city or class to giving for the poor (Blowers 2009, 1–27).

54 Scrib. *Comp.* Praef. par. 3.

55 Ferngren 2009, 110.

56 See on medical sects Chapter 5, pp. 123–125.

adds that apart from abortion, exposure of babies and suicide, the medical ethics of the Christian physician would not have been very different from those of his pagan colleagues, 'except perhaps a greater willingness to help the poor'.[57] Compassion, so characteristic of Christian values, would have complemented Greco-Roman practices, not supplanted it. A difference could perhaps be added: that Christian doctors would continue health ministration even if the patient's prognosis was poor, while such a patient would probably have been abandoned by Hippocratic doctors, as in the examples given above.[58]

Christian Schulze compiled a list of every physician who could be identified as a Christian, and came to the amazing count of 150 during the Imperial period, or 194 if one adds those of uncertain status.[59] In North Africa, four *medici* are mentioned in literature, and four in inscriptions.[60] We also know for certain that Maximus, who had converted from Arianism,[61] and Gennadius were Christian doctors: Augustine describes the latter as a man 'of devout mind, kind and generous heart, and untiring compassion, as is shown by his care for the poor'.[62]

The four North African physicians

Cassius Felix (*discussed in Chapter 7*)

Of the medical authors discussed in this book, we know for certain that Cassius Felix was a Christian – not only does he openly confess that he is a Christian in the first lines of his *On medicine*, but a hagiographic text, the

57 Ferngren 2009, 107–109. See the Codex Theodosianus, in which the emperor Valentinian I (a Christian) states that the doctors of the newly established College of Physicians were salaried as a way to 'relieve' them of obsequious service to the rich and make them available for honorable service to the poor (Chapter 5 on Vindicianus).

58 See however, Van der Eijk (1999) who argues that Hippocratic doctors did not leave their patients alone when they had a bad prognosis but assisted them until the end.

59 Schulze 2005, 46–134 *passim*.

60 In North Africa Schulze (2005) identified four mentioned in literature: Aemilianus (in *Martyrologium Romanus* par. 373), Cassius Felix (Nutton 1997, 1016), Dioscurus (Aug. *Ep.* 117) and Vindicianus (Aug. *Conf.* 7.6 and *Ep.* 138). The four mentioned in inscriptions were Flabius Quintus (Mactar), Rozonus (Cartenna in Mauretania), Filiossus (Carthage) and an anonymous *medicus* of a synod in Carthage. Schulze (2005, 138) also mentions nine inscriptions of women doctors; it appears that they made up 10 percent of physicians.

61 Aug. *Ep.* 170.10.

62 Aug. *Ep.* 159.3.

De miraculis Sancti Stephani protomartyris, mentions a renowned *archiater* from Carthage called Felix who could be Cassius Felix. When he was summoned to a sickbed, he confided in the course of his consultation that he was guided in his work by the Almighty God.[63] There are no indications in his book of a specifically Christian approach or therapy.

Theodorus Priscianus (*discussed in Chapter 6*)

In the preface of his *Physica* it seems that Theodorus Priscianus believed in the concept of *natura/physis*. In the first book of his *Euporiston*, the *Phaenomenon* (c. 2), he invokes Nature to reprimand the physicians who are pretentiously parading their knowledge at a sickbed instead of treating the dying patient, and continues by pointing out that Nature has provided all the necessary remedies, in seeds, in fruit, in herbs – in short, in most plants that are freely available and easily obtainable; that is the reason why he is writing the *Euporiston*, a book of easily obtainable remedies. The work does not reveal a Christian approach.[64]

Caelius Aurelianus (*discussed in Chapter 7*)

Caelius Aurelianus, the translator/adapter of some of the works of Soranus, could have known Q. Aurelius Symmachus (c. 345–402), a prominent statesman and man of letters, who happened to be proconsul of Africa Proconsularis in 373.[65] Symmachus, one of the last pagans in high positions in Rome, sought to preserve the traditional religion of Rome at a time when the aristocracy was converting to Christianity and laws were promulgated to eradicate paganism. Since Caelius shared Symmachus' literary interest, it is probable that he could also have been a pagan. It should also be mentioned that Praetextatus, to whom Caelius' Greek letters were written, was a pagan.[66]

63 *Patristica Latina* 41.833–854. See also Chapter 7. Scarborough (2008, 208–9) mentions that this corresponds with a funerary inscription from Cirta (*CIL* VIII.7566), 'attesting an ancestral home, where he probably became a respected practitioner before going to Carthage'.
64 See also Chapter 6 on Theodorus for more details.
65 He was, *inter alia*, City Prefect of Rome in 384–5 and consul in 391 (Cameron 2011 *passim*). This is the person who recommended Augustine to the post in Milan (see Chapter 8 on Augustine).
66 Cameron 2011, 372–373. See Chapter 7 regarding the Greek letters used for the dating of Caelius.

Helvius Vindicianus (*discussed in Chapter 5*)

Vindicianus spent a number of years at the court of the emperor Valentinian and his son Gratian in Treviri (now Trier). It was here that Vindicianus, thanks to many years of meritorious service, was appointed Count of the College of Physicians. Valentinian was a Christian, and one would expect that an official appointed to such a prestigious post would also be a Christian, or at least have sympathy with the Christian cause. One must, however, remember that the court was not yet wholly Christianized – the religious views of the famous poet Ausonius, who had great influence at the court by virtue of being the tutor of the young emperor, Gratian, and who also probably played a role in Vindicianus' appointment as proconsul of Africa Proconsularis, were 'notoriamente controversa'.[67] Fiorucci thus, after having considered all possible aspects of the problem, comes to the conclusion that Vindicianus was probably not a Christian, but as many of the other members of the intellectual circle at the court, a pagan, with empathy for the Christian cause.[68]

The origin of the hospital

Inspired by the parable of the Good Samaritan and by compassion and *agapê*, caring for those in need started gaining momentum, and was taken over by local churches; it was organized on greater scale, so that by the third century the church in Rome, for instance, was caring for 1500 widows and disabled people.[69] Initially only Christians were assisted medically, but during the plague of 250, Cyprian, bishop of Carthage, ordered that all the sick, Christians and pagans alike, should be helped. Thereafter medical care became more outwardly focused. This parochial work of charitable assistance – not in the first instance curing, but caring – prepared the way for larger non-parochial institutions, such as hospitals. And after the

67 Fiorucci 2011, 225 n.2.

68 Fiorucci's arguments (2011, 225–235), which can unfortunately not be discussed in detail here, are based on Vindicianus' advice to Augustine not to waste time on astrology in which he, *inter alia*, explains coincidences as 'the power of chance which pervades the whole of nature', and his letter to the emperor Valentinian in which he displays typical Hippocratic values – even his philanthropy is that advised in the Hippocratic treatise *On the Physician*. Vindicianus' reference to the 'Divine Providence' in his letter to the emperor (par. 7) can, due to the brevity of the remark, not be regarded as proof that he is a Christian (a reference to a similar concept also occurs in Cicero and Galen, Fiorucci 2011, 233 notes 22 and 23).

69 Ferngren 2009, 115. The church had a considerable staff of 46 presbyters, seven deacons, seven sub deacons and 42 acolytes.

legalization of Christianity in 313, charitable projects could be organized more easily. The Roman state still shunned the obligation of caring for the poor, and was thus more than grateful to assign public funds to bishops for Christian projects in return for, for example, tax exemption – an excellent example of the 'Christianization of euergetism'.[70]

The concept of an institution providing charitable care, and in particular long-term health care, to the ordinary citizen, was unknown in the Greco-Roman world in the early Empire. It was a distinctively Christian concept. Well-off patients were visited at home by doctors, and the temples of Asclepius were visited for incubation sleep and healing dreams, but there was no long-term care. On large estates, provision was made for sick slaves, and with the extension of the empire when sick and wounded soldiers could no longer be sent home for treatment, military hospitals or *valetudinaria* were erected near the borders. They were, however, built for a specialized group (slaves and soldiers) and not for the public, and were therefore not precursors of the hospital as we know it.[71]

After the legalization of Christianity in 313, charitable organizations proliferated; there was often no differentiation between assistance for paupers, pilgrims, orphans and the diseased.[72] From the late fourth century on, hospices, called *xenodochia*, arose in the mainly Greek-speaking East, initially built to shelter pilgrims and messengers between the various bishops, but eventually housing disadvantaged and mentally infirm people as well as the diseased. About a generation later *xenodochia* were established in the western part of the empire, as well, mainly because the pagan emperor Julian the Apostate (r. 361–363) realized that these institutions attracted potential converts; he thus ordered that *xenodochia* also be established by pagan bishops to attract pagan converts.[73]

Monasteries, which became established in the fourth century, also provided health care. Infirmaries that initially provided health services for the monks later took in civilian patients, as well. One of the duties of the monks in these monasteries was copying the medical manuscripts of the Greek masters, in this way ensuring the survival of Greco-Roman medicine.

Reference has already been made in Chapter 2 to 'health facilities in the cities of Roman North Africa, and to the hospitals establishedby St. Basil

70 Ferngren 2009, 123.

71 Cilliers & Retief 2002, 60–66.

72 Nutton 1984, 9; Ferngren & Amundsen 1996, 2971–2975.

73 Jul. *Ep.* 40. In this letter to Arsacius, the pagan high priest in Galatia, Julian wrote: 'In every city establish *xenodochia* in order that strangers may profit by our benevolence.'

the Great and that by St. Ephraim in Edessa. The role of Christian women such as Fabiola, Pulcheria and Pauline and even the empress Eudoxia in founding hospitals has been noted. North Africa could also boast of three hospitals of which one was in Hippo Regius; furthermore the military camp at Lambaesis possibly also had a hospital with an Aesculapium attached to it.

The third, fourth and fifth centuries – the development of tensions

From the third century on, a gradual shift in Christian theological thinking set in, with growing emphasis on supernatural healing, demonic possession and exorcism as a cure. Until then miraculous cures were thought to have been confined to the Gospel era. Magic, which had been universally condemned by Christians, also made its appearance in the form of amulets, charms and healing incantations.[74] It must of course be kept in mind that even after the legalization of Christianity by Constantine in 313, large parts of the empire still remained pagan.[75]

In the third century, the martyrdom of the twin Christian brothers Cosmas and Damian, both excellent physicians, led to the proliferation of healing saints, healing shrines and the belief in the healing power of relics associated with the saints.[76] These circumstances had a negative influence on orthodox secular medicine. Thus, in order to accommodate the growing belief in supernatural and magical healing, secular orthodox doctors became less 'scientific' in their approach to medicine. Alexander of Tralles, the renowned Lydian physician of the fifth and sixth centuries, for instance, recommended the use of, *inter alia*, amulets and charms in his treatment.[77]

Conclusion

In the changing world of late Antiquity, it is inevitable that Greco-Roman and Christian views on healing would have influenced each other. It has in the course of this chapter been mentioned that the Greek concept of *philanthropia* (Latin *humanitas*), love of mankind in general, had acquired

74 Ferngren & Amundsen 1994, 2968.
75 Nutton 1984, 7.
76 Ferngren & Amundsen 1994, 2969.
77 Nutton 1984, 6.

a new name with a new content: *agapê*, love of one's neighbour, compassion and personal concern for those in need. The two contrasting documents written by Cassiodorus, mentioned above, are a shining example of the influence of Christianity on Greco-Roman views on healing. Galen's view that the ideal physician shows *philanthropia* by healing suffering, and that compassion is not a necessary virtue, is in stark contrast with Cassiodorus' directive to his monks to show compassion and to put their trust in the Lord rather than in the art of medicine.

Furthermore, the Roman custom of *euergesia*, civic beneficence in the form of public donations, was also beginning to change in the Christianized world, in that citizens' obligation to the state was replaced by private charity. The idea that everybody shared in the image of God was a radical departure from the Greco-Roman view that the disabled and the poor had no worth, and gave impetus to the Christian idea that charity should extend beyond one's own class.

But it was not a one-way street. As indicated above, there are numerous examples of Christian borrowings from pagan healing views. Not only were pagan medical terms and analogues taken over by the Christians in theological exegesis, but Christian iconography also reflected the Greco-Roman influence, and pagan sites and buildings were taken over, renamed and re-built. However, the establishment of caring communities, which eventually developed into hospitals, was a uniquely Christian initiative, and arguably their greatest contribution to medicine.

10. The role of Roman North Africa in the preservation and transmission of medical knowledge

Introduction

Oswald Spengler, in his famous book *The decline of the West*, postulated that any civilization 'is a super organism with a limited and predictable lifespan'.[1] Looking at the history of the world in a broad perspective, he rejected the usual linear division of history into ancient, medieval, and modern epochs, and instead believed that meaningful units in history are whole cultures which develop as organisms; the lifespan of such a culture is about a thousand years. Events such as the decline or fall of a culture do not happen fortuitously, he believed, but are a historical change of phase within a greater world picture. One of the eight cultures that he identified is 'Classical' (Greek and Roman). If one were to look at this culture, and take as a starting year 480 BCE, the beginning of the Fifty Golden Years of Greek civilization (also known as the *Pentekontaetia*) and as an end point take 476 CE, the traditional date of the fall of Rome, it does add up to nearly a thousand years. Spengler's cyclic theory could thus apply to this culture.[2] In the first chapter of this book, where the environment, population and cultural life of specifically Roman North Africa were discussed, it was stated, à la Spengler, that the history of Roman North Africa is interesting because it encapsulates, as it were, the rise and fall of a civilization. The period in this case was half a millennium, from c. 146 BCE to 439 CE. But the history of Roman North Africa, although inextricably linked to that of the Roman Empire as a whole, ran its own course, and had its own reasons for its decline, which do not necessarily coincide with the reasons for the decline of Rome.[3]

An account of the preservation and transmission of medical texts is linked to events forming part of the decline of Roman North Africa. Possible reasons for that decline will be discussed, followed by the role of the five

1 Spengler 1991 (Vols. I and II published in German in respectively 1918 and 1922).

2 One of the criticisms of Spengler's model is that the Greco–Roman model does not fit the other cultures.

3 See Ward-Perkins 2005 and Heather 2005 for reasons for the fall of Rome.

important medical authors who form the core of this book. Some repetition in these two sections of information discussed in detail in former chapters is inevitable, the intention being to bring all the strands together in this final chapter to present a complete picture. The vicissitudes of a text of one of these authors, Cassius Felix, in the ensuing centuries, will then follow, since it exemplifies the phases in the transmission of most of the medical texts written in North Africa in the fourth to sixth centuries CE. The medical contribution of Roman North Africa fortunately did not end with its demise after the Arab conquest – in the eleventh century, Constantine the African, a brilliant Carthaginian merchant, took his knowledge and books to southern Italy, where his translation of Arabic medical texts into Latin proved to be an enormous contribution to the furthering of medical knowledge in Europe in the Middle Ages.

Circumstances leading to the demise of Roman influence in North Africa, fifth and sixth centuries CE

At least two centuries before 476 CE, Rome had been experiencing serious political and economic problems, while Roman North Africa had already made its debut, as it were, on the stage of the Mediterranean world. From the second century until it was overrun by the Vandals in the fifth century, the country had experienced unequalled prosperity, thanks mainly to its production and export of agricultural products, especially olive oil.[4] Roman influence still endured to some extent – one could even call it a brief renaissance – after the Byzantine conquest and settlement in the sixth century, but vanished completely after the Arab invasion in the seventh century.

When looking for reasons for the decline of Roman North Africa, more specifically for the complete disappearance of Roman influence in the country after the Arab conquest, a question arises. Why is it that no trace of the culture and language of the Romans remains in North Africa, whereas there is still so much evidence of the Roman heritage in the Roman provinces in Europe (for instance, France, Spain, Belgium)? It should be noted that when these provinces were overrun by the barbarians, they were much less Romanized and developed than North Africa. There, all that remains after nearly 600 years of Roman occupation (c. 146 BCE – 439 CE) are the ruins of massive amphitheatres and other public buildings, silent witnesses of a period of unequalled prosperity in Roman provincial administration.

4 See Chapter 1 and Cilliers 2007, 39–43, for more detail.

Foreign invasions

The Vandals

A reason for the demise that immediately springs to mind is the Vandal invasion in the fifth century.[5] The Vandals entered North Africa from Spain in 429, and marched eastwards, seizing towns as they went along. After defeating a Roman army, they arrived at the gates of Carthage, where, according to the Bishop Quodvultdeus, the populace was still cheering their teams in the circus.[6] The city was easily taken. Life went on under the new regime, and the local people were still active in the city. The Vandals are accused of being destructive – 'vandalistic' – but it has been pointed out that this view is a later misrepresentation.[7] Attracted by the wealth of North Africa, they came to settle and to enjoy the benefits of the Roman amenities – the baths, the spectacles in the arena and the amphitheatre. Although they did plunder rich Christian churches, confiscate rural properties and dispossess – and sometimes even exile – aristocratic landlords, it was in their interest to maintain administrative systems that were effective: Latin, for instance, remained the official language, and Roman coins were still used. The Vandals respected Rome's rich cultural heritage, and some even converted to Christianity. In short, 'they conquered the province, but kept it Roman and would leave it Roman'.[8]

However, in their enjoyment of all the Roman amenities, the Vandals used and abused everything without replacing anything. They did not take up the financial burdens of the cities, with the result that the already fragile municipal system, which had hitherto been maintained by the rich upper classes, rapidly declined in the fifth century, especially since many of the rich aristocrats who could afford it had fled the country. A second problem was the order of the Vandal king, Geiseric, to dismantle the protective city walls, which left the inhabitants defenceless against the depredations of the local Berber tribes. This caused the abandonment of many of the frontier towns by the end of the fifth century.

5 See Chapter 1 and Cilliers 2007, 43–45, for more detail.

6 Quodvultdeus, *Sermo de tempore barbarico* 1.1, Patristica Latina 40, 700. The addiction of the city to the pleasures of the circus and the theatre was regarded as a scandal by the Gallic monk Salvian (*On the government of God*, 6.69).

7 See Chapter 1.

8 Cilliers 2007, 44.

The Byzantines

A second invasion of North Africa followed in 533, scarcely a century later, this time by an army sent from Byzantium by the emperor Justinian, who wished to reunite the eastern and western halves of the empire. The Byzantines easily defeated the Vandals, 'enervated by a century of Roman luxury'.[9] After their defeat, the Vandals simply disappeared – some became integrated into the local population, others fled to Spain. No trace remains of their sojourn in North Africa, not even any words from their language. Only the undeserved term 'vandal' remains, as invective.

Under the Byzantines there was a short revival, especially during the 30 years of peace when Heraclius was emperor (r. 610–641). North Africa remained Roman but Greek was introduced as the official language. Buildings, roads, aqueducts and public buildings were repaired; there was even an intellectual revival. To protect the cities against the Berbers, who had grown audacious during Vandal rule, the emperor ordered the city walls to be rebuilt; because of the urgency, the Byzantine soldiers simply made use of the neglected Roman temples and monuments. The sad condition in which the Roman remains are today must therefore be ascribed to the Byzantines, not the Vandals. Corrupt administration under Byzantine governors made the situation worse and lead to civil unrest and uprisings, leaving many inhabitants worse off than under Vandal rule.

The Arabs

The brief Byzantine occupation only postponed the Arab conquest. Shortly after the death of the emperor Heraclius in 647, the Muslims invaded North Africa. Their enemies were no longer the Byzantines, who had vanished from history, but the Berbers. Within half a century the Muslims had occupied the whole of Roman North Africa; in 698 Carthage was captured and annihilated. A new capital, Kairouan, was built near the ruins of Carthage, and would become one of the Muslims' holy places. The mass conversion of the Berbers to Islam after the Arab conquest greatly strengthened the burgeoning Islamic culture, which completely replaced the Roman culture and language.

9 Cilliers 2007, 44.

Romanization

There is another reason for the demise of Roman culture. Scholars such as Frend (1952), Courtois (1955) and Shaw (1980) have argued that the Romanization of North Africa was only a veneer, a fragile superstructure affecting only the upper classes of a society, which at its roots remained faithful to its pre-Roman traditions (the Berber customs and tribal structures). Lepelley corroborates this view, pointing out that systematic Romanization and urbanization only took place in what is now northern and central Tunisia and eastern Algeria; elsewhere, it was limited.[10] Roman cities were enclaves in the world of the rural Berber tribes. The fact that the gap between the Romanized upper class and the Berbers was never bridged explains the eventual disintegration of the province.

Linked to the three invasions, when the many thousands who could afford to leave fled the country, it becomes clear that the already small number of Romans and their descendants in Roman North Africa became smaller with each wave of invaders. As they were vastly outnumbered, it would have become impossible to preserve the Roman cultural heritage. After the Arab conquest, North Africa became more and more isolated from the outside world – it turned its back, as it were, to Europe and faced the East.

The role of five North African authors in the preservation of medical texts

The disruption caused by the successive waves of invaders was, paradoxically, the main reason so much medical literature from North Africa survived at all. Monica Green points out that Carthage was still an open harbour and a regular stopping point for ships.[11] Among those who fled the country to Italy and Spain would have been scholars and clerics, whose most precious possessions would have been books.

The common contribution of the five writers was the translation of the works of Greek authors of old from Greek into Latin, making them available to the ordinary doctor and all others who were interested in medical matters

10 Lepelley 1979, 20–21. See also Heather's remark (2005, 519 n. 40) that 'the number of immigrants from Italy in the towns in North Africa in the third century must not be overstated'.
11 Green 1985, 139–141.

but could no longer understand Greek. What exactly the impulse was that led to the translations cannot be pinpointed, apart from the statement of Vindicianus that he was translating Greek works for those who no longer understand the language, perhaps worried that within a generation or two there would not be anybody left with enough knowledge of Greek to do it.[12] Vindicianus' example was followed by his student Theodorus, although the latter first wrote his *Euporiston* in Greek to gain recognition in the larger medical community, and then translated it into Latin himself. Caelius Aurelianus, Cassius Felix and Muscio wrote their texts in Latin without any explanation. In short, the works of all five authors had as aim the dissemination of medical knowledge among those of the laity who were interested but could not understand Greek.

Langslow's remark that Vindicianus' works herald the beginning 'of what may be seen as a "Golden Age" of ancient Latin medical compendia [...] produced by practicing doctors in the period c. AD 370– 450' deserves repeating.[13] Temkin adds to this that 'their efforts to salvage the tremendous treasures of the past can be seen as the historical achievement of the first half of the millennium'.[14]

Our five authors lived at the turning point in the history of Roman North Africa. The disruption caused by the Vandal invasion was, paradoxically, the main reason medical texts were preserved. And among the texts the refugees took with them would have been the translations of Vindicianus, Theodorus, Caelius and Cassius Felix.[15] Thereafter, the centre of translation shifted to Ravenna in northern Italy.[16]

Vindicianus, fourth and fifth centuries

The disasters thus had as side effect the dissemination of the medical texts translated in the fourth and fifth centuries. Of Vindicianus we know that as early as the first decades of the fifth century, Marcellus of Bordeaux quoted one of his remedies for coughs.[17] There are, furthermore, many passages

12 Five of the manuscripts that contain his *Gynecology* state in the first chapter that he is translating the work from Greek into Latin because of the 'ignorance' (of the readers) of Greek (Rose 1894, 429).

13 Langslow 2000, 63.

14 Temkin 1977a, 168.

15 Cilliers 2008, 60–63; Green 1985, 209.

16 Green 1985, 140–141.

17 In Niedermann & Liechtenhan 1968, 292.

in the *Etymologies* of the Archbishop Isidore of Seville (c. 560–636)[18] in Spain that resemble Vindicianus' *Gynecology,* and his letter to his nephew Pentadius is quoted in the seventh and eighth century by the Venerable Bede in the Anglo-Saxon world. Vindicianus' three short works (*Gynecology,* and the letters to Pentadius and the emperor Valentinian) were, according to Langslow, among the most widely excerpted medical works throughout post-Classical times and the Middle Ages.[19]

Theodorus Priscianus, fifth century

Since Theodorus' work was practical rather than theoretical, he was known and often cited in later ages, in the Greek-speaking East as well as in the Roman West.[20] He is, for instance, quoted by the renowned physician Alexander of Tralles in Lydia in the sixth century with regard to a diagnosis of epilepsy. His *Gynecology,* the third book of the *Euporiston,* was so popular that it was transmitted independently of the main work.[21] Due to its applicability, it was excerpted on numerous occasions.[22]

Caelius Aurelianus, fourth and fifth centuries

By the middle of the sixth century, Caelius was known in Italy since he was quoted in the *Institutions* of Cassiodorus (485–585). Cassiodorus was the minister in the government of the Ostrogothic king, Theoderic, who became a monk and founded a monastery at Vivarium in southern Italy. He compiled a work, one part of which was a compendium of such secular knowledge as he thought necessary for the monks, among which there were some medical texts – *inter alia,* Latin translations of Hippocrates, Galen and possibly Caelius Aurelianus.[23] Caelius was also excerpted in Isidore of Seville's *Etymologies.*[24]

18 An encyclopedia in twenty volumes dealing with the arts, law, religion, medicine, and the like. The work contains excerpts of many authors, its intention being to trace the origin of words and concepts. This encyclopedia was one of the main routes by which learning was transmitted to the Middle Ages. From Spain copies were sent to abbeys all over Europe (Sabbah 1998, 149 n. 83).

19 Langslow 2000, 65. See also Cilliers (2008, 56 n. 36) for further references to Vindicianus' works mentioned or used in later centuries.

20 Cilliers 2008, 57.

21 Hanson & Green 1996, 1057.

22 Langslow 2000, 55 n. 36.

23 Nutton 2004, 300.

24 Sabbah 1998, 149 n. 83.

Cassius Felix, fifth century

Due to its brevity and practical approach, Cassius Felix' *On medicine* was known and used throughout the Middle Ages. In an insightful article, the French scholar Guy Sabbah traced the vicissitudes of the manuscripts of Cassius Felix's work until the early Middle Ages, thereby throwing some light on 'the unbroken usefulness of the late Latin medical texts'.[25] In broad outlines, the phases in the transmission of the various manuscripts of Cassius' text replicate those of the other North African authors. It should be pointed out that texts that were for some reason not transmitted during the critical centuries – from the time when the first copy of the text was made until the eleventh century, when the first complete text was written down – were forever lost. It was not inevitable that a valuable work would somehow find its way to Europe.[26]

In the first phase (c. 446/447 CE) Cassius would have had his slaves make copies for students or friends. None of these copies survive. Thereafter, c. 620 CE, we find unacknowledged quotes of his work in Isidore's *Etymologies*, which had as aim to trace the etymology of words and concepts. The manuscripts could have been brought to Spain by the second wave of refugees – derelict monks of plundered churches in North Africa might have brought them to the Archbishop's Abbey in Seville during and after the Byzantine invasion.

The second phase was the reproduction of some pages of the *On medicine*, found in the eighth century at a principality under the control of the bishop of Coire, in the west of France. There is also evidence at this time of the work in the Abbey of St. Gall in eastern Switzerland.

The following phase comprises the modification and adaptation of the work in medical compilations with a practical aim. Cassius Felix was still well known and respected, regarded as on the same level as Hippocrates and Galen. A section of his *On medicine* thus emerges in the ninth century in the *Tereoperica*[27] in a manuscript in Paris that contains at least 38 chapters of Cassius' work; in the beginning, the *Tereoperica* is quite close to the *On medicine,* but more and more irregularities occur in the later chapters until, at c. 66 of the 108 chapters, the *On medicine* is completely abandoned in

25 Sabbah 1994, English abstract.

26 Sabbah 1994, 11–28.

27 For *Therapeutica*, one can see that the text has been transcribed many times, and not always by the brightest monks! Yet Sabbah (1994, 23) dryly remarks that at least the text survived, thus everything is not lost due to the ignorance or laziness (or bad handwriting, one could add) of the monks transcribing the manuscripts in the *scriptoria*!

favour of a nosological order with emphasis on fevers (one of the favourite topics of Antiquity in the Mediterranean). Thus it appears that in some form or other, determined by the intellectual characteristics and needs of the time, the *On medicine* was transmitted through many centuries (and other manuscripts in much the same way).[28]

We see in the *Tereoperica* an interesting change: fifth-century North Africa was not ninth-century France. There were differences in climate, in *materia medica* and in the tableau of diseases, but it was the terminology, pathology and, to a lesser extent, the symptomology of Cassius Felix, as an author of the Logic/Dogmatic sect, that attracted the compilers of the ninth-century work. Two movements, seemingly contradictory but actually complementary, take place in the *Tereoperica*: 'la reconnaissance de la force et de la dignité de la tradition, l'ouverture à l'appel et à la nécessité de l'innovation' ('The recognition of the strength and dignity of tradition, <but also> an opening to the appeal and necessity for innovation').[29]

Muscio, fifth or sixth centuries

Of Muscio we only know that he is probably from African origin, and lived in the fifth or sixth century. But his Latin catechism on women's diseases and midwifery, the *Gynecology*, was well known in the Middle Ages. The work is written for midwives, with the explicit aim to raise their level of expertise; the text is thus simplified so that the 'weaker minds' of the midwives may more easily understand it (the question-and-answer format of the catechism also helps to remember the important facts). The text is generally based on Soranus' *Gynecology*, but after Muscio's reworking, it can actually be regarded as an independent new commentary.[30] Thirteen complete or near complete manuscripts are extant, and in the late medieval period the work was also translated into various new vernaculars – evidence of its popularity.

North Africa in the eleventh century: Constantine the African

The history of Roman North Africa closes on a dismal note – the country partially survives two invasions, but after the Arab conquest Roman influence completely disappears. Only the ruins of once impressive buildings

28 Green (1985, 61) states that 'there is nothing inevitable about the transmission of knowledge'.

29 Sabbah 1994, 28.

30 Maire 2001, 321.

Figure 10.1 Monte Cassino

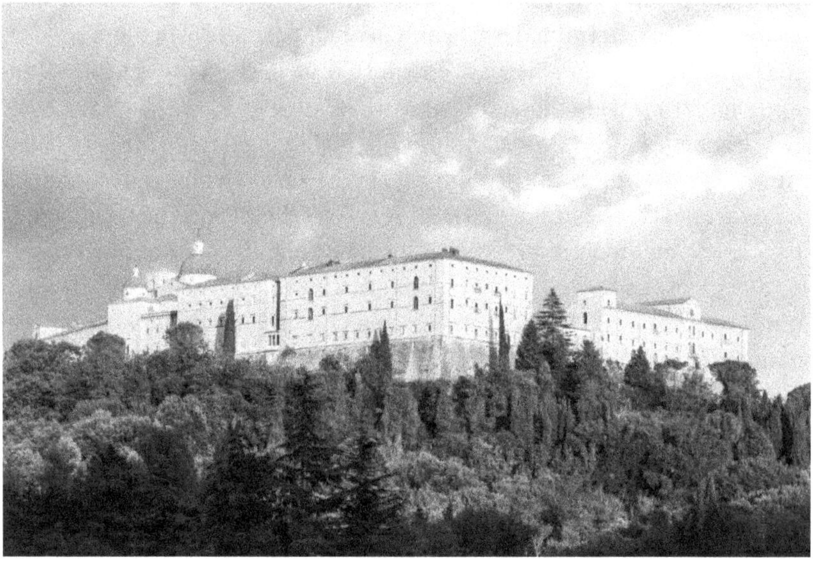

and aqueducts remain, but no trace of the culture and language of the Romans, despite so many centuries of rule. And yet life went on, and North Africa did, in accordance with Spengler's theory, rise again. Kairouan, the new capital, replaced Carthage, which finally fell in 698, and eventually became one of the holiest places of Islam thanks to the Great Mosque of Uqba, built in c. 670. Ironically, it was almost wholly built of the debris of Roman and Byzantine buildings nearby.[31]

While Islamic North Africa was in the centuries to come ruled by successive warring dynasties, medicine in various guises – Hippocratic, Galenic and folk medicine – was still practiced in Italy. During the fifth to eleventh centuries, a tenuous but continuous thread of learning and practice connected the last phase of Roman medicine with the dawn of science in the late Middle Ages.[32] In this troubled period, the monasteries were the repositories of learning – not that they advanced science, but they saved it from oblivion through the copying of manuscripts. The monastery of Monte Cassino in southern Italy, founded by St. Benedict in 529, played an especially critical role in this transmission. The copying of manuscripts was one of the most important tasks of the monks, and fragments of Latin and translated Greek manuscripts of whatever kind were copied there.

31 Wood & Wheeler 1966, 156.

32 McKitterick 2015, 1902.

This thin thread – actually, the life artery – of medical knowledge was unexpectedly strengthened by an infusion of fresh blood when a Muslim drug merchant from Tunis in North Africa named Constantine (later called Constantine the African), arrived in southern Italy in the 1060s or 1070s. It is difficult to disentangle legend from fact in his peregrinations, but this seems to have been Constantine's second visit to Italy – during his first, he realized that the knowledge of theoretical medicine in Italy was practically non-existent, that it was limited to simple practical knowledge, and lagged far behind the level of medicine prevailing in the Islamic world of the time.[33] On Constantine's return to North Africa from Italy he seems to have practiced in Carthage for some time before returning to Italy with a precious cargo, consisting not of drugs and spices, in which he had traded before, but of Arabic books on medicine and *materia medica*. Constantine, a native speaker of Arabic, who was described as 'erudite' by one of his early biographers, had, during his travels the world over, studied the arts and sciences of, *inter alia*, the Arabs, Persians and Indians. After first suffering a shipwreck near the coast of Italy, he arrived at Salerno in southern Italy, having salvaged most of his cargo. Salerno in the eleventh century had a famous medical school known far beyond the Alps, to which people flocked from all over the world – the sick to be healed, and students to study medicine. It is possible that Constantine, after his arrival, could have taught at this school for some years, but after conversion to Christianity, he became a monk and spent the rest of his life at the Abbey of Monte Cassino, where he translated the books that he had salvaged from the shipwreck from Arabic into Latin.[34] At his death, some time before 1099, this merchant-turned-monk had translated at least twenty books into his adopted tongue, among which some works of Hippocrates and Galen that had previously been translated into Arabic. His best-known work is the *Liber Pantegni* ('The whole [medical] art'), a handbook of general medicine written by a famous Arab scholar, Ali ibn al-Abbas al-Majusi. Also influential was his translation of a handbook that in translation has the title *Provision for the traveller and sustenance for the settled* – a *viaticum*; this contains all the basics of medicine (in seven volumes!)

33 According to Green (1985, 47), the Latin medical corpus in the eleventh century 'consisted of a diverse array of writings, mainly on practical matters, manuscripts which furthermore had suffered many corruptions in the course of the transmission'. Numerous Greek medical texts – those of Aristotle, Hippocrates, Galen and Dioscorides, for example – that would otherwise have been lost were, during the eighth and ninth centuries, translated from Greek into Arabic by, *inter alia*, the Christian Nestorians in Syria, and became part of Arab medical theory and practice.

34 Green 2001, 10.

that a traveller or people who did not have a physician nearby needed to know. Several smaller works on specialized subjects also survive, covering diets, fevers, urines, leprosy, melancholy and even sexual intercourse. Like the work of his Roman North African predecessors, Constantine's works are not mere translations; he had to adapt the medical information from the original Arabic sources in a way that was relevant and accessible to his European readers.[35]

Constantine was one of a number of translators of Arabic texts into Latin during the eleventh, twelfth and thirteenth centuries: the Spanish scholar L. M. A. Cambra identifies schools of translation in, *inter alia*, North West Africa, Sicily and Spain.[36] These translations were of immense value to Roman medicine and to Western science in general. Many of the works translated by Constantine became 'the core of medical instruction and practice for the next four generations'.[37] Green adds that the transmission of Arab knowledge by way of these translations was 'an achievement whose later ramifications for Western science and medicine have still not been fully assessed'.[38]

Conclusion

Although the history of Roman North Africa ends on a dismal note, the fall of Carthage did not signify the end of the civilized world. The fact that Constantine was an erudite man, and that his shipment did not contain the usual drugs and spices but learned books, affirms that Kairouan, where he probably studied medicine, was an important centre of Islamic scholarship and learning.[39] Susan Raven's remark that North Africa would flourish again after the fall of Carthage, 'but not in a Roman way', is thus verified by the (Arabic) provenance of the immense (medical) contribution of Constantine the African.[40]

35 Green 1990.

36 Cambra (2016, 425) distinguishes three stages in the transmission of the Greek texts: translations from Greek into Arabic, works in Arabic, and translations from Arabic into Latin. Islamic civilization thus acted as an intermediary in the transmission of ancient Greek medical knowledge to western Europe during the Renaissance.

37 Green 1990, 47.

38 Green 1990, 47.

39 McKitterick 2015, 696 states that scholars from all over the world flocked to Kairouan, second only to Mecca and Medina. Kairouan remained the principal holy city even after the political capital had been transferred to Tunis in the twelfth century.

40 Raven 1993, 230.

Bibliography

Primary sources

Augustine

Epistles:

Sancti Aurelii Augustini Epistulae. I-LV pars 3, 1. Kl.-D. Daur (ed.). 2004. Corpus Christianorum. Series Latina 31. Turnhout.

Sancti Aurelii Augustini Epistulae. LVI-C pars 3, 2. Daur, Kl.-D. (ed.) 2005. Corpus Christianorum. Series Latina 31A. Turnhout.

Sancti Aurelii Augustini Epistulae. CI-CXXXIX pars 3, 3. Daur, Kl.-D. (ed.). 2009. Corpus Christianorum. Series Latina 31B. Turnhout. http://www.augustinus.it/latino/lettere/index2.htm

Sermons. Nuova Biblioteca Agostiniana. Opere di Sant'Agostino, a cura della Cattedra Agostiniana. Vol. 34. Presso l''Agostinianum' di Roma. https://www.augustinus.it/latino/discorsi/index2.htm

City of God: *The city of God against the pagans. In seven volumes.* W. McAllen (ed.). 1972. Loeb Classical Library series. London.

On the soul: www.newadvent.org/fathers/1508.htm

On the Trinity: Sancti Aurelii Augustini De Trinitate libri XV. W. J. Mountain & F. Glorie, F. (eds.). 1968. www.newdvent.org/fathers/1301.htm

On marriage: F. J. Thonnard, E. Bleuzen, A. C. de Veer (eds.). 1974. www.traditionalcatholic.co/tag/augutine-on-marriage

Premières polémiques contre Julien. Œuvres de Saint Augustin 23. Paris. Content: *De nuptiis et concupiscentia; Contra duas epistulas pelagianorum.* www.newadvent.org/fathers/1309.htm

Against Faustus: *Sancti Aureli Augustini De utilitate credendi; De duabus animabus; Contra Fortunatum; Contra Adimantum; Contra epistulam fundamenti; Contra Faustum.* Sect. VI, pars 1. I. Zycha (ed.). 1891. Corpus Scriptorum Ecclesiasticorum Latinorum. Vol. 25. Vienna.

On Christian doctrine: *Sancti Aurelii Augustini De doctrina christiana, De vera religione.* Pars 4,1. J. Martin (ed.). 1962. Corpus Christianorum. Series Latina 32. Turnhout.

De genesi ad litteram: *The literal meaning of Genesis.* J.H. Taylor (transl. and ann.). 1982. New York.

Confessions: *Saint Augustine. Confessions.* H. Chadwick (transl.). 1992.Oxford

Augustinus' Confessiones. *Latijnsche tekst met vertaling.*

Sizoo. 1948. Delft.

Aëtius of Amida: *Tetrabiblon/Libri Medicinales.* A. Olivieri (ed.). 1935. Leipzig, Berlin.

Anonymous: The *expositio totius mundi et gentium.* J. E. Woodman (transl.). MA Thesis. 1964. The Ohio State University.

Apuleius. *The Apologia and Florida.* C. P. Jones (transl.) Loeb Classical Library, 2010. London.

Caelius Aurelianus:

Acute diseases and *Chronic diseases*

Ein Brüchstück des Caelius Aurelianus. V. Rose, V. 1870. *Hermes* 4, 141–144.

Celeres passiones, Akute Krankheiten. Buch I-III; *Tardae passions, Chronisches Krankheiten.* Buch I–V. G. Bendz (ed.). 1990–1993. Übersetz von I. Pape. Corpus Medicorum Latinorum VI.I. Berlin.

Caelius Aurelianus on acute diseases and on chronic diseases. I. E. Drabkin (ed. & transl.). 1950. London.

Caelius Aurelianus 607. K.-D. Fischer 2019. In: R. Herzog & P. L. Schmidt (eds.). *Handbuch der lateinischen Literatur.* Bd. VI. Munich.

Gynaecia: Caelius Aurelianus. Gynaecia. *Fragments of a Latin version of Soranus'* Gynaecia *from a 13th-century manuscript.* M. F. Drabkin & I. E. Drabkin (eds.). 1951. Baltimore.

Medicinalium responsionum libri. In: V. Rose (ed.). *Anecdota Graeca et Graecolatina* II, pp. 163–260.

Cassiodorus. *Cassiodorus. Variae.* S. J. B. Barnish (ed.). 1992. Liverpool.

Cassius Felix. *Cassius Felix. De la Médicine.* A. Fraisse (transl. & comm.). 2002. Paris.

Codex Iustinianus. *The Codex of Justinian. A new annotated translation with parallel Latin and Greek text.* B. W. Frier (ed.). 2016. Cambridge

Codex Theodosianus. *The Theodosian Code and Novels.* C. Pharr *et al.* (ed. and transl.). 1952. Pennsylvania.

Cyprian. *De mortalitate.* In: P. Campbell (ed.). *The complete works of Saint Cyprian of Carthage.* 2013. Merchantville, NJ.

Dioscorides. *Pedanius Dioscorides of Anazarbus. De materia medica.* Beck, L. (transl.). 2005. Hildesheim, Zürich, New York.

Fontes Iuris Romani ante-Iustiniani. S. Riccobono *et al.* (eds. & transl.). 1968. Florence.

Fracastoro. *De contagione, contagiis morbis et eorum curatione Libri III.* In: *Hieronymus Fracastorius. Contagion, contagious diseases and their treatment.* W. C. Wright (transl.). 1930. New York.

Galen: Kühn, C. G. 1821–1833 (reprint Hildesheim 1964–1965). *Claudii Galeni Opera Omnia I-XX.* Leipzig.

On sects for beginners. Vol. I.

On the anatomy of the uterus. Vol. II.

Anatomical Procedures. Vol. II.

On bones for beginners. Vol. II.

On the utility of the parts. Vol. III.

On the construction of the embryo. Vol. IV.

On plenitude. Vol. VII.

On the cause of diseases. Vol. VII.

On the pulse for beginners. Vol. VIII.

On the therapeutic method. Vol. X.

On the method of healing. Vol. X.

On the powers of simple drugs. Vol. XII.

On the composition of drugs according to kind. Vol. XIII.

On the composition of drugs according to places. Vol. XII and Vol. XIII.

On prognosis. Vol XIV.

Antidotes. Vol. XIV.

On easily available remedies. Vol. XIV.

Commentary on Hippocrates' On the nature of man. Vol. XV.

On my own books. Vol. XIX

The best doctor is also a philosopher. In: P. N. Singer (transl.). 1997. *Galen. Selected works.* Oxford, pp. 30–34.

On habits. 1941. Leipzig.

De semine. P. De Lacy (ed., transl. & comm.). 1992. Corpus Medicorum Graecorum V.3.1. Berlin.

On examinations by which the best physicians are recognized. A. Z. Iskandar (transl. & comm.). 1988. Berlin.

Gargilius Martialis. B. Maire (ed., transl. with comm.). *Gargilius. Les remedies tirés des legumes et des fruits*. 2002. Budé, Paris.
Hippocrates. *The Hippocratic Treatises 'On Generation,' 'On the Nature of the Child' and 'Diseases IV'.* I..M. Lonie (ed. & transl.). 1981. Berlin, New York.
Homer. *The Odyssey*. R. Fagles (transl.). 1996. Penguin Books.
Isidore of Seville. *The Etymologies of Isidore of Seville*. S..A. Barney, W..J. Lewis, J..A. Beach, O. Berghof (transl.). 2006. Cambridge.
Jerome. *Select Letters*. F..A. Wright (transl.) 1933. Loeb Classical Library. Cambridge, Mass.
Jordanes. *The origin and deeds of the Goths*. C. Mierow (transl.). http://wikipedia.org/wiki/goths
Justinian. *The Digest or Pandects of Justinian*. See Codex Justinianus above.
Juvenal. *Satires*. S. M. Braund (transl.) 2004. Loeb Classical Library. Cambridge, Mass.
Livy. *The war with Hannibal*. A. de Sélincourt (transl.). 1965. Penguin Classics.
Marcellus. *Marcellus über Heilmittel*. M. Niedermann, E. Lichtenhan, J. Kollesch & D. Nickel (eds.). 1968. Corpus Medicorum Latinorum V. Berlin.
Muscio/Mustio. *Gynaecia* Muscionis ex Graecis Sorani in Latinum translata sermonem. In: V. Rose (ed.). 1882. *Sorani gynaeciorum vetus translatio Latina*. Leipzig.
Nicander. *Nicander. The poems and poetical fragments*. A. S. Gow & A. F. Scholfield (ed., transl. & notes). 1953. Cambridge.
Oribasius. *Oribasius. Synopsis*. Vols. V and VI. A. Molinier (ed.). In: U. Bussemaker & C. Daremberg. *Oeuvres d'Oribase*. 1873–1876. Paris.
Oribasius. *Letter to Eunapius*. CMG VI.3. 1926 Leipzig.
Oribasius. *Oribasii collectionum medicorum reliquiae*. CMG 6.1–2. J. Raeder (ed.). 1928–1933.
Paul of Aegina. *The seven books of Paulus Aegineta*. F. Adams (transl.). 1844–1847.
Pontius Diaconus of Carthage. *Life of and passion of Cyprian, bishop and martyr*. R. E. Wallis (transl.). In: *Ante-Nicene Fathers*. Vol. 5. A. Roberts, J. Donaldson, A. Coxe (eds.). 1886. Buffalo, NY.
Procopius. *History of the Vandal War*. H. B. Dewing (transl.). 1916. Loeb Classical Library. Cambridge Mass.
Rufus Ephesius. Medicus gratiosus. Haak. H. L. 2013. Leiden.
Rufus of Ephesus. *Rufus d'Ephese. Du nom des parties du corps humain*. Ch. Daremberg & Ch. E. Ruelle (eds. & transl.). 1879. Paris.
Salvian. *On the government of God*. E..M. Sanford (transl.). 1930. New York.
Scribonius Largus. *Scribonii Largi Compositiones*. S. Sconnochia, (ed. & comm.). 1983. Leipzig.
Sextus Aurelius Victor. *Epitome de Caesaribus*. T. M. Banchich (transl.). 2000. Buffalo, NY.
Silius Italicus. *Punica*. J. D. Duff (transl.). 1934. Loeb Classical Library. Cambridge, Mass.
Soranus. *Soranus' Gynecology*. O.Temkin (transl., comm.). 1956. Baltimore, London.
St. Cyprian. *Epistles*. In: *The complete works of Saint Cyprian of Carthage*. P. Campbell (ed.). 2013. Merchantville, NJ.
Strabo. *The geography of Strabo. An English translation with introduction and notes*. D. W. Roller (ed.). 2014. Cambridge.
Tertullian. *Tertullian. De anima*. Waszink, J. H. (ed. & comm.). 1947. Amsterdam.
Tertullian. *Ad nationes*: www.tertullian.works_nationes.htm
The Digest or Pandects of Justinian. See Codex Iustinianus above.
Theodorus Priscianus. *Theodori Prisciani Euporiston libri tres. Cum Physicorum fragmenta et additamenta Pseudo-Theodoreis. Accedunt Vindiciani Afriquae feruntur reliquiae*. Rose, V. (ed.). 1894. Leipzig.
Thessalus of Tralles. *Thessalus of Tralles*. H. Friedrich (transl.). 1968. Meisenheim am Glan, Hain.
Trotula. *On womens'diseases. A medieval compendium of womens' medicine*. M. H. Green (ed. & transl.). *The 'Trotula'*. 2001. Philadelphia: University of Pennsylvania Press.

Ulpian. In: *The Digest or Pandects of Justinian*. 1985. See Codex Iustinianus above.
Victor of Vita. *History of the Vandal Persecution*. J. Moorhead (transl.). 1992. Liverpool.
Vindicianus:
Gynaecia. Vindicianus's *Gynaecia*. text and translation of the Codex Monacensis (Clm 4622). L. Cilliers (transl. & comm.). 2005. *The Journal of Medieval Latin* 15, 153–236.
Ein deutscher anatomischer Vindiciantext. C. Ferckel. 1914. *ZWG* 7, 306–318.
Theodori Prisciani Euporiston libri III accedunt Vindiciani Afri quae feruntur reliquae. V. Rose (ed.). 1894. Leipzig.
Ein neuer Text der Gynaecia *des Vindician aus einer Münchener Handschrift des 12. Jahrhunderts* (*Cod. Lat. 4622, Blatt 40–45*). Schipper, J. 1921. Erlangen. Diss. Med. Leipzig.
Letter to Pentadius. *Die* Epistula Vindiciani ad Pentadium nepotem *und ihre Einordnung in die Geschichte der Humoraltheorien*. M. Schoch. 1996. Inaugural-Dissertation, Würzburg.
Letter to the emperor Valentinian. In: M. Niedermann & E. Liechtenhan. *Marcellus. Über Heilmittel*. 1968. Berlin, pp. 46–52.

Secondary studies

Adair, M. J. 1996. Plato's view of the 'wandering uterus'. *The Classical Journal* 91.2, 153–163.
Adam, F. 1856. *The extant works of Aretaeus, the Cappadocian*. London.
Allan, N. 1990. Hospice to hospital in the Near East, an instance of continuity and change in late antiquity. *Bull. Hist. Med.* 64, 447–450.
Avalos, H. 1999. *Health care and the rise of Christianity*. Peabody, Mass.
Arbesmann, R. 1954. The concept of 'Christus Medicus' in St. Augustine. *Tradition* 10, 1–28.
Boyce, J. 2014. *Born bad. Original sin and the making of the Western World*. Collingwood, Australia.
Baader, G. 1991. Der Hebammenkatechismus des Muscio – ein Zeugnis frühmittelalterlicher Geburtshilfe. In: N. Affeldt (ed.). *Frauen in Spätantike und Frühmittelalter. Lebensbedingungen, Lebensnormen, Lebensformen*. Sigmaringen, pp. 115–125.
Bascombe. E. 1851/2013. *A History of epidemic pestilences*. London.
Beck, L. Y. (ed. and transl.) 2005. *Pedanius Dioscorides of Anazarbus. De materia medica*. Hildesheim, Zürich, New York.
Becker, C. 1967. Der Octavius des Minucius Felix. In: *Realencyclopaedie der Altertumswissenschaft* Suppl. II, 952 ff.
Benseddik, N. 1988. La pratique médicale en Afrique au temps d'Augustin. *Atti de VI Convegna di Studio Africa Romana*. Sassari, pp. 663–682.
Beschaouch, A. 1968. *Mustitana. Recueil des nouvelles inscriptions de Mustis, cité Romaine de Tunisie*, Tome I. Paris. In: *Karthago* XIII (1965–66), pp. 117–224.
Birley, A. R. 1996. Septimius Severus. In: Hornblower & Spawforth 1996, pp. 1390–1391.
Blowers, P. M. 2009. Pity, empathy and the tragic spectacle of human suffering. Exploring the emotional culture of compassion in late ancient Christianity. *Journal of Early Christian Studies* 18.1, 1–27.
Boak, A. E. R. & Sinnigen, W. R. 1977. *A history of Rome to 565 A.D.* Sixth edition. New York.
Boyce Gibson, W. R. 1924. Problems of spiritual experience. III. Love. The ideal and the one. *Australasian Journal of Psychology and Philosophy* 2.4, 258–271.
Brett, M. & Fentress, E. 1996. *The Berbers*. Oxford.
Brown, P. 2000. *Augustine of Hippo*. New edition with Epilogue. Paperback. Oakland, CA.
Brown, P. 2012. *Through the eye of a needle. Wealth, the fall of Rome, and the making of Christianity in the West, 350–550 AD*. Princeton, Oxford.
Bujan, M. E. V. 1982. Vindiciano y el tratado *De natura generis humani*. *Dynamis*, 25–56.

Cadden, J. 1993. *Meanings of sex difference in the Middle Ages. Medicine, science and culture.* Cambridge.

Cambra, L. M. A. 2016. The intermediary role of the Arabs during the Middle Ages in the transmission of ancient scientific knowledge to Europe. *International Journal of Innovative Science and Technology* 3.3, 422–426.

Cameron, A. 1993/2012. *The Mediterranean world in late Antiquity AD 395–700.* Second Edition. London, New York.

Cameron, A. 2011. *The last pagans of Rome.* Oxford.

Canizares, P. P. 2010. The importance of having medical knowledge as a layman. The Hippocratic treatise *Affections* in the context of the Hippocratic Corpus. In: Horstmanshoff 2010, pp. 87–99.

Cilliers, L. 2007. Some thoughts on the demise of Roman influence in North Africa, 5th/6th century AD. *Akroterion* 52, 37–48.

Cilliers, L. 2008. Roman North Africa in the 4th century AD. Its role in the preservation and transmission of medical knowledge. In: L. Cilliers (ed.). *Asklepios. Studies in Ancient Medicine.* Acta Classica Supplement. II, pp. 49–63.

Cilliers, L. 2010. The didactic letters prefacing Marcellus' *On Drugs* as evidence for the expertise and reputation of doctors in the late Roman Empire. In: Horstmanshoff 2010, pp. 401–418.

Cilliers, L. 2014. The contribution of the 4th century AD North African physician, Helvius Vindicianus. In: D. Michaelides (ed.). *Medicine and healing in the ancient Mediterranean world.* Oxford, Philadelphia, pp. 122–128.

Cilliers, L. & Retief, F. P. 1999. Die rol van die vrou in die antieke Geneeskunde (The role of women in ancient medical science). *Acta Classica* 42, 47–65.

Cilliers, L. & Retief, F. P. 2002. The evolution of hospitals from antiquity to the Renaissance. *Curationis* 25.4, 60–66.

Cilliers, L. & Retief, F. P. 2006. City planning in Graeco-Roman times with emphasis on health facilities. *Akroterion* 51, 43–57.

Cilliers, L. & Retief, F. P. 2013. Dream healing in the Asklepieia in the Mediterranean. In: S. Oberhelman (ed.). *Dreams, healing and medicine in Greece from antiquity to the present.* Burlington, pp. 69–92.

Coulmas, F. 2014. *The Blackwell Encyclopedia of writing systems.* Oxford.

Courtois, C. 1955. *Les Vandales et l'Afrique.* Paris.

Craik, E. M. 2006. *Two Hippocratic treatises.* On sight *and* On anatomy. Leiden, Boston.

Craik, R. 2010. The teaching of surgery. In: Horstmanshoff 2010, pp. 223–234.

Crawford, R. 1914. *Plague and pestilence in literature and art.* Oxford.

De Labriolle, P. 1924/1968. *The history and literature of Christianity from Tertullian to Boethius.* London.

Deichgräber, K. 1934. Theodoros 46. In: *Reallexikon der Altertumswissenschaft.* Vol. V A, pp. 1866–1868.

Dennis, Holmes van Mater. 1970. *Hippo Regius. From the earliest times to the Arab conquest.* Amsterdam.

Diepgen, P. 1937. *Die Frauenheilkunde der alten Welt.* Munich.

Drabkin, I. E. 1944. On medical education in Greece and Rome. *Bulletin of the history of medicine* 15, 246–247.

Dunbabin, K. M. D. 1978. *The mosaics of Roman North Africa. Studies in iconography and patronage.* Oxford.

Edelstein, E. J. & Edelstein, L. 1945/1998. Vol II. *Asclepius. Collection and interpretation of the testimonies.* Baltimore, London.

Edelstein, L. 1967a. The Hippocratic Oath. Text, translation and interpretation. In: O. and C. L. Temkin 1967, pp. 4–63.

Edelstein, L. 1967b. The history of anatomy in antiquity. In: O. & C. L. Temkin 1967, pp. 247–302.
Edelstein, L. 1967r. The Methodists. In: O & C. L. Temkin 1967, pp. 173–194.
Edelstein, L. 1967d. The relation of ancient medicine to philosophy. In: O. and C. L. Temkin 1967, pp. 349–366.
Edwards, J. 2000. *The mystery of the imperial dyes*. Historical Dye Series no. 7. J. M. Castagno (ed.). *Encyclopedia Americana*. Vol. III.
El-Abbadi, Mostafa A. & Omnia M. Fathallah (eds.). 2008. *What happened to the ancient library of Alexandria?* Leiden, Boston.
Ennabli, E. A. 1992. *Pour sauver Carthage. Exploration et conservation de la cité punique, romaine et byzantine*. Tunis.
Ensslin, W. & Deichgräber, K. 1961.Vindicianus. G. Wissowa (ed.). *Paulys Realencycläpedie der classischen Altertumswissenschaf*Vol. IX A.1. Stuttgart, pp. 29–36. .
Fentress, E. 2006. Romanizing the Berbers. *Past and Present* 190, 3–34.
Ferngren, G. B. & Amundsen, D. W. 1996. Medicine and Christianity in the Roman Empire. Compatibilities and tensions. In: W. Haase (ed.). *Aufstieg und Niedergang der römischen Welt. Geschichte und Kultur im Spiegel der neueren Forschung*. Vol. II. 37.3. Berlin, pp. 2957–2979.
Ferngren, G. B. 2009. *Medicine and health care in early Christianity*. Baltimore.
Fiorucci, F. 2011. Elvio Vindiciano. Pagano o Cristiano? *Giornale Italiano di Filologia* 2, 225–235.
Fiorucci, F. 2009. Osservazioni sulla Epistula ad Pentadium. *Appunti Romani di Filologia* 11, 67–90.
Fiorucci, F. 2012. Elvio Vindiciano. Aspetti storici. *Klio* 94, 482–497.
Fischer, K.-D. 1998a. Beiträge zu den pseudosoranischen *Questiones Medicinales*. In: K.-D. Fischer, D. Nickel & P. Potter (eds.). *Text and tradition. Studies in ancient medicine and its transmission. Presented to Jutta Kollesch*. Leiden, pp. 1–54.
Fischer, K.-D. 1998b. Der *Liber Byzantii*. Ein unveröffentliches griechisches therapeutisches Handbuch in lateinischer Übersetzung. In: C. Deroux (ed.). *Maladie et maladies dans les textes latins antiques et médiévaux. Revue d'Etudes Latines*, pp. 276–294.
Fischer, K.-D. 1999. Bisher unberücksichtigte Handschriftenfunde zur Überlieferung der Werke des Caelius Aurelianus. In: Ph. Mudry, O. Bianchi D. Castaldo (eds.). *Le traité des* Maladies aiguës *et des* Maladies chroniques *de Caelius Aurelianus. Nouvelles approaches*. Nantes.
Fischer, K.-D. 2019. Caelius Aurelianus. In: P. L. Schmidt (ed.). *Handbuch der lateinische Literatur*. Vol. VI.607.5. Munich.
Fischer, K.-D. 2019. Theodorus Priscianus. In: P.L. Schmidt (ed.). *Handbuch der lateinische Literatur*. Vol. VI.607.5. Munich.
Flemming, R. 2000. *Medicine and the making of Roman women. Gender, nature, and authority from Celsus to Galen*. Oxford.
Flemming, R. 2007. Women, writing and medicine in the Classical World. *Classical Quarterly* 57.1, 257–279.
Forbes, R. J. 1955. *Studies in ancient technology*. Leiden.
Formisano, M. 2004. The 'natural' medicine of Theodorus Priscianus. Between tradition and innovation. *Philologus* 148, 126–142.
Fraisse, A. 2002. *Cassius Felix. De la médicine*. Paris.
Frank, T. (ed.). 1938/1975. *An economic survey of ancient Rome*. Baltimore.
Frend, W. H. C. 1952. *The Donatist church. A movement of protest in Roman North Africa*. Oxford.
Gagarin, M. (ed.). 2010. *The Oxford Encyclopedia of ancient Greece and Rome*. Oxford.
George, J. W. 2004. Vandal poets in their context. In: Merrills 2004a, pp. 133–144.
Gibbon, E. 1776, repr. 1909 and 1974. *The rise and fall of the Roman Empire*. London.
Goodall, W. 1933. On infectious diseases and epidemiology in the Hippocratic Collection. *History of Medicine* 1, 533.

Gourevitch, D. 1975. La gynécologie et l'obstétrique. In: H. Temporini (ed.). *Aufstieg und Niedergang der römischen Welt. Geschichte und Kultur im Spiegel der neueren Forschung.* Vol. II.37.3. Berlin, pp. 2084–2146.

Gourevitch, D. 1984. *Le mal d'être femme. La femme et la médicine dans la Rome antique.* Paris.

Gourevitch, D. 1991. La pratique méthodique. Definition de la maladie, indication et traitement. In: P. Mudry & J. Pigeaud (eds.). *Les écoles médicales à Rome.* Genève, pp. 57–82.

Gourevitch, D. 1998. The paths of knowledge. Medicine in the Roman world. In: Grmek 1998, pp. 104–138.

Graham, A. 1902. *Roman Africa. An outline of the history of the Roman occupation of North Africa.* New York.

Green, M. 1985. *The transmission of ancient theories of female physiology and disease through the early Middle Ages.* Unpublished dissertation, Princeton University. Ann Arbor, Mich.

Green, M. 1990. Constantinus Africanus and the conflict between religion and science. In: G. R. Dunstan (ed.). *The human embryo. Aristotle and the Arabic and European traditions.* Exeter, pp. 47–75.

Green, M. 2000. From 'Diseases of women' to 'Secrets of women'. The transformation of gynecological literature in the later Middle Ages. In: *Women's healthcare in the medieval West. Texts and contexts.* Ashgate.

Green, M. (ed. and transl.). 2001. *The Trotula. An English translation of the medieval compendium of women's medicine.* Philadelphia.

Grmek, M. D. 1984. Les vicissitudes des notions d'infection, de contagion et de germe dans la médicine antique. In: *Mémoires V. Textes médicaux latins antiques.* Université Saint-Etienne, pp. 53–70.

Grmek. M. D. & Gourevitch. D. 1988. L'école médicale de Quintus et de Numesianus, *Mémoires du Centre Jean-Palerme* 8, 43–60.

Grmek, M. D. 1989. *Diseases in the ancient Greek world.* M. & L. Muellner (transl.). Baltimore, London.

Grmek, M. D. 1998. *Western medical thought from Antiquity to the Middle Ages.* Cambridge, Mass.

Gruen, E. S. 2006. Romans and Others. In: N. Rosenstein & R. Morstein-Marx (eds.). *A Companion to the Roman Republic.* Hoboken, NJ, pp. 459–477.

Hansen, E. (ed.). 2005. *Groot Studiebybel.* Kaapstad/Capetown.

Hanson, A. 1991. Continuity and change. Three case studies in Hippocratic gynecological therapy and theory. In: S. B. Pomeroy (ed.). *Women's history and ancient history.* Chapel Hill, London, pp. 73–110.

Hanson, A. 1992. Conception, gestation and the origin of female nature in the *Corpus Hippocraticum. Helios* 19, 31–71.

Hanson, A. 2010. Doctors' literacy and papyri of medical content. In: Horstmanshoff 2010, pp. 187–204.

Hanson, A. & Green, M. 1996. Soranus of Ephesus. *Methodicorum Princeps.* In: W. Haase (ed.). *Aufstieg und Niedergang der römischen Welt. Geschichte und Kultur im Spiegel der neueren Forschung.* Vol. II.37.2. Berlin, New York, pp. 968–1075.

Harrison, S. 1996. Apuleius. In: Hornblower & Spawforth 1996, pp. 131–132.

Hays, G. 2004. 'Romuleis Libicisque litteris': Fulgentius and the 'Vandal renaissance'. In: Merrills 2004a, pp. 101–132.

Heather, P. 2005. *The fall of the Roman Empire. A new history.* London.

Hemingway, C. & S. 2000. Ancient Greek colonization and trade and their influence on Greek art. In: *Heilbrunn Timeline of Art History.* New York.

Hodge, A. T. 1992. *Roman aqueducts and water supply.* London.

Honoré, T. 1996. Salvius Iulianus. In: Hornblower & Spawforth 1996, p. 778.

Hopkins, K. 1965. Contraception in the Roman World. *Comparative Studies in Society and History* 8, 124–151.

Hornblower, S. & Spawforth, A. (eds.). 1996. *The Oxford Classical Dictionary.* Third Edition. Oxford, New York.

Horstmanshoff, H. F. J. 1995. Galen and his patients. In: Ph. J. Van der Eijk, H. F. J. Horstmanshoff, P. H. Schrijvers (eds.). *Ancient medicine in its socio-cultural context* Vol. I. Amsterdam, Atlanta, pp. 83–99.

Horstmanshoff, M. 1999. Les émotions chez Caelius Aurelianus. In: Ph. Mudry, O. Bianchi. D. Castaldo (eds.). *Le traité des maladies aiguës* et *des maladies chronique de Caelius Aurelianus. Nouvelles approches.* Nantes, pp. 259–290.

Horstmanshoff, H. F. J. & Van Everdingen, J. J. E. 2003. *De eed van Hippokrates.* Alphen aan den Rijn.

Horstmanshoff, M. (ed.). 2010. *Hippocrates and medical education. Selected papers read at the XIIth International Hippocrates Colloquium.* University of Leiden. Leiden, Boston.

Horstmanshoff, Manfred & Rosen, Ralph M. 2003. The *andreia* of the Hippocratic physician and the problem of incurables. In: Rosen, R. M. & Sluiter, I. (eds.). *Andreia. Studies in manliness and courage in Classical Antiquity. Mnemosyne* Suppl. 238. Leiden, pp. 95–114.

Isichei, E. 1995. *A history of Christianity in Africa from antiquity to the present.* Grand Rapids Mich.

Iskandar, A. Z. 1976. An attempted reconstruction of the late Alexandrian medical curriculum. *Medical History* 2.3, 235–258.

Israelowich, I. 2015. *Patients and healers in the high Empire.* Baltimore.

Jackson, R. 1988. *Doctors and diseases in the Roman Empire.* Norman, London.

Jones, A. H. M. 1964. (Vol. I) and 1973 (Vol. II). *The later Roman Empire 284–602. A social, economic and administrative survey.* Oxford.

Jones, W. H. S. 1957. Ancient Roman folk medicine. *Journal of the History of Medicine and Allied Sciences* 12, 459–472.

Jouanna, J. 1999. *Hippocrates.* M. B. DeBevoise (transl.). Baltimore, London.

Jouanna, J. 2005. La théorie des quatre humeurs et des quatre tempéraments dans la tradition latine (Vindicien, Pseudo-Soranos) et une source retrouvée. *Revue des études grecque* 118, 138–167.

Jouanna, J. 2006. Le postérité du traité hippocratique de la *Nature de l'homme.* La théorie des quatre humeurs. In: W. von C. Müller, C. Brockmann, C. W. Brunschön (eds.). *Ärzte und ihre Interpreten. Medizinische Fachtexte als Forschungsgegenstand der klassischen Philologie.* Leipzig, pp. 117–142.

Keenan, M. E. 1936. Augustine and the medical profession. *TAPA* 67, 168–190.

Keyser, P. 2008. Pelops (p. 634), Numisianus (p. 584), Quintus (p. 717), Marinus (p. 532), Satyrus (p. 728). In: Keyser, P. T. & Irby-Massie, G. L. (eds.). *The encyclopedia of ancient natural scientists. The Greek tradition and its many heirs.* London, New York.

King, H. 1995. Medical texts as a source for women's history. In: A. Powell (ed.). *The Greek World.* London, pp. 199–218.

King, H. 1998. *Hippocrates' woman. Reading the female body in ancient Greece.* London, New York.

Kollesch, J. 1966. Therapeuthische Grundsätze im Werk des Vindician. *NTM. Schriftenreihe für Geschichte der Naturwissenschaften, Technik und Medizin* 3, Heft 7, 27–31.

Korpela, J. 1987. *Das Medizinalpersonal im antiken Rome.* Helsinki.

Kudlien, F. 1970. Medical education in classical antiquity. In: *UCLA Forum in Medical Studies* 12, 3–37.

Kühn, C. G. (ed.). 1821–1833, reprint 1964/5. *Claudii Galeni opera omnia.* Hildesheim.

Kumar, P. & Clark, M. (eds.). 2002. *Clinical Medicine.* Fifth ed. Elsevier Science.

MacKendrick, P. 1980. *The North African stones speak.* London.

Laes, C. 2010. The educated midwife in the Roman Empire. An example of differential equations. In: Horstmanshoff 2010, pp. 261–287.

Lancel, S. 1995. *Carthage. A history.* Oxford.

Langslow, D. R. 2000. *Medical Latin in the Roman Empire*. Oxford.

Last, J. M. (ed.). 2007. *A dictionary of public health*. Oxford: Oxford University Press.

Lee, A. D. 2013. *From Rome to Byzantium AD 363 to 565. The transformation of ancient Rome*. Edinburgh.

Legewie, B. 1931. Die körperliche Konstitution und die Krankheiten Augustins. *Miscellanea Agostiniana* II. Rome, pp. 5–21.

Lennox Manton, E. 1988. *Roman North Africa*. London.

Leone, A. 2007. Changing townscapes in North Africa from late Antiquity to the Arab conquest. *Munera* 28. Bari.

Lepelley, C. 1979. *Les cités de l'Afrique romaine au bas-empire. Tome I. La permanence d'une civilisation municipale*. Paris.

Lepelley, C. 1981. *Les cités de l'Afrique romaine au bas-empire. Tome II. La permanence d'une civilisation municipale*. Paris.

Lepelley, C. 2001. The survival and fall of the Classical city in late Roman Africa. In: *Aspects de l'Afrique Romaine. Les cités, la vie rurale, le Christianisme*. Bari.

Leven, K.-H. 2010. Athumia and philanthropia. Social reactions to plagues in late antiquity and early Byzantine society. In: Horstmanshoff 2010, pp. 393–407.

Liddell, H. G., Scott, R., Jones, H. S., 1953. *A Greek-English Lexicon*.

Lloyd, G. E. R. 1962. Right and left in Greek philosophy. *Journal of Hellenic Studies* 82, 56–66.

Lloyd, G. E. R. 1979. *Magic, reason and experience. Studies in the origins and development of Greek science*. Indianapolis, Cambridge.

MacDonald, A. H. 1996. Aurelius Victor. In: Hornblower & Spawforth 1996, p. 222.

MacKendrick, P. 1980. *The North Africa stones speak*. London.

Maire, B. 2001. *Gynaecia* Muscionis. Réincarnation des *Gynaikeia* des Soranos ou naissance d'un traité? In V. Dasen (ed.). *Naissance et petite enfance dans l'Antiquité*. Göttingen.

Maire, B. 2002. Le triangle méthodique. Soranos, Caelius Aurelianus et Mustio. In: N. Palmieri (ed.). *Rationel et irrationel dans la médicine ancienne et médiévale*. Mémoires XXVI. Saint-Étienne, pp. 215–230.

Manton, L. E. 1988. *Roman North Africa*. London.

Marasco, G. 1998. I medici di corte nell' Impero Romano. Prosopografia e ruolo culturale. *Prometheus* 24: 243–263.

Marasco, G. 2000. *Littérature et réalité dans l'oeuvre de Vindician*. Actes du VIe colloque international sur les textes médicaux latins du 1er au 3 Septembre 1998 à Nantes.

Marasco, G. 2010. The curriculum of studies in the Roman Empire and the cultural role of physicians. In: Horstmanshoff 2010, pp. 205–222.

Mattern, S. P. 2008. *Galen and the rhetoric of healing*. Baltimore.

Matthews, J. 1975. *Western aristocracies and imperial court AD 364–425*. Oxford.

Matthews, J. F. 1996a. Manichaeism. In: Hornblower & Spawforth, p. 917.

Matthews, J. F. 1996b. Cyprian. In Hornblower & Spawforth, p. 419.

Mattingly, D. J. & Hitchner, R. B. 1995. Roman Africa. An archaeological review. *Journal of Roman Studies* 85, 165–213.

McKitterick, R. (ed.). 2015. *The New Cambridge Medical History, r. 700–r. 900*. Vol. 2. Cambridge.

Meijer, F. J. 1984. Cato's African Figs. *Mnemosyne* 37, 117–124.

Merrills, A. H. (ed.). 2004a. *Vandals, Romans and Berbers. New perspectives on late antique North Africa*. Vermont.

Merrills, A. H. 2004b. Vandals, Romans and Berbers. Understanding Late Antique North Africa. In: Merrills 2004a, pp. 3–28.

Meyer-Steinegg, Th. 1909. *Theodorus Priscianus und die römische Medizin*. Jena.

Migliorini, P. 1991. Elementi metodi in Teodoro Prisciano. Les ecoles médicales à Rome. In: *Actes du 2ème Colloque international sur les textes médicaux latins antiques.* Lausanne 1986. Published Conference Proceedings. Geneva, pp. 232–240.
Miller, G. L. 1990. Literacy and the Hippocratic art. Reading, writing and epistemology in ancient Greek medicine. *Journal of the History of Medicine and Allied Sciences* 45, 11–40.
Mudry, P. 2006a. Caelius Aurelianus ou l'anti-romain. Un aspect particulier du traité des Maladies aigués et des Maladies chronique. In: *Medicina, Soror Philosophiae.* Lausanne, pp. 179–192.
Mudry, P. 2006b. Sur l'étiologie des maladies attribueés à Hippocrate par Celse. *De Medicina*, pref. 15. In: *Medicina, Soror Philosophiae.* Lausanne, pp. 483–489.
Mumford, L. *The city in the Greek and Roman world.* London, New York.
Niedermann, M. & Liechtenhan, E. 1968. *Marcellus. Über Heilmittel.* Berlin.
Nutton, V. 1971. Two notes on immunities. *Journal of Roman Studies* 61, 52–63.
Nutton, V. 1972. Ammianus and Alexandria. *Journal of Roman Studies* 7, 165–176.
Nutton, V. 1977. Archiatri and the medical profession in antiquity. *PBSR* 45, 191–226.
Nutton, V. 1983. The seeds of disease. An explanation of contagion and infection. *Medical History* 17, 1–34.
Nutton, V. 1984a. From Galen to Alexander. Aspects of medicine and medical practice in Late Antiquity. In: J. Scarborough (ed.). *Dumbarton Oaks Papers* 38, 1–13.
Nutton, V. 1984b. Galen in the eyes of his contemporaries. *Bulletin of the History of Medicine* 58, 315–324.
Nutton, V. 1988a. The perils of patriotism. Pliny and Roman medicine. In: V. Nutton. *From Democedes to Harvey. Studies in the History of Medicine.* Variorum Reprints, VII. London, pp. 30–58.
Nutton, V. 1988b. Murders and miracles. Lay attitudes to medicine in classical antiquity. In: Nutton 1988a, VIII.23–52.
Nutton, V. 1988r. Archiatri and the medical profession in antiquity. In: Nutton 1988a, pp. 191–226.
Nutton, V. 1988d. Continuity or rediscovery. The city physician in Classical antiquity and medieval Italy. In: Nutton 1988a, VI, pp. 9–46.
Nutton, V. 1997. Cassius Felix. In: H. Cancik & H, Schneider (eds.). *Der neue Pauly.* Vol. II, 4. Chicago, p. 1016.
Nutton, V. 1998. To kill or not to kill. Caelius Aurelianus on contagion. In: K.-D. Fischer, D. Nickel, P. Potter (eds.). *Text and tradition.* Leiden, pp. 233–242.
Nutton, V. 2000. Did the Greeks have a word for it? Contagion and contagion theory in Classical Antiquity. In: L. I. Conrad and D. Wujastyk (eds.). *Contagion. Perspectives from pre-modern Societies.* Burlington.
Nutton, V. 2004, second edition 2013. *Ancient Medicine.* London, New York.
Ogilvie, R. M. 1980. *Roman literature and society.* London.
Önnerfors, A. 1993. Das medisinische Latein von Celsus bis Cassius Felix. In: H. Temporini (ed.). *Aufstieg und Niedergang der römischen Welt.* Vol. II. 37.1: 227–392.
Oser-Grote, 2005. Ätiologie. In: K.-H. Leven, *Antike Medizin. Ein Lexikon.* Munich, pp. 17–19.
Paoli, U. E. 1963. *Rome. Its people, life and customs.* Bristol.
Pigeaud, J. 1982. Pro Caelio Aureliano. In: *Médecins et médecine dans l'Antiquité.* Mémoires 3. Saint Étienne, pp. 105–117.
Pohl, W. 2004. The Vandals. Fragments of a narrative. In: Merrills 2004a, pp. 31–48.
Pormann, P. E. 2008. Paulos of Aegina. In: Keyser & Irby-Massie 2008, p. 629.
Pormann, P. E. 2010. Medical education in late antiquity. From Alexandria to Montpelier. In: Horstmanshoff 2010, pp. 419–442.
Porter, A. J. 2016. Compassion in Soranus' *Gynecology* and Caelius Aurelianus' *On Chronic Diseases.* In: *Homo Patiens. Approaches to the patient in the ancient world.* G. Petridou and C. Thumiger (eds.). Leiden, Boston, pp. 285–303.

Power, K. 1999. Family, relatives. In: A. D. Fitzgerald (ed.). *Augustine through the ages. An Encyclopedia.* Grand Rapids, pp. 353–355.

Quilici, L. 2008. Land Transport. Part 1: Roads and Bridges. In: J. P. Oleson (ed.). *The Oxford handbook of engineering and technology in the Classical world.* New York, Oxford.

Raven, S. 1969 (repr. 1993). *Rome in Africa.* London.

Rebillard, E. 2012. *Christians and their many identities in late antiquity. North Africa 200–450 CE.* Ithaca, London.

Retief, F. P. & Cilliers, L. 1998. The epidemic of Athens, 430–426 BR. *South African Medical Journal* 88, 50–53.

Retief F. P. & Cilliers, L. 2000a. Epidemics of the Roman Empire, 27 BC–AD 476. *South African Medical Journal* 90(3), 267–272.

Retief, F. P. & Cilliers, L. 2000b. Loodvergiftiging in antieke Rome [Lead poisoning in ancient Rome], *Acta Academica* 13.2, 167–184.

Retief, F. P. & Cilliers, L. 2000c. The epidemic of Justinian, A.D. 542. Prelude to the Middle Ages. *Tydskrif vir Geesteswetenskappe* 40.3, 249–254.

Retief, F. P. & Cilliers, L. 2004. Malaria in the Graeco-Roman world. *Acta Classica* 47, 127–138.

Retief F. P. & Cilliers 2006. Periodic pyrexia and malaria in antiquity. *South African Medical Journal* 96.6, 684–688.

Retief, F. P. & Cilliers, L. 2009. Aretaeus of Cappadocia. The forgotten physician. *Acta Academica* 41.3, 23–39.

Retief, F. P. & Cilliers, L. 2009. Melaatsheid in the antieke tyd (Leprosy in antiquity). *Tydskrif vir Natuurwetenskap en Tegnologie* 28.2, 1–11.

Retief, F. P. & Cilliers, L. 2011. The role of Asclepius in the evolution of medicine, *S. A. Tydskrif vir Natuurwetenskap en Tegnologie*, 30.1. Art. # 26.

Riché, P. 1995. *Éducation et culture dans l'Occident barbare VIe–VIIIe siècle.* Éditions du Seuil.

Riddle, J. M. 1987. Folk tradition and folk medicine. Recognition of drugs in Classical Antiquity. In: J. Scarborough (ed.). *Folklore and folk medicine.* Wisconsin, pp. 33–61.

Riddle, J. M. 1991. Oral contraceptives and early-term abortifacients during Classical Antiquity and the Middle Ages. *Past and Present* 132, 3–32.

Riddle, J. M. 1984. Gargilius Martialis as a medical writer. *Journal of the History of Medicine and Allied Sciences* 4, 408–429.

Rose, V. 1894. *Theodori Prisciani Euporiston libri III accedunt Vindiciani Afri quae feruntur reliquae.* Leipzig.

Rosen, R. M. & Horstmanshoff, H. F. J. 2003. *The* andreia *of the Hippocratic physician and the problem of incurables.* Departmental paper, University of Pennsylvania. Retrieved from http:// repository.upenn.edu/classics_papers/10 on 17/11/2017.

Rostovtzeff, M. 1957. *The social and economic history of the Roman Empire.* Second edition. Oxford.

Sabbah, G. 1994. Le *De medicina* de Cassius Felix à la charnière de l'Antiquité et du Haut Moyen Age. In: *Tradición e innovación de la medicina Latina le la Antigüedad y de la Alta Edad Media.* Universidade de Santiago de Compostela.

Sabbah, G. 1998. Notes sur les auteurs médicaux Africains de l'Antiquité Tardive (IVe–Ve siècles). In: P. Colombat & P. Mattei (eds). Recherches et Travaux. *Curiosité historique et intérêts philologiques. Hommage à Serge Lancel.* Grenoble, pp. 131–150.

Sallares, R. 1991. *The ecology of the ancient Greek world.* Ithaca, New York.

Scarborough, J. 1969. *Roman medicine.* London.

Scarborough, J. 2008a. Cassius Felix. In: Keyser & Irby-Massie 2008, pp. 208–209.

Scarborough, J. 2008b. Caelius Aurelianus. In: Keyser & Irby-Massie 2008, pp. 201–202.

Scarborough, J. 2010. The pharmacy of Methodist medicine. The evidence of Soranus' *Gynecology.* In: J. Scarborough. *Pharmacy and drug lore in Antiquity.* Ashgate, pp. 204–216.

Scarborough, J. 2013. Theodora, Aëtius of Amida, and Procopius. Some possible connections. *Greek, Roman and Byzantine Studies* 53.4, 742–762.

Schwartz, A. 2004. The settlement of the Berbers in North Africa. In: Merrills 2004a, pp. 49–58.

Scobie, A. 1986. Slums, sanitation and mortality in the Roman world. *Klio* 68: 399–433.

Schulze, C. 2005. *Medizin und Christentum in Spätantike und frühem Mittelalter: Christliche Ärtze und ihr Wirken*. Tübingen.

Shaw, B. D. 1980. Archaeology and knowledge. The history of the African provinces of the Roman Empire. *Florilegium* 2, 28–60.

Shaw, B. 1995. The noblest monuments and the smallest things. Wells, walls and aqueducts in the making of Roman Africa. In: *Environment and Society in Roman North Africa. Studies in History and Archaeology*. Ashgate.

Shaw, B. D. 2011. *Sacred violence. African Christians and sectarian hatred in the age of Augustine*. Cambridge.

Sigerist, H. E. 1958. The Latin medical literature of the early Middle Ages. *Journal of the History of Medicine and Allied Sciences* 13, 127–146.

Sigerist, H. E. 1967. *A history of medicine. Vol. I. Primitive and archaic medicine*. Oxford.

Spencer, W. G. (transl.). 1953. *Celsus. De medicina*. Loeb Classical Series. Cambridge Mass.

Spengler, O. (repr.). 1991. *The decline of the West*. A. Helps & H. Werner (eds.). C. F. Atkinson (transl.). New York.

Stannard, J. 1961. Hippocratic pharmacology. *Bulletin of the History of Medicine* 35, 497–518.

Stannard, J. 1982. Rezeptliteratur als Fachliteratur. In: W. Eamon (ed.). *Studies on medieval Fachliteratur*. Brussels, pp. 59–73.

Stark, R. 1992. Epidemics, networks and the rise of Christianity. *Semeia* 5, 162.

Stegers, F. 2004. *Asklepiosmedizin. Medizinische Alltag in der romischen Kaiserzeit*. Stuttgart.

Stevenson, J. 1996. Lactantius. In: Hornblower & Spawforth 1996, p. 811.

Stok, F. 1012. Fonte e datazione dell' Epistola du Vindiciano a Pentadio. *Technai* 3, 137–143.

Strootman. R. 2011. Alexandrië, een wereldstad. *Lampas* 44, 292–310.

Temkin, O. (transl., intr. and comm.). 1956. *Soranus'* Gynecology. Baltimore.

Temkin, O. & Temkin, C. L. (eds.). 1967. *Ancient medicine. Selected papers of Ludwig Edelstein*. Baltimore, London.

Temkin, O. 1971. *The falling sickness*. Baltimore, London.

Temkin, O. 1977a. *The double face of Janus and other essays in the history of medicine*. Baltimore, London.

Temkin, O. 1977b. The history of Hippocratism in late antiquity. The third century and the Latin West. In: Temkin 1977a, pp. 167–177.

Temkin, O. 1977c. The scientific approach to disease. Specific entity and individual. In: Temkin 1977a, pp. 441–455.

Temkin. O. 1977d. An historical analysis of the concept of infection. In: Temkin 1977a, pp. 456–471.

Temkin, O. 1991. *Hippocrates in a world of pagans and Christians*. Baltimore, London.

The Princeton Encyclopaedia of Classical sites in http://perseus.tufts.edu

Thesaurus Linguae Latinae. 1900. Leipzig.

Thieling, W. 1911. Die griechische Einflüsse in der Literatur. In: W. Thieling (ed.). *Der Hellenismus in Kleinafrika. Der griechisches Kulturinfluss in den römischen Provinzen Nordwestafrikas*. Leipzig.

Tieleman, T. 2011. Herophilus en de Alexandrijnse geneeskunde. De herontdekking van een wetenschappelijke bloeiperiode. *Lampas* 44, 368–376.

Totelin, L. M. V. 2009. *Hippocratic recipes. Oral and written transmission of pharmacological knowledge in fifth- and fourth-century Greece*. Leiden, Boston.

Totelin, L. M. V. 2010. Teaching the Hippocratic gynecological recipes. In: Horstmanshoff 2010, pp. 287–300.

Van der Eijk, P. 1999. *Ancient histories of medicine. Essays in medical doxography and historiography in Classical Antiquity.* Leiden, Boston, Cologne.

Van der Eijk, P. 1999a. Historical awareness, historiography and doxography in Greek and Roman medicine. In: Van der Eijk 1999, pp. 1–31.

Van der Eijk, P. 1999b. Antiquarianism and criticism. Forms and functions of medical doxography in Methodism (Soranus and Caelius Aurelianus). In: Van der Eijk, pp. 397–452.

Van der Eijk, P. J. 1999c. The systematic status of therapy in the Hippocratic Corpus and in the work of Diocles of Crystus. In: D. Manetti & A. Roselli (eds.). *Aspetti della terapia nel Corpus Hippocraticum*. Florence.

Van der Eijk, P. 2005. The Methodism of Caelius Aurelianus. Some epistemological issues. In: P. van der Eijk. *Medicine and philosophy in Classical Antiquity. Doctors and philosophers on nature, soul, health and disease,* pp. 299–327. Cambridge.

Van der Eijk, P. J. 2014. Galen and early Christians on the role of the divine in the causation and treatment of health and disease. *Early Christianity* 5, 337–370.

Van Tilburg, C. 2013. A healthy mistake. The excrement problem from ancient Greece to nineteenth-century Holland. In: A. Karenberg, D. Groß & M. Schmidt (eds.). *Forschungen zur Medizingeschichte. Beiträge des 'Rheinischen Kreises der Medizinhistoriker'*. Kassel, pp. 103–117.

Van Tilburg, C. 2014. Greek and Roman ideas about healthy drinking-water in theory and practice. *Journal of Medical Humanities & Social Studies of Science and Technology/ Rivista de Humanidades Médicas & Estudios Sociales de la Ciencia la Tecnologia* 5.1, 1–30.

Van Tilburg, C. 2015. *Streets and streams. Health conditions and city planning in the Graeco-Roman world.* Leiden.

Von Staden, H. (ed., transl. and notes). 1989. *Herophilus. The art of medicine in early Alexandria.* Cambridge.

Von Staden, H. 1992. Spiderwoman and the chaste tree. The semantics of matter. *Configurations* 1, 23–56.

Van Geest, P. 2002. 'Inveni medicum, qui in caelo habitat et in terris spargit medicinam'. Augustinus van Hippo over ziekte en genezing. *Leidschrift. Historisch Tijdschrift. Mens sana in corpore sano? Aspecten uit de medische geschiedenis* 17.1, 29–50.

Wallis, E. (transl.). 1885. Pontius of Carthage. *Life of Cyprian.* Online at Christian Classics Bible Society.

Ward-Perkins, B. 2005. *The fall of Rome and the end of civilization.* Oxford.

Wasserman, H. P. 1997. *Geneeskunde in die Bybel.* Pretoria.

Waszink, J. H. 1947. *Tertullliani* De anima. Amsterdam.

Weiskotten, H. T. 2008. *The life of St. Augustine. A translation of the Sancti Augustini Vita by Possidius.* Merchantville, NJ.

Wilson, A. 1995. Running water and social status in North Africa. In: M. Horton (ed.). *Published Conference Proceedings.* Bristol.

Wilson, A. 1998. Water supply in ancient Carthage. *Journal of Roman Archaeology.* Supplementary Series, pp. 65–102.

Wilson, A. G. 2014. *Augustine, wannabe philosopher. The search for* otium honestum. Knoxville.

Wood, R. & Wheeler, M. 1966. *Roman Africa in colour.* London.

Xella, P., Quinn, J., Melchiorri, V., Van Dommelen, P. 2013. Phoenician bones of contention. *Antiquity* 87, 1191–1199.

Zinsser, H. 1935. *Rats, lice and history. A chronicle of disease, plagues and pestilence.* London.

Index Locorum

Abbreviations derived from:
- C.T. Lewis & C.S. Short, *A Latin Dictionary*. Oxford 1993.
- S. Hornblower, A. Spawforth, E. Eidinow, *Oxford Classical Dictionary*, 4th edition. Oxford 2012
- R.J. Hankinson, *The Cambridge Companion to Galen*. Cambridge 2008.
- G. Fichtner, *Corpus Hippocraticum: Verzeichnis der hippokratischen und pseudohippokratischen Schriften*. Tübingen 1992.

Index

For Product Safety Concerns and Information please contact our EU
representative GPSR@taylorandfrancis.com
Taylor & Francis Verlag GmbH, Kaufingerstraße 24, 80331 München, Germany

www.ingramcontent.com/pod-product-compliance
Lightning Source LLC
LaVergne TN
LVHW010549300926
849162LV00002B/278

* 9 7 8 9 4 6 2 9 8 9 9 0 0 *